# FROM SOCIAL SILENCE TO SOCIAL SCIENCE

SAME-SEX SEXUALITY, HIV & AIDS AND GENDER IN SOUTH AFRICA

CONFERENCE PROCEEDINGS EDITED BY VASU REDDY, THEO SANDFORT, LAETITIA RISPEL

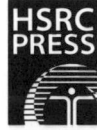

*For everyone who has died of HIV and AIDS.*
*For everyone who lives with HIV and AIDS.*
*For everyone who works to make a difference for those living with HIV and AIDS.*

*From Vasu,*
*for the late Ronald Louw, my mentor, my friend and my comrade*

*From Theo,*
*for all women and men who relentlessly put same-sex sexuality*
*on the African map of HIV/AIDS*

*From Laetitia,*
*for all the courageous researchers who dare to push the boundaries*
*of public health and social science research*

Published by HSRC Press
Private Bag X9182, Cape Town, 8000, South Africa
www.hsrcpress.ac.za

First published 2009

ISBN (soft cover) 978-0-7969-2276-2
ISBN (pdf) 978-0-7969-2277-9
ISBN (epub) 978-0-7969-2295-3

© 2009 Human Sciences Research Council

The views expressed in this publication are those of the authors. They do not necessarily reflect the views or policies of the Human Sciences Research Council ('the Council') or indicate that the Council endorses the views of the authors. In quoting from this publication, readers are advised to attribute the source of the information to the individual author concerned and not to the Council.

Copyedited by Barbara Hutton
Typeset by Baseline Publishing Services
Cover design by Karin Miller and FUEL Design
Printed by Logo Print, Cape Town, South Africa

Distributed in Africa by Blue Weaver
Tel: +27 (0) 21 701 4477; Fax: +27 (0) 21 701 7302
www.oneworldbooks.com

Distributed in Europe and the United Kingdom by
Eurospan Distribution Services (EDS)
Tel: +44 (0) 20 7240 0856; Fax: +44 (0) 20 7379 0609
www.eurospanbookstore.com

Distributed in North America by Independent Publishers Group (IPG)
Call toll-free: (800) 888 4741; Fax: +1 (312) 337 5985
www.ipgbook.com

# Contents

| | | |
|---|---|---|
| Foreword | | vii |
| Messages of support | | viii |
| Acknowledgements | | ix |
| Introduction<br>*Vasu Reddy, Theo Sandfort and Laetitia Rispel* | | xi |

**Theory, methodology, context**

| | | |
|---|---|---|
| 1 | Researching same-sex sexuality and HIV prevention<br>*Peter Aggleton* | 2 |
| 2 | Sexuality research in South Africa: The policy context<br>*Robert Sember* | 14 |
| 3 | Same-sex sexuality and health: Psychosocial scientific research in South Africa<br>*Juan Nel* | 32 |
| 4 | Homosexual and bisexual labels: The need for clear conceptualisations, operationalisations and appropriate methodological designs<br>*Theo Sandfort and Brian Dodge* | 51 |
| 5 | Gender, same-sex sexuality and HIV/AIDS in South Africa: Practical research challenges and solutions<br>*Pierre Brouard* | 58 |
| 6 | From social silence to social science: HIV research among township men who have sex with men in South Africa<br>*Tim Lane* | 66 |

**History, memory, archive**

| | | |
|---|---|---|
| 7 | Gay AIDS activism in South Africa prior to 1994<br>*Mandisa Mbali* | 80 |
| 8 | Sexing women: Young black lesbians' reflections on sex and responses to safe(r) sex<br>*Zethu Matebeni* | 100 |
| 9 | Creating memory: Documenting and disseminating life stories of LGBTI people living with HIV<br>*Ruth Morgan, Busi Kheswa and John Meletse* | 117 |

## Perspectives from sub-Saharan and southern Africa

10  What we know about same-sex practising people and HIV in Africa  126
    *Cary Alan Johnson*

11  Same-sex sexuality and HIV/AIDS: A perspective from Malawi  137
    *Daveson Nyadani*

12  A bird's-eye view of HIV and gay and lesbian issues in Zimbabwe  143
    *Samuel Matsikure*

13  Epidemiological disjunctures: A review of same-sex sexuality and
    HIV research in sub-Saharan Africa  147
    *Kirk Fiereck*

## Needs, programming, policy and direction for future research

14  Mobilising gay and lesbian organisations to respond to the political
    challenges of the South African HIV epidemic  168
    *Nathan Geffen, Zethu Cakata, Renay Pillay and Paymon Ebrahimzadeh*

15  Are South African HIV policies and programmes meeting the needs of
    same-sex practising individuals?  176
    *Laetitia Rispel and Carol Metcalf*

16  Lessons learned from current South African HIV/AIDS research among
    lesbian, gay and bisexual populations  190
    *Dawie Nel*

17  Observations on HIV and AIDS in Cape Town's LGBT population  198
    *Glenn de Swardt*

18  Some personal and political perspectives on HIV/AIDS in Ethekwini  207
    *Nonhlanhla 'MC' Mkhize*

19  Health for all? Health needs and issues for women who have sex
    with women  216
    *Vicci Tallis*

## Conclusions

20  Taking research and prevention forward  228
    *Theo Sandfort, Vasu Reddy and Laetitia Rispel*

Contributors  242
Index  246

# Foreword

To be same-sex oriented and South African, to live in the age of AIDS, and in a time of struggle for democracy, freedom and social justice is exciting, challenging, painful and often bewildering. These are some of the energies behind this book.

Our Constitution proudly safeguards gay and lesbian equality, and renounces discrimination on the ground of disability. But its vaunting promises fall far short of reality in too many lives in our country. Despite constitutional protection on the ground of sexual orientation, hatred, phobia and discrimination are still rife.

From the mid-1980s, as the fearsome African demography of the disease became apparent, AIDS was neither seen nor labelled as a 'gay disease'. As a proudly and openly gay man, one who not long after my sexual coming-out had to come to terms with being infected myself, I felt some obscure relief to think that I was one in a mass heterosexual epidemic. The 'non-gay' shape of the epidemic would protect me, and other gay men, from the worst homophobic reactions to AIDS.

And in many ways it did. But too often heterosexual predominance meant that same-sex sexuality and gender were eclipsed. In our national response, both governmental and organisational, gay people have been under-served, under-informed, and under-treated.

The harm-sowing myth that homosexuality is 'unAfrican' has played its part in obscuring and stifling responses to the epidemic amongst gay people in Africa. The result has been a partially 'hidden epidemic'.

*From Social Silence to Social Science* offers important new thought and understanding. The volume raises visibility about vulnerable and marginal groups. Its varied chapters – by scholars, programme workers and activists – light the obscure corners of the epidemic, and suggest practical action.

A striking feature of the volume is that its contributions address both local and continental research and programming.

It is my hope that the authors' expertise and insights, and their collation in this volume, will foster real thought and real action. The diversity of contributions is impressive, and many authors proffer important ideas. So the text is timely.

We have yet a long journey ahead with same-sex equality in Africa, and perhaps an even longer journey with AIDS. This volume will, I hope, help light our way with both.

Edwin Cameron
Justice of the Constitutional Court of South Africa

# Messages of support

In May 2007, a varied group of sociologists, epidemiologists, social workers and HIV/AIDS activists gathered in Pretoria for a ground-breaking conference entitled Gender, Same-sex Sexuality and HIV/AIDS. The conference was jointly convened and funded by the Human Sciences Research Council (HSRC) and the HIV Center for Clinical and Behavioral Studies at the New York State Psychiatric Institute and Columbia University.

In an address to conference delegates, Dr Olive Shisana, president and CEO of the HSRC, emphasised that, 'while we know the epidemic is pronounced among our heterosexual population, we also know that our lesbian and gay communities are not immune to HIV/AIDS. Over and above people who self-identify as lesbian, gay or bisexual, HIV and AIDS also impacts on men who have sex with men [MSM] and women [WSW] who have sex with women – categories of sexual practice that are often erased from studies and interventions.

'We also know that we live in a society where prejudice runs deep about homosexuality, fuelled in part by perceived ideas about gender, belief systems, stigmatisation and socialisation. Despite the commendable Constitution of South Africa, sadly attitudes and stereotypes prevail about homosexuality and same-sex sexuality'. She concluded that 'work on MSM and WSW in relation to HIV/AIDS is long overdue in South Africa…This conference will stimulate all of us to explore challenges and find potential solutions for research on same-sex sexual practices and HIV/AIDS'.

Dr Anke Erhardt, director of the HIV Center for Clinical and Behavioral Studies at the New York State Psychiatric Institute and Columbia University also addressed delegates, noting that 'while the AIDS epidemic started in South Africa as a gay epidemic, gay men disappeared from view as soon as it became clear how devastating the epidemic was going to be in the heterosexual population. These developments are understandable, but not acceptable. This event will help to increase the political attention for same-sex sexuality and HIV/AIDS'.

Dr Erhardt went on to note: 'I am pleased that the conference does not only deal with men. It is my understanding that, contrary to what usually is thought, HIV/AIDS is a major concern for lesbian women as well. It deserves balanced attention… [This event will form] the basis for future collaborative projects, in the field of research, prevention, advocacy and policy, and ultimately contribute to the end of the HIV/AIDS epidemic and the stigma and injustice that is furthered by this gruesome epidemic…I am pleased that, with the Center's expertise in these areas, we were able to contribute to the organisation of this conference. I would like to congratulate the organisers on the stimulating programme they were able to put together…I want you to know that the HIV Center is committed to working with you after the conference is over.'

# Acknowledgements

Expressing thanks and appreciation should not be just an empty ritual, and because we feel it sincerely, it is not possible to make too much of it.

First, we acknowledge the individual contributions of our authors who helped move *From Social Silence to Social Science* from the spoken text at a conference to the published version now before us. Many of the authors originally presented their papers at the conference – Gender, Same-sex Sexuality and HIV/AIDS in South Africa: An International Conference of Researchers, Community Leaders and Activists – which was held in Pretoria from 9 to 11 May 2007. As co-editors, we relied heavily on each other to carefully peer-review each contribution. We very much appreciate the patience and willingness of our contributors to revise and sometimes rewrite sections. Tim Lane in particular must be thanked for his wonderful collegiality in agreeing to us appropriating his invention as the title of this volume. We are confident that what we have assembled here is highly relevant and contributes to improving our understanding of HIV/AIDS in South and southern Africa in its complex relationship to gender and same-sex sexuality.

Second, our funders were crucial to our thinking about, and implementation of, the project. In no particular order, our special thanks to Aids Fonds Netherlands, HIVOS (Humanistisch Instituut voor Ontwikkelingssamenwerking) and the Royal Netherlands Embassy in Pretoria for resources that principally funded the conference. More directly, without the generous financial support of Atlantic Philanthropies, this book would not have been published.

Third, we acknowledge and appreciate the partnerships we as editors have collectively developed and strengthened, which emerged first with the conference, then with this book and subsequently with other local and internationally-driven research projects. The Human Sciences Research Council (HSRC) of South Africa, together with the HIV Center for Clinical and Behavioral Studies, Columbia University, have firmly consolidated partnerships in research. Within the HSRC we thank Dr Olive Shisana (president and CEO) for her support for the work we have embarked on through this conference, and at the HIV Center we express to the director, Dr Anke Erhardt, our appreciation for her ongoing wisdom and collegiality in strengthening our work in the field. These partnerships are also significantly consolidated through our collaboration with community partners, including OUT LGBT Well-being (Pretoria) and the Durban Lesbian and Gay Community and Health Centre. And here we thank Dawie Nel (OUT) and Nonhlanhla Mkhize for their continued support, enthusiasm and willingness to collaborate with us.

Vasu would like to acknowledge the work and example of his co-editors for their personal support, friendship, patience and intellectual advice. He maintains that while the theoretical perspectives and disciplinary backgrounds of his co-editors (and the many authors in the book) may be diverse and multifaceted, the final manuscript demonstrates how difference can strengthen the cohesiveness of the final product. He also thanks colleagues within the HSRC (particularly staff within the Gender & Development Unit, Annette Gerber and Ella Mathobela for administrative support in the lead-up to the conference) and especially our editor at the HSRC Press for her patience and perspicacity in the editing process.

Without loved ones, writing would certainly be lonely.

Vasu would like to thank Sudeshan who, as always, continues to nourish with companionship, affection and support, and to inspire by example. Through all stages of this project, my father especially, and my mum, sisters and niece, and a small circle of friends provided comfort, love and advice.

Theo would like to express his thanks to all people who made the conference and this book a success. It is amazing what people are able to accomplish together, when they decide that change is needed. While same-sex sexuality was virtually off the map, the conference seemed to have induced an enthusiasm about much-needed research activities. In the meantime, new contacts are made and friendship circles are built. He thanks his colleague Vasu for the deep friendship which has developed through the process. Special thanks also go to Laetitia, as co-editor, and to his colleague Robert Sember, with whom he started this journey and whose valuable insights and critical skills have helped sharpen his focus. Finally, Theo especially thanks his sometimes worrying but always supportive and proud partner Jeff.

Laetitia would like to acknowledge Vasu and Theo for their comradeship, and for giving her an opportunity to climb an exciting and steep learning curve and to explore largely unchartered terrain. Thanks to Nico Jacobs for administrative support. Edward Hank is thanked for his support, wisdom and encouragement, and her children Andrew and Nadine are thanked for their understanding and the many cups of tea.

# Introduction

Vasu Reddy, Theo Sandfort and Laetitia Rispel

> We all died
> Coughed and died
> We died of TB
> That was us
> Whispering it at funerals
> Because nobody ever said AIDS
>
> *Eddie Vulani Maluleke*[1]

## Because nobody ever said AIDS

Maluleke's poem 'Nobody Ever Said AIDS' conveys a sense of sorrow and loss in an intimate vision of what it may mean to live in the time of HIV and AIDS. But a more purposeful meaning is that collectively we must counter the stigma and pain by 'crossing from solitude' (to borrow the title of Rustum Kozain's poem). This 'crossing' may spur a shift away from silence towards challenging denial and creating a better understanding of how HIV and AIDS affect the way we live, love and express our desires. If we resist the crossing, denial could result in the erasure of the lived experiences of people who are infected and affected by HIV, and the epidemic will continue to feed on fear, blame, ignorance and inequality.

HIV/AIDS is a disease of the global world that is shaped by local factors, contexts and ideologies (see Adams & Pigg 2005; Altman 2001). And it is the African continent that carries the largest human burden of the pandemic (Barnett & Whiteside 2002; Baylies et al. 2000; Kalipeni et al. 2004; Mendel et al. 2001; UNAIDS 2008). HIV has changed the way we think about sex, gender, life and death, compelling us to confront topics and issues that ordinarily many of us choose to avoid. Despite the increase in knowledge about HIV (largely through medicine and public health, but also through the activism of movements such as the Treatment Action Campaign), mortality rates remain high, people have not fully modified their sexual behaviour toward safer sex, and the disease remains stubbornly non-discriminatory in a world where inequalities persist. It spares no colour, no age, no creed, no geography, no religion or spiritual belief, and not least sexual orientation. Poor people carry the burden of transmission and women are more vulnerable than men, suggesting that not only the virus but also socio-economic and cultural conditions have an impact on transmission rates.

The ways in which HIV and AIDS are profiled and represented are part of a powerful body of beliefs and assumptions concerning the supposed causes and effects of HIV infection and related illnesses. Schoepf (2001: page) for example, reinforcing the idea that 'disease epidemics are social processes', maintains that 'AIDS in many cultures is weighted with extraordinary symbolic and emotional power, including ideas about social and spiritual "pollution"' (see also Aggleton 1999; Aggleton et al. 1999; Altman 1994; Crimp 2004; Herdt 1997; Sontag 1991; Treichler 1999; Waldy 1996). HIV has a close proximity to fundamental questions of sexuality and sexual pleasure. It requires us to focus on the sexual behaviours and practices that underpin the epidemic – questions which call for 're-sexualising the epidemic' (Berger 2004: page).

For approximately three decades HIV and AIDS have harnessed deep-seated sexual fears and have shored up public anxiety about social problems (see Duggan & Hunter 1995), displacing these fears and anxieties onto certain groups (often sex workers, usually homosexuals, and increasingly women). HIV and AIDS have induced a sex panic that exists in many quarters of our society, reinforced by stereotypes, perceptions and myths that are socially and culturally founded. Although a common myth is that HIV is a homosexual disease which is prominent in Western settings, this myth is not fully operative in African contexts given that homosexual bodies and practices are often stigmatised. The bodies of gay men in particular have become sexed in relation to AIDS (Watney 1997, 2000. See also Ruel and Campbell (2006) for a more contemporary argument about the link between homophobia and HIV/AIDS.

## A timeline of the AIDS epidemic

The pre-history of the HIV epidemic contributed to the perception and politicisation of it being a homosexual disease, especially when it was first identified in 1981 as a disease with no name. Initially doctors diagnosed it as pneumocystis carinii pneumonia and a 'rare cancer' (kaposi sarcoma in gay men).[2] In the same year, the US-based Centers for Disease Control declared the new disease an epidemic. In 1982, when doctors found that many homosexual men were dying without explanation, they labelled the disease Gay Related Immune Deficiency or GRID.

French scientists isolated the HI virus in 1983, and around 1984/85 the medical establishment named the syndrome of illnesses it causes as Acquired Immune Deficiency Syndrome (AIDS). In 1985 AIDS was reported in 51 countries, with Africa reflecting the largest number of infections. By 1987 that number had risen to 127 countries. In 1988 women were named as the fastest growing group of people living with AIDS. On 1 December of that year the first annual World AIDS Day was commemorated. Ten years later, Simon Nkoli, an icon of the lesbian and gay struggle in South Africa, died of HIV/AIDS. Since then many South Africans have died of HIV and AIDS, some of whom publicly disclosed their sexual orientation while many others chose not to.

And like many South Africans who have died of HIV and AIDS, the history of the global epidemic shows many who have died and many who continue to live with the virus. By the end of the first decade there were around 8 to 10 million people living with AIDS worldwide; by 1997 this number had escalated to 30 million. In 2000, the year in which South Africa hosted the thirteenth International AIDS Conference in Durban, it was announced that AIDS was the number one killer in Africa. In 2003 evidence emerged that HIV vaccine trials reported poor results; at the same time new evidence confirmed that antiretroviral medications can be effectively used in developing world settings. By 2004, 95 per cent of those with AIDS were living in the developing world. In 2007 it was estimated that more than 25 million people had died of AIDS since it was first identified in 1981, with current rates of about 3 million deaths per year.

## South Africa then and now

Although the first case of AIDS was reported in South Africa in 1982 and started with gay men, little is known about the current prevalence of HIV among largely LGBT (lesbian, gay, bisexual and transgender) South Africans (see the conclusion to this book for a brief epidemiological profile of the epidemic). The size of the global epidemic and the fact that the dominant mode of transmission is now seen as heterosexual have eclipsed the gay male epidemic, with women now identified as the most at risk. Important and often cited epidemiological studies, such as the *Nelson Mandela HSRC Study of HIV/AIDS* (Shisana & Simbayi 2002), did not report on homosexual transmission. Other key studies, such as *AIDS: The Challenge for South Africa* (Whiteside & Sunter 2000), *The Moral Economy of AIDS in South Africa* (Nattrass 2004), *HIV/AIDS in South Africa* (Abdool Karim & Abdool Karim 2005), and *Waiting to Happen: HIV/AIDS in South Africa – The Bigger Picture* (Walker et al. 2004), review and/or take stock of key aspects of HIV/AIDS in South Africa. However, they pay cursory attention to questions of homosexual transmission.

A thorough review of the epidemiological literature shows that there is little current information available on homosexual/same-sex transmission of HIV in South Africa. This is despite the fact that as early as the mid-1980s the impact of AIDS on the homosexual community was a matter of concern for South Africans (Isaacs & Miller 1985; see also Philips [2004] for an argument about HIV, homosexuality and rights in southern Africa). Mention is made of the fact that AIDS started in South Africa in the early 1980s as a homosexually-based illness, but that in the early 1990s it became known as a heterosexually transmitted epidemic. Originally, these two areas of concern were independent, involving different HIV subtypes: subtype B found in homosexual men at the beginning of the epidemic, and subtype C associated with the epidemic in the heterosexual population (Williamson & Martin 2005). It is not known whether the two subtypes are still firmly divided between the heterosexual and homosexual populations.

It remains unclear what homosexual transmission (including men who have sex only with men [MSM] or with both men and women, and women who have sex with women [WSW] exclusively or with both men and women) currently contributes to the overall epidemic in South Africa. Given the relatively small estimated size of this population, it is unlikely that this contribution is extensive. That does not, however, mean that it is insignificant. Little is known about whether homosexual and bisexual men adequately protect themselves and their partners against HIV transmission, and whether they are sufficiently informed, skilled and motivated to do so. It is also unclear how lesbian and bisexual women are affected by the HIV epidemic. Sexual violence against lesbian and bisexual women, especially the phenomenon of 'corrective rape' of black lesbians, could well compound HIV transmission among lesbians (Reddy et al. 2007). There is thus no indication of how the 'heterosexual' and 'homosexual' epidemics interact, although an interaction seems unavoidable given information gathered by NGOs and other community groups that work with these populations.

The absence of homosexuality in the health sciences, public health and behavioural sciences literature about HIV/AIDS in South Africa stands in sharp contrast to scholarly work in law, anthropology, history, gender studies, cultural studies and other humanities-oriented disciplines, where homosexuality is the focus of a significant body of literature (see for example Elder 2003; Epprecht 2004; Germond & De Gruchy 1997; Gevisser & Cameron 1994; Hoad 2007; Hoad et al. 2005; Isaacs & McKendrick 1992; Luirinck 2000; Morgan & Wieringa Spurlin 2006; Van Zyl & Steyn 2005). This disparity in focus could be attributed to the inherently conservative influence of funding for large behavioural sciences research projects and the epidemiology of the AIDS epidemic in South Africa, which is predominantly heterosexual. The little research that has been done in this area in recent years has been undertaken by NGOs with extremely limited resources (in this regard the ground-breaking work of OUT LGBT Well-being is key – see OUT 2004a, 2004b, 2004c, 2004d). The work done by scholars in disciplines that traditionally do not undertake funded research is evidence that the absence of homosexuality in health-related research does not represent a lack of homosexual activity or activism in South Africa. While representative of the diverse and active sexual cultures in South Africa, the currently available literature does not provide information necessary for the formulation of initiatives to address the HIV-related risk behaviours, risk contexts, and treatment needs of homosexual South Africans (see the concluding chapter of this book).[3]

## Homosexuality in South Africa

As noted, the historical interpretation of homosexuality in South Africa is fairly extensively documented. Criminalisation and legal sanctions against homosexuality characterised apartheid, crystallising the homosexual into a model of illness and disease. In marked contrast, post-apartheid South Africa (with its promise of broad constitutional reform under a bill of rights culture) facilitated the protection of rights, and guaranteed rights to produce identities for homosexuals. Where apartheid policed, politicised and criminalised the 'sexual acts' of homosexuals, post-apartheid, in turn, sexualised lesbian and gay identities, thereby freeing homosexuality from the clutches of a pathological discourse.

The political gains for homosexuals would not have been possible without the mobilisation, lobbying, advocacy and leadership of many stalwarts in the lesbian and gay struggle (notable among them Zackie Achmat, Edwin Cameron, Sheila Lapinsky, Ronald Louw, Ivan Toms, Simon Nkoli, Pumi Mtetwa, Jonathan Berger, and some who are not gay, such as Mazibuko Jara). The Gay and Lesbian Organisation of the Witwatersrand and the regional coalitions of the National Coalition for Gay and Lesbian Equality played a dominant role in the 1990s. At the level of community-based mobilisation many organisations – such as the Triangle Project (Cape Town), OUT LGBT Well-being (Pretoria), the Durban Lesbian and Gay Community & Health Centre, including also the Forum for the Empowerment of Women (Johannesburg) and Behind the Mask (Johannesburg) – have played and continue to assert an important role in the national landscape in South Africa for lesbian and gay equality. In recent years, especially in the decriminalisation campaign for same-sex marriage equality in South Africa, the Joint Working Group (a network of lesbian and gay organisations in South Africa) has emerged as a key player in respect of hate crimes against sexual minorities, and the development of programming in respect of HIV/AIDS for same-sex sexuality.

While the promise of legal reforms has brought benefits for the homosexual, the translation of constitutional equality into material terms and protections remains a critical task for civil society actors committed to advancing and securing rights in a context where homophobia still persists. Such homophobia is fuelled in part by cultural, religious and general social conservatism toward homosexuality. Certainly one of the most violent manifestations to date in South Africa remains the deliberate and premeditated rape of black lesbians by men who want to 'discipline' and 'punish' women who they believe to be non-conforming and unwomanly, so they are to be made 'straight'. The deaths of Zoliswa Nkonyana, Sizakele Sigasa, Salome Masooa and several others demonstrate that violence and oppression within heteropatriarchal contexts confirm societal causes of HIV risk and vulnerability (see OUT LGBT Well-being 2004b; Reddy et al. 2007).

The organisation and arrangement of same-sex desires and practices (as is the case elsewhere in the world) is replete with diversity across race, ethnicity, class, generation, networks, resources, opportunities, and degrees of marginalisation from resources and power. Such structural factors equally determine how persons might exercise and organise their personal lifestyles, identities and sexual practices. Economic differences are also intimately connected to racial differences and together these define a variety of spaces and resources for organising sexual desire, identity and practice. Given the historical and racialised over-determination of privilege in South

Africa, it may be the case that there are more white men and women who have the luxury of access to private space in comparison to black men and women. This does not rule out the reality that a slowly emerging black middle class has also facilitated privileged access for upwardly mobile black lesbians and gays. Over and above these differences, access to resources for both white and black lesbians and gays does not necessarily ensure that such individuals see or experience the oppressed position of homosexuals, nor do they actively express solidarity with those who are oppressed. In the last few years, since major constitutional victories have been won, there has been a marked decline in political mobilisation by lesbians and gays against broad societal injustices. This could be the effect of general complacency, or the possibility that inequalities only matter if they infringe on lesbian and gay equality. Thus, there is no fully-fledged organised and mobilised leadership of lesbians and gays in South Africa to tackle issues in a sustained way at either the macro or micro level. The recent mobilisation of gays and lesbians in South Africa to support the establishment of the Civil Union Bill that now provides legal recognition of same-sex partnerships was the last full-scale organised campaign by the sector.

In turning to sexual practice and naming, we find some complications. There are many men and women who, while engaging in same-sex sexual practices, refrain from labelling themselves as 'gay', 'lesbian' or 'bisexual' (see Reid 2006). It is increasingly becoming apparent through community-based research work and sexual health programmes by lesbian and gay organisations that there are many who reject conventional labels of identity (studies that highlight some of these issues are Dowsett 1996; King 2004; Loue 2007; studies that address the issue from the perspective of lesbian health and sexuality are Dolan 2005; Munson & Stelboum 1999). While the meanings of specific labels are not fully explored, it is evident, through anecdotal evidence and work within lesbian and gay organisations, that the distribution of same-sex practices, independently and in relation to heterosexual sex, may reflect a hidden population and, by extension, a hidden epidemic to which we must turn (in some cases, where earlier campaigns in parts of the Western world showed a decline in HIV, new research seems to demonstrate a re-emergence among same-sex populations – see Jaffe et al. [2007]). More importantly, the health of LGBT populations (usually conceived as sexual minorities) is often overlooked and erased, eclipsed usually by focusing on the heterosexual epidemic (see Meyer and Northridge [2007] for an extensive series of arguments that prioritise a spectrum of health issues).

## Sub-Saharan Africa in 2008: Epidemiological trends and modes of transmission

The 2008 *Report on the Global AIDS Epidemic* (UNAIDS 2008) confirms that in the three decades of AIDS, the incidence has peaked, the generalised epidemic is nearing saturation, and mortality is rising.[4] In 2007, 67 per cent of all people living with

HIV were in sub-Saharan Africa, with southern Africa sharing a disproportionate proportion of the global burden: 35 per cent of HIV infections and 38 per cent of AIDS deaths. The disease continues to take its toll on young women (15–29), on children, on inadequate health services, resulting in rapidly rising death rates and an increase in orphans. The report also indicates that the global percentage of adults living with HIV has levelled off since 2000, but that there were 2.7 million new HIV infections and 2 million HIV-related deaths.[when?] While the rate of new HIV infections had fallen in several countries, globally the positive trend was partially offset by increases in new infections in other countries. In 14 of 17 African countries with adequate survey data, the percentage of young pregnant women (ages 15–24) who live with HIV had declined since 2000/01. Importantly, as treatment access increased in the last decade, the annual number of AIDS deaths decreased. Globally, the percentage of women among people living with HIV remained stable (at 50 per cent) although women's share of infections is increasing in several countries. Also reported is that in most regions outside sub-Saharan Africa, HIV continues to disproportionately affect injecting drug users, sex workers and MSM.

The UNAIDS report outlines that an estimated 1.9 million people were newly infected with HIV in the sub-Saharan region in 2007, bringing to 22 million the number of people living with HIV in this region. Given the heterogeneity of the region, epidemics vary from country to country in terms of scale and scope. Epidemiological trends show that in a growing number of countries there is a decline in HIV prevalence, with women remaining disproportionately affected in comparison to men. In Zimbabwe there was a decline in HIV prevalence among pregnant women attending antenatal clinics (from 26 per cent in 2002 to 18 per cent in 2006). In Botswana there was also a drop in HIV prevalence among pregnant 15–19-year-olds (25 per cent in 2001 to 18 per cent in 2006). The epidemic appears to have stabilised in Malawi and Zambia in the midst of evidence suggesting favourable behaviour change. While HIV data from antenatal clinics in South Africa suggest the possibility of the epidemic stabilising, there is no evidence yet of major changes in HIV-related behaviour. HIV prevalence found in adults in Swaziland in 2006 showed the highest prevalence documented in a national population-based survey anywhere in the world. In Lesotho and parts of Mozambique, HIV prevalence among pregnant women is increasing.

While heterosexual intercourse remains the dominant force in the region, epidemiological evidence suggests that the region's epidemic is more diverse than was previously thought. Apart from evidence in modes of transmission with heterosexual intercourse related to serodiscordant couples, sex workers and injecting drug users[check wording], recent studies demonstrate that unprotected anal sex between men is another factor in the regional epidemic. Evidence showing HIV transmission between MSM revealed some important data: 1) in Zambia, one in three (33 per cent) surveyed MSM tested HIV-positive; 2) in the city of Mombasa (Kenya), 43 per cent of men who said they had sex with other men were found to be living with HIV; 3) in Dakar, Senegal, an HIV prevalence of 22 per cent was found among the 463 surveyed MSM. These data suggest that anal sex between men is a mode of transmission that should be investigated and examined, albeit against the grain of sexual orientation and cultural interdictions against homosexuality.

Such an investigation must take place in a context in which the myth that AIDS is a gay-related disease still prevails. 'Silence' and 'invisibility', tokens of diminution, have been the characteristic obstacles in the path of lesbian and gay struggles worldwide. The association with homosexuality as a plague, and by deduction a 'disease', is closely connected to the view that the homosexual (usually the negative is directed toward male homosexuals) is a person who has the potential to 'transmit' his sexuality, if not 'infect' the public with both disease and sexual orientation. The corollary of this view is that if the homosexual is pathologised, it is therefore possible to find a 'cure' for the problem. The language of pathological discourse also suggests that homosexuality, as abnormal sexual behaviour, could be corrected in order for the homosexual to re-enter the heterosexual world as a patriotic, moral and obedient citizen.

## The critical literature on HIV/AIDS

The literature on HIV/AIDS is vast, and rather than retrace the key themes to motivate the context of our current argument, it is appropriate to summarise some of its central features by drawing on recent studies.[5] Parker (2001) highlights the fact that in the west in the mid to late 1980s, social science research around HIV/AIDS focused on collecting quantifiable data on sexual partners, frequency of different sexual practices, and previous sexual history in terms of sexually transmitted diseases (data here were directed toward the development of prevention and intervention programmes to reduce behaviours associated with heightened risk). According to Parker, in the 1990s a shift occurred with the influence of anthropology, with social science research now challenging the biomedical and epidemiologically-driven behavioural model of the 1980s, and focusing rather on the interpretation of cultural meanings as 'central to a fuller understanding of the sexual transmission of HIV in different social settings' (Parker 2001: page).

Following Parker, another dimension, possibly a third feature of research, developed out of cultural analysis. This concerned the structural, political and economic factors that shape sexual experience, and which in turn influence behaviour change in the context of HIV/AIDS (some of these social factors are poverty, economic exploitation, gender power, sexual oppression, racism and social exclusion). Underlining these aspects is a further confirmation that AIDS, like sexuality, is embedded in local social contexts. This implies that social and cultural rules and conditions are factors that determine the circumstances under which people engage in sexual practice. It would therefore seem plausible that a common feature of the critical literature is that HIV/AIDS opens up both epistemological and epidemiological questions, confirming that biological and social conditions shape the way we learn about the disease.

The pandemic also challenges response efforts by communities and countries, and the complex relations between culture and HIV and AIDS have been particularly well documented over the decades. A critical body of literature exists, which could be distinguished in terms of two interrelated aspects in the human and social sciences literature (including public health studies): 1) the *micro* and *macro* approaches to culture; and 2) cultures of prevention and care that underline responses to the epidemic. Explanations with regard to the former notably focus on the cultural understanding of how power shapes the lives of individuals and communities in the arena of HIV and AIDS in its relation to: a) gender roles and power relations; b) sexual violence and HIV/AIDS; c) sexuality and identity; d) population structure and dynamics (e.g. sexual relationships and family structure) in relation to orphans and vulnerable children and migration; and e) the organisation of culture into communities of worship, bodily practices and healing traditions.

Explanations with regard to point 2 above focus on cultures of prevention and care. The following trends can be identified: a) biomedical responses focus on technologies that attempt to stem the spread of HIV, such as testing, sexual technologies such as condoms, microbiocides, circumcision, and antiretroviral therapy and vaccines; b) a behavioural response concerns what the literature terms 'high-risk groups' and the strategies used to target and intervene; c) human rights responses interrogate HIV-associated stigma and discrimination. Within this approach there is also a focus on 'addressing broader systemic and social determinants' (UNESCO 2008: page); d) pedagogic and educative responses focus on addressing prevention. There are also studies that focus on: e) health systems reform and policy responses to HIV/AIDS; f) the role and impact of civil society'(UNESCO 2008: page) and community groups; g) 'national responses to HIV' (UNESCO 2008: page); and h) HIV and AIDS 'in post-conflict situations' (UNESCO 2008: page), highlighting the link between HIV/AIDS and security issues. Beyond the trends, the issue of policy and practice remains central and it is to this that we now turn.

## Policy and practice: HIV risk and vulnerability

Motivated largely by the knowledge gap referred to previously, the conference around which this book emerged posed a number of future-oriented questions. Structured around 'gender', 'same-sex sexuality' and 'HIV/AIDS' as the organising frames for the arguments, we asked the following questions: 1) How are same-sex sexual expressions and practices organised and networked? 2) What is the prevalence of HIV among same-sex practising populations? and 3) what is the contribution of homosexual transmission to the South African epidemic? The answers to these questions lie beyond the scope of this book. However, they are developed from the conference consensus that to administer any meaningful HIV intervention for same-sex practising populations, it is crucial to determine HIV prevalence, behavioural correlates, psychosocial contexts, sexual networks and virological aspects. In the absence of valid data in respect of what the contribution of homosexual (including men who have sex with men or with both men and women, and women who have sex with women or with both men and women) transmission is to the overall epidemic in South Africa, further research serves a valuable purpose.

Clearly this whole enterprise is predicated on the utility and validity of research that will help to: 1) develop appropriate narratives about relevant public health issues in relation to understanding the networks, arrangements and organisation of same-sex sexuality; and 2) provide information (epidemiological data) to be able to advocate for funding and policies (without information it is difficult to make a case for resources).

Scaling up prevention and treatment requires a sound policy framework too. However, this requires a response to the epidemic through a sustained understanding of gender inequalities and the lack of empowerment of women and girls, as well as through challenging discrimination, stigma and social marginalisation.

In positive terms, the Department of Health's *HIV and AIDS and STI National Strategic Plan for South Africa 2007–2011* (DoH 2007) (hereafter NSP) recognises the absence of MSM in national interventions. From a policy perspective there is finally an attempt to mitigate the possible impact of HIV through homosexual transmission. The NSP states that MSM have not been considered to any great extent in national HIV and AIDS initiatives and that there is currently very little known about the HIV epidemic (DoH 2007: page). The NSP notes further that 'MSM practices are more likely to occur in particular institutional settings, such as prisons' and that 'MSM behaviours and sexualities are wide-ranging and include bisexuality', with the possibility that 'the HIV epidemic amongst MSM and the heterosexual HIV epidemic' are interconnected (DoH 2007: page).

While it is evident that some important work is beginning to emerge on the continent of Africa (see concluding chapter in this book),[6] including in South Africa, we want to stress that the focus should be on vulnerable populations and the themes they represent in relation to HIV/AIDS, in order to address the absence in the South African literature and to encourage broader critical analysis of same-sex sexual practices in the context of HIV/AIDS in South Africa. This brings us to the organisation of the book.

## An overview of *From Social Silence to Social Science*

All research endeavours should ideally reflect a collective history, demonstrating a process in which researchers, subjects, their histories, identities, contexts and experiences impact on the 'new knowledge' that emerges out of gaps identified when questions are posed. This volume has such a history. *From Social Silence to Social*

*Science: Perspectives on Same-Sex Sexuality, HIV/AIDS and Gender in South Africa* is a project with its history in an international conference which took place in 2007. The conference was co-hosted and organised by the Human Sciences Research Council's Gender and Development Unit, the HIV Center for Clinical and Behavioural Studies at the New York State Psychiatric Institute, and the Department of Socio-medical Sciences at Columbia University Mailman School of Public Health in New York, in partnership with two community-based organisations: the Durban Lesbian and Gay Community and Health Centre and OUT LGBT Well-being (Pretoria).

Overall, the conference had a threefold purpose: 1) to review the history of research strategies on homosexuality in South Africa and to evaluate available research pertaining to same-sex sexual practices in South Africa, in general and as it relates to HIV/AIDS; 2) to identify research needs and priorities related to same-sex sexual practices and HIV/AIDS; and 3) to explore challenges and potential solutions to research on same-sex sexual practices and HIV/AIDS. The gathering brought together researchers, health professionals, community leaders and activists who took stock of available knowledge, established research priorities, and explored ways of resolving challenges related to undertaking such research as well as ways of creating a basis for innovative, community-supported research activities.

The title of the book suggests multiple and sometimes conflicting meanings, purposes and audiences. Yet there is a common denominator. At face value, if 'social silence' implies that homosexual transmission is absent from epidemiological studies, then the 'social science' envisaged in this book offers a corrective to that erasure. The title therefore signifies the recognition that there are shifts, movements and developments to the way knowledge is made and remade. Many of our contributors persistently ask, challenge and pose some answers to whether we are paying sufficient attention to the health needs, aspirations and concerns of same-sex practising individuals in South Africa, especially in the absence of research-based targeted HIV interventions.

## Multiple authors, audiences and purposes

Chapters assembled here represent in their individual capacity focused interventions with a broad appeal to both specialist and non-specialist audiences. (It is our ambitious aim that this book will be read by many.) The text presents a varied intersection of theoretical, empirical and practical contributions in a collection intended to describe, review, analyse, inform and pose further questions warranting answers. It is thus relevant to academic debates about HIV/AIDS, and is equally important to programming, policy-making, advocacy and community development in the field of HIV/AIDS.

The chapters range across wide terrains of concern, are infused by interdisciplinary energy, and draw on the expertise of research psychologists, historians, epidemiologists, sociologists, literary scholars and so forth. Our vision was to reflect the perspectives of a broad range of stakeholders and to provide authors (irrespective of their background and location) a space in which to think critically about key issues pertinent to developing our understanding of the complex relationship between gender, same-sex sexuality and HIV/AIDS in South Africa. Our contributors draw on the best insights based on their experience in the sector. While focusing on specific issues, they keep the historical context in which they write in clear view. Through this multidisciplinary lens, with its focus on HIV/AIDS and same-sex sexuality, we hope to bridge the chasm between policy, needs, service provision, research, practice and, ultimately, prevention; and we hope to direct debate and discussion to developing research-based *interventions* that assist in changing sexual practices that will reduce and ultimately end HIV infection.

## The gender framework

Our scholarly goal with this book is to lay a foundation for other scholars, researchers and practitioners to chart a new theoretical and empirical terrain for understanding same-sex sexuality in the context of the HIV/AIDS epidemic, through the recognition of the salient category of gender (see Albertyn 2003; Baylies et al. 2000; Meerkotter 2005; Patton 1994; Roth & Hogan 1998; Wilton 1997). As is evident, gender matters in the policies, processes and practices of HIV/AIDS. Gender is pervasive and deeply embedded and embodied in all aspects and processes of society, culture, sexual relations and social institutions. It is central to better understanding the epidemiological and social and sexual networks within which same-sex sexual practices are organised.

It is also axiomatic that gender is implicated in all aspects concerning sexuality. By extension, same-sex sexuality is also gendered. We know that our sexualities disclose an uneven process, principally between the sexes. Women and men are differently situated through a range of cultural, social, economic, unequal relations, and access to and consumption of power. The statistical invisibility of women's participation and representation in many arenas within our society and the globalising world is widely evident and we know that change is slow. Patriarchal struggles continue and the spectre of gender-based violence still poses a threat for full equality for women and girl children in particular. But the promise of equality is complicated by the reality that it is women, especially African women between the ages of 15 and 24, who are most vulnerable to the disease. And when it concerns same-sex sexual expression and, indeed, identity, heteronormative biases prevail (heteronormativity, we know, is a facet of patriarchal power).

## Same-sex sexuality

At the risk of being overambitious, we believe this volume inaugurates a new vigour into the literature on same-sex sexuality and HIV/AIDS in South Africa, drawing our collective attention to focused ways in which HIV/AIDS (particularly HIV-related risk behaviours, risk contents and treatment needs) is understood within same-sex sexual practices (which is broader than simply being gay or lesbian self-identified). The volume therefore deliberately foregrounds the question of *same-sex sexuality* (and lesbian and gay identity to a lesser extent) as central to HIV prevention, treatment, policy-making and programming. If our collective argument suggests that it is time to focus on the 'surveillance' of homosexual transmission to uncover what we do not know about the epidemic, we do so by not negating the importance of 'sex' and questions of identity formation.

We therefore purposefully chose the concept 'same-sex sexuality'. Our use of this category is not intended to minimise the significance of identity-based labels, but to rather broaden the frame in the recognition that there are those persons who engage in same-sex sexual practices but who do not allocate labels (or linguistic identities) to themselves. 'Same-sex sexuality' in broad terms encompasses a set of ideas, meanings and values that either consciously or unconsciously structure the social and sexual lives of people in either positive or negative ways (depending on the way it is organised, arranged and managed; see Robertson [2005]). Basically, the category of 'same-sex sexuality' should comprise all men and women with same-sex desires or practices, either exclusive or including sex with the other gender. As indicated earlier, these populations are heterogeneous: some openly visible, others hidden. So, arising out of the configuration called 'same-sex sexuality', the terms 'men who have sex with men' and 'women who have sex with women' grew out of the global response to the HIV/AIDS epidemic since the late eighties. The terms in this usage describe behaviour rather than identity (although in many contexts people who self-identify as MSM may use the term as an identity descriptor).

Central to the meaning of these terms is that within the epidemic there were many men (less the case with women) who were having sex with men and who were not part of the mainstream of gay communities. The terms themselves also problematise identity labels, confirming the possibility that identities (sexual identities in particular) could be fluid and dynamic. Either way, the terms open up limitations despite their broad location within sexual cultures, and function as a point of departure for us to begin to understand that we may need to conceptualise sexual cultures with caution. It is with this understanding that we have gathered here a selection of ideas that draw on a range of intertwined domains – sexuality, sexual practice, identity, policy, HIV/AIDS, service delivery – all of which enable us to see the cross-cutting meanings of sexual expression in relation to HIV.

## Some precautions

While the collection as a whole represents an exploratory effort to examine what we know about homosexual transmission in the context of HIV/AIDS, the chapters do not provide a detailed account of everything relevant to gender, same-sex sexuality and HIV/AIDS (understandably a rather tenuous and broad relationship exists in same-sex sexuality). Rather, chapters are meant to offer both descriptive and analytic insights into issues that could (and should) lead to an improved understanding of same-sex sexuality and HIV/AIDS from the frame of individual or organisational experiences.

While we ensured broad representation of 'voice', location and gender, several chapters were not included in the final manuscript (mainly to eradicate duplication, although some authors chose not to submit). But despite these precautions, we are aware that some overlap on matters of facts and interpretation is nevertheless present in the book. In order to maintain coherence of argument within individual chapters, it was necessary at times to allow for overlap while ensuring the delicate balance of broad representation. It is also inevitable that there will be some gaps and limitations in a project of this scope and especially in respect of the diversity of sites and disciplinary spaces in which our authors are located. While completing this introduction, we are also perfectly aware of the fact that this book reflects a specific moment in time. Since the start of our work on this book, several new projects have started and are delivering their first outcomes.

## Organisation of the book

This book contains an overview introduction, followed by four main parts which consist of 19 chapters. The concluding chapter (Chapter 20) abstracts some of the key ideas emanating from the various strands of the argument and turns some of these points into practical recommendations. However, the various parts of the book are not watertight, so debates and issues can be traced within and between the sections. Parts and chapters therefore need not be read in sequence. Chapters move around and take directions of their own that reflect, in large measure, the conference from which they emerged. Also, because this volume is not offering a core theory regarding what is happening in terms of homosexual transmission in respect of HIV/AIDS in South Africa, chapters circle around a handful of themes, approaching them from different vantage points and with different interpretive tools.

### Part 1: Theory, methodology, context

Part 1 offers a first immersion into some key conceptual aspects. It examines and locates some of the immediate theoretical, contextual and methodological factors that are central to thinking about same-sex sexuality. It reflects some of the significant future terms of debates on studying and researching sexualities through the filters of policy, HIV/AIDS, category formation, and community practice.

Chapter 1 by Peter Aggleton locates the meaning, interpretation and researching of same-sex sexuality within the context of HIV prevention and through the lens of the Universal Declaration of Rights. Aggleton emphasises the interconnectedness between gender and meanings about masculinity and femininity in relation to how same-sex sexualities and relationships are defined, lived and understood, particularly in the global South. The chapter highlights a progressive agenda for action, one which encompasses policy research, social research, epidemiological research and programme evaluation, in order to move HIV prevention forward.

Chapter 2 by Robert Sember reviews the meaning of sexuality, identities and practices in the context of the South African Bill of Rights. He makes the case that rights are not normative. Sember assesses the limitations of rights by examining the possible tensions between the aspirations espoused by the Constitution and the reality of lived experience. The chapter concludes with the value of what Sember terms 'engaged research' and the value of appropriate 'method' in the advancement of sexual and reproductive rights.

In Chapter 3, Juan Nel reviews current psychosocial scientific research in South Africa. Nel emphasises the declassification of same-sex sexual orientation as psychopathology in Euro-American psychiatry and psychology, but also cautions against the risk and vulnerability to potential secondary victimisation that LGBTI (lesbian, gay, bisexual, transsexual and intersexual) persons face at the hands of healthcare providers, communities and individuals in South Africa.

Chapter 4 by Theo Sandfort and Brian Dodge challenges some of the underlying assumptions that inform labels and categories in the context of AIDS research and their value in understanding the meaning of sexuality within sexual practices. MSM as a concept is interrogated to the extent that it is important for researchers, but also insofar as it presents limitations.

In Chapter 5, Pierre Brouard reviews research challenges and solutions in the context of same-sex sexuality, noting that questions of identity versus practice need to be debated and explored. Brouard also suggests that what is key to the methods employed in conducting HIV/AIDS research is a willingness to be reflexive, flexible, respectful, ethical and consultative, while at the same time remaining committed to high standards, unrelenting curiosity and healthy wariness.

Chapter 6 by Tim Lane reviews some of the important emerging literature on MSM in the context of Africa, and also discusses some of the ethical challenges and barriers to conducting MSM HIV research. He ends the chapter with some crucial suggestions on overcoming the difficulties in conducting such research.

*Part 2: History, memory, archive*

Part 2 illuminates in creative, historical and anthropological terms a set of ideas about experience, activism and identities. If an archive is viewed as a repository that represents the *active* forces of the past, which disclose how cultural events construct and participate in reconfiguring knowledge, it also discloses resistance to silencing and erasure. The three chapters in this section yield important insights into social change through the lens of experience, identity and 'voice'.

Chapter 7 by Mandisa Mbali provides a detailed and cogent socio-historical analysis of how HIV/AIDS entered into a complex same-sex social and organisational world in the early 1980s in South Africa. She outlines how the freer political climate in South Africa's transition era provided spaces for advocating for non-discriminatory approaches to sexual orientation and AIDS.

In Chapter 8 Zethu Mathebeni offers important insights into the views of a group of young (aged 18–35) self-identified black lesbian women, who share experiences and thoughts on lesbian sex, pleasure, performance, safer sex and how they continue to relate sexually with other women in the time of HIV and AIDS.

In Chapter 9 Ruth Morgan, Busi Kheswa and John Meletse describe how their work in the Gay and Lesbian Memory in Action HIV Oral History Project uses memory to document life histories that break the silence and stigma surrounding living with HIV.

*Part 3: Perspectives from and on sub-Saharan and southern Africa*

In the third part, authors use case studies to analyse the state of knowledge in service delivery, research and programming across a selection of African countries. Any future research into understanding homosexual transmission in the HIV epidemic can only benefit from what we can learn from other sites.

Chapter 10 by Cary Alan Johnson, aptly titled 'What we know about same-sex practising people and HIV in Africa', summarises research that was conducted up until 2007 on same-sex practices and HIV in Africa. Johnson argues that despite the paucity of research, policy-makers and implementers can draw on best practices from successful programmes for MSM in Ghana, Senegal and other countries in Africa, as well as initiatives in the African diaspora.

In Chapter 11 Daveson Nyadani outlines the context in Malawi, where denial and stigmatisation of same-sex sexuality is rife; because of these realities, little is known about how people with same-sex desires shape their lives. Written from the perspective of an active campaigner for lesbian and gay rights, and as a researcher, Nyadani demonstrates the steps that should be taken to improve the situation around same-sex sexuality in relation to HIV/AIDS in Malawi.

In Chapter 12 Sammy Matsikure outlines the situation in Zimbabwe from an activist and service delivery perspective. Over the years Zimbabwe has stood out on the African continent for the most virulent verbal attacks against homosexuals by President Robert Mugabe. Representing the work of Gays and Lesbians of Zimbabwe, Matsikure outlines some of the key challenges, compounded by persistent denial and stigmatisation of homosexuals, and identifies some key recommendations in the area of research, training and HIV prevention.

Chapter 13 by Kirk Fiereck provides a detailed, critical overview of five survey studies of same-sex practising men in Ghana, Kenya, Senegal and Nigeria. His chapter draws on appropriate historical and anthropological literature to comment on the central themes of the survey. Fiereck suggests that future research and public health interventions targeting same-sex practising individuals must critically account for epidemiological categories in programme development.

*Part 4: Needs, programming, policy, and directions for future research*

Part 4 provides broad and necessary interventions focused on the policy–practice mismatch, the lesbian and gay service delivery sector in South Africa, the health needs of WSW, and the important role of political mobilisation in building social movement in respect of HIV/AIDS. Research and policy-making in the area of HIV/AIDS is vast, and the chapters in this section zoom in on the South African experience to suggest how innovative work could lead to a renewed understanding through an epidemiological, practical and advocacy lens.

Chapter 14, by Nathan Geffen and colleagues, offers a trenchant critique of the response by lesbian and gay organisations in relation to HIV/AIDS. While the chapter acknowledges the achievements of LGBT organisations in achieving equality for lesbians and gays, the central argument is that such organisations are insufficiently mobilised to deal with the political factors exacerbating the HIV epidemic. Recommendations are offered for interventions by lesbian and gay organisations in response to the HIV epidemic, asserting the urgency for 'campaign politics' to be a necessary part of service delivery provision.

Chapter 15 by Laetitia Rispel and Carol Metcalf analyses the current South African response to HIV in relation to the needs of same-sex practising people and makes valuable recommendations on the critical role of government in ensuring the provision of sexual and reproductive health services in a supportive and non-discriminatory environment for vulnerable populations. The authors recommend greater LGBT participation in the national HIV response. Such a response requires research to improve understanding of the HIV epidemic among the LGBT community, and to support programme development to improve access to, and coverage with, prevention, treatment and care services.

In Chapter 16 Dawie Nel profiles the work of OUT LGBT Well-being, a service provider in Pretoria. He utilises relevant health data from various studies to argue that important research work has already commenced in the service provider sector. He also suggests that collaborative research between community structures, academics and policy-makers is necessary to obtain national HIV prevalence rates among LGB people, as well as to better understand risky behaviours and programmatic impacts.

In Chapter 17 Glenn de Swardt offers a personal narrative of observations and anecdotal evidence of the realities of HIV and AIDS among select groupings of Cape Town's LGBT populations. De Swardt lists a number of challenges in addressing HIV and AIDS within the sector, identifies various research needs, and outlines the HIV-related services offered by Triangle Project, one of the oldest lesbian and gay service providers specialising in health services in the country.

Nonhlanhla Mkhize, in Chapter 18, describes the work of the Durban Lesbian and Gay Community and Health Centre. Based on the principles and context of fighting homophobia, the chapter describes the importance and relevance of HIV/AIDS through the lens of the historical formation of the Centre. Mkhize shares personal and political perspectives on the Centre's work, mission and vision, and offers some statistics that reinforce why future programmatic work requires appropriate research-based interventions.

In Chapter 19 Vicci Tallis brings together the insights and experiences of a researcher and feminist activist who has worked extensively in the HIV/AIDS sector in South Africa. Tallis motivates that the health needs of women (particularly WSW, including lesbian, bisexual and non-lesbian identifying women) have long been neglected by both service providers and researchers. Health, Tallis argues, is gendered, and she calls on the lesbian community to define a research agenda which will develop understanding and better health services for WSW.

As a compilation, all of the chapters form a nucleus that address a selection of areas, issues and problems relevant to understanding same-sex sexuality in the context of HIV/AIDS. However, as editors, we are aware that the conversation opened up in the book is not a consistently scholarly one in that the chapters vary in substance, formulation and address. As stated earlier, there is sometimes repetition without apparent gain and there is no single streamlined argument. It is for these reasons that we have designed a conclusion that offers a streamlined overview of key issues emerging in the arguments of the chapters.

The concluding chapter reflects, raises further questions, probes issues and stitches central threads of the book together, and hopefully takes us beyond the ideas espoused in the pages of this project.

Working on this volume has been empowering for us as co-editors, who, like our authors, are engaged in the process of the production of knowledge. We hope it has been equally empowering for those who are being studied and for those who will potentially benefit from the work. This volume serves as an invitation to policy-makers, researchers, activists and programmers to join forces to further the work that many of the authors have passionately articulated. We return to the opening epigraph in which Maluleke claimed, 'We all died/Because nobody ever said AIDS.' If we search for meaning in these statements, we might collectively ask, is it not time that we should take stock of the possibility of a 'homosexual epidemic'? We will not know if we do not ask the appropriate questions.

## A note on terminology

In this introductory chapter we regularly used the term same-sex sexuality; when we did so we implied a range of erotic orientations and practices that involve persons of the same biological sex. While 'homosexuality' would be an adequate label as well (as it is indeed used by some of the authors), we prefer the use of 'same-sex sexuality' because it is less loaded with pre-existing values and perspectives. We did not explicitly state to the contributors to this volume that same-sex sexuality was the only label they could use. Other labels – such as MSM, WSW, bisexual gay, lesbian – are used as well. Whenever such labels are used the context usually makes clear what, in terms of sexual orientation, gender role orientation and identity, authors are referring to.

## Acknowledgement

A special thanks to Jane Bennett (and other reviewers) for reading and offering comment on an initial draft of this chapter.

## Notes

1   This is a stanza from Eddie Maluleke's poem 'Nobody Ever Said Aids'. Also cited is Rustum Kozain's poem 'Crossing from Solitude'. Both texts feature in *Nobody Ever Said AIDS: Stories & Poems from Southern Africa* (Rasebotsa et al. 2004).

2   The narrative motivating the timeline of the AIDS epidemic discussed in this paragraph is in part drawn from the HIV Center for Clinical and Behavioural Studies brochure outlining a timeline of the AIDS epidemic (from 1981–2007).

3   The concept of 'risk' is often used when investigating sexual behaviour in the context of HIV/AIDS. Usually referred to as 'the probability of a generally negative outcome, accompanied by the magnitude of the damage it will do' (Joffe 1999: 4), the meanings of risk could have the potential of allocating blame and shame, and reinforcing the already stigmatised sexual identity of the homosexual (see also Douglas 1992). In contrast, some commentators have also explored how intentional risk-taking could have pleasurable outcomes within the context of sexual negotiation and may assist in a person's 'self-development, self-actualisation, self-authenticity and self-control' (see Lupton & Tulloch 2002: 122).

4   This section offers a summative paraphrase of key issues contained in the 2008 *Report on the Global AIDS Epidemic* (UNAIDS 2008) and relies principally on chapters 2 and 3 (pages 30–93).

5   This section draws on summary notes extracted from *Culture, HIV & AIDS: An Annotated Bibliography* (UNESCO 2008). For readers wanting to pursue the critical literature, this study provides a fairly detailed annotated bibliography of academic and policy literature in English, French and Spanish. Critical reviews of the literature focused on South Africa also exist (see CADRE 2000a, 2000b). It should be emphasised that beyond the social science and medical literature on HIV/AIDS, and beyond statistical arguments, there is also a significant body of literature in the human sciences (poetry, fiction, drama, cinema, art) and critical studies exist. (See Parker 2001 for a detailed explication of HIV/AIDS research focused on the relationship between sexuality, culture and power.)

6   See also a recent special report by AmFAR AIDS Research (2008), which focuses on MSM and HIV and contains recent epidemiological data (128 countries) of HIV among MSM, showing an increased high rate of infection in countries where the epidemic appears to be fuelled by denial, indifference and inaction. Some important community-driven initiatives focused on same-sex populations are also currently under way in the form of collaboration between LGBT partners in southern Africa, Latin America and the Schorer Foundation (Netherlands). The aim is to upscale HIV/AIDS prevention programmes between 2007 and 2010, targeting LGBT people. The southern African partnering organisations are OUT LGBT Well-being (Pretoria), the Durban Lesbian and Gay Community and Health Centre, the Triangle Project (Cape Town), the Rainbow Project (Namibia), Lesbians and Gays in Botswana and the Gay and Lesbian Association of Zimbabwe. The southern African project is called PRISM (Prevention Initiative for Sexual Minorities). Preliminary conclusions from a needs assessment focused on men indicate that 'HIV and STIs are seen as serious health problems confronting gay men', and 'casual sex seems to be occurring in a context where anal sex is a preference', indicating that 'these men (are) at a high risk of contracting and transmitting an STI or HIV' (OUT LGBT Well-being 2008a: 29). In respect of resourced and under-resourced women who have sex with women, indications are that 'HIV, STIs and alcohol abuse are serious health problems', 'there is no regular testing for STIs or HIV, no consistent barrier methods during casual sexual encounters' (OUT LGBT Well-being 2008b: 19).

## References

Abdool Karim Q & Abdool Karim SS (Eds) (2005) *HIV/AIDS in South Africa*. Cape Town: Cambridge University Press

Adams V & Pigg SL (Eds) (2005) *Sex in development: Science, sexuality and morality in global perspective*. Durham: Duke University Press

Aggleton P (Ed.) (1999) *Men who sell sex: International perspectives on male prostitution and HIV/AIDS*. London: University College of London Press

Aggleton P, Davies G & Hart G (Eds) (1999) *Families and communities responding to AIDS*. London: University College of London Press

Albertyn C (2003) Contesting democracy: HIV/AIDS and the achievement of gender equality in South Africa. *Feminist Studies* 29(3): 595–615

Altman D (1994) *Power and community: Organizational and cultural responses to AIDS*. London: Taylor and Francis

Altman D (2001) *Global sex*. Chicago & London: University of Chicago Press

amFAR AIDS Research (2008) *MSM, HIV and the road to universal access: How far have we come?* (Special Report). New York: amFAR

Barnett T & Whiteside A (2002) *AIDS in the twenty-first century: Disease and globalization*. New York: Palgrave Macmillan

Baylies C, Bujra J & The Gender AIDS Group (2000) *AIDS, sexuality and gender in Africa: Collective strategies and struggles in Tanzania and Zambia*. London & New York: Routledge

Berger J (2004) Re-sexualising the epidemic: Desire, risk and HIV prevention. *Development Update* 5(3): 45–68

CADRE (Centre for AIDS Development, Research and Evaluation) (2000a) *The economic impact of HIV/AIDS on South Africa and its implications for governance: A bibliographic review* (Compiled by S Gelb, K Kelly, U Kistner, M O'Donovan, W Parker & A van Niekerk on behalf of USAID through the Joint Centre for Political and Economic Studies). Johannesburg: CADRE

CADRE (2000b) *The economic impact of HIV/AIDS on South Africa and its implications for governance: A literature review*. Johannesburg: CADRE

Crimp D (2004) *Melancholia and moralism: Essays on AIDS and queer politics*. Cambridge, Massachusetts: MIT Press

DoH (Department of Health, South Africa) (2007) *HIV and AIDS and STI National Strategic Plan for South Africa 2007–2011*. Pretoria: Department of Health

Dolan KA (2005) *Lesbian women and sexual health: The social construction of risk and susceptibility*. Binghamton, New York: Routledge

Douglas M (1992) *Risk and blame: Essays in cultural theory*. London: Routledge

Dowsett GW (1996) *Practicing desire: Homosexual sex in the era of AIDS*. Stanford, CA: Stanford University Press

Duggan L & Hunter ND (1995) *Sex wars: Sexual dissent and political culture*. London & New York: Routledge

Elder GS (2003) *Hostels, sexuality and the apartheid legacy: Malevolent geographies*. Athens, Ohio: Ohio University Press

Epprecht M (2004) *Hungochani: The history of a dissident sexuality in southern Africa*. Montreal: McGill-Queen's University Press

Germond P & De Gruchy S (Eds) (1997) *Aliens in the household of god: Homosexuality and Christian faith in South Africa*. Cape Town & Johannesburg: David Philip

Gevisser M & Cameron E (Eds) (1994) *Defiant desire: Gay and lesbian lives in South Africa*. Johannesburg: Ravan Press

Herdt G (Ed.) (1997) *Sexual cultures and migration in the era of AIDS: Anthropological and demographic perspectives*. London: Claredon

Hoad N (2007) *African intimacies: Race, homosexuality and globalization*. Minneapolis: University of Minnesota Press

Hoad N, Martin K & Reid G (Eds) (2005) *Sex & politics in South Africa: The equality clause/gay & lesbian movement/the anti-apartheid struggle*. Cape Town: Double Storey

Isaacs G & McKendrick B (1992) *Male homosexuality in South Africa: Identity formation, culture and crisis*. Cape Town: Oxford University Press

Isaacs G & Miller DE (1985) AIDS: Its implications for South African homosexuals and the mediating role of the medical practitioner. *South African Medical Journal* 68(5): 327–330

Jaffe HW, De Cock KM & Valdiserri RO (2007) The re-emerging HIV/AIDS epidemic in men who have sex with men. *JAMA* 298(30): 2412–2414

Joffe H (1999) *Risk and 'the other'*. Cambridge: Cambridge University Press

Johnson CA (2007) *Off the map: How HIV/AIDS programming is failing same-sex practicing people in Africa*. New York: International Gay and Lesbian Human Rights Commission

Kalipeni E, Cradock S, Ghosh J & Oppong JR (Eds) (2004) *HIV and AIDS in Africa: Beyond epistemology*. Oxford: Blackwell

King JL (2004) *On the down low: The lives of 'straight' black men who sleep with men*. New York: Broadway Books

Loue S (Ed.) (2007) *Health issues confronting minority men who have sex with men*. New York: Springer

Luirinck B (2000) *Moffies: Gay life and lesbian life in southern Africa*. Cape Town: David Philip

Lupton D & Tulloch J (2002) 'Life would be pretty dull without risk': Voluntary risk-taking and its pleasures. *Health, Risk and Society* 4(2): 113–124

Meerkotter A (2005) The impact of the HIV/AIDS epidemic on women's citizenship in South Africa. In A Gouws (Ed.) *(Un)Thinking citizenship: Feminist debates in contemporary South Africa*. Landowne: University of Cape Town Press

Mendel G, Byamugisha Rev G & Kaleeba N (2001) *A broken landscape: HIV & AIDS in Africa*. Auckland Park: M & G Books

Meyer IN & Northridge ME (Eds) (2007) *The health of sexual minorities: Public health perspectives on lesbian, gay, bisexual and transgender populations*. New York: Springer

Morgan R & Wieringa S (Eds) (2005) *Tommy boys, lesbian men and ancestral wives: Female same-sex practices in Africa*. Johannesburg: Jacana Media

Munson M & Stelboum JP (Eds) (1999) *The lesbian polyamory reader: Open relationships, non-monogamy and casual sex*. Binghamton, New York: The Haworth Press

Nattrass N (2004) *The moral economy of AIDS in South Africa*. Cape Town: Cambridge University Press

OUT (OUT LGBT Well-being) (2004a) *Gay and lesbian people's experiences of the health care sector in Gauteng: Prevalence and risk factors*. Arcadia, Tshwane: OUT LGBT Well-being

OUT (2004b) *Hate crimes against gay & lesbian people in Gauteng*. Arcadia, Tshwane: OUT LGBT Well-being

OUT (2004c) *Reporting practices to the police among gay & lesbian people in Gauteng*. Arcadia, Tshwane: OUT LGBT Well-being

OUT (2004d) *Suicide among gay & lesbian people in Gauteng: Prevalence and risk factors*. Arcadia, Tshwane: OUT LGBT Well-being

OUT (2008a) *PRISM project: Needs assessment report (resourced gay men in Tshwane aged 18–40)*. Arcadia, Tshwane: OUT LGBT Well-being

OUT (2008b) *PRISM project: Needs assessment report (resourced and under-resourced women who have sex with women (WSW in Tshwane aged 18–40)*. Arcadia, Tshwane: OUT LGBT Well-being

Parker R (2001) Sexuality, culture and power in HIV/AIDS research. *Annual Review of Anthropology* 20: 163–179

Patton C (1994) *Last served? Gendering the HIV pandemic*. London: Taylor & Francis

Philips O (2004) The invisible presence of homosexuality: Implications for HIV/AIDS and rights in southern Africa. In E Kalipeni, S Craddock, J Ghosh & JR Oppong (Eds) *HIV and AIDS in Africa: Beyond epistemology*. Oxford: Blackwell

Reddy V, Mkhize N & Potgieter C-A (2007) Cloud over the rainbow nation. *HSRC Review* 5(1): 10–11

Reid G (2006) How to become a 'real' gay: Identity and terminology in Ermelo, Mpumalanga. *Agenda. Empowering women for gender equality* 67(13): 137–145

Robertson J (Ed.) (2005) *Same sex cultures and sexualities: An anthropological reader*. Oxford: Blackwell Publishing

Rasebotsa N, Samuelson M & Thomas K (Eds) (2004) *Nobody ever said AIDS: Stories & poems from southern Africa*. Cape Town: Kwela Books

Roth NL & Hogan K (Eds) (1998) *Gendered epidemic: Representations of women in the age of AIDS*. New York: Routledge

Ruel E & Campbell RT (2006) Homophobia and HIV/AIDS: Attitude change in the face of an epidemic. *Social Forces* 84(4): 2167–2178

Schoepf BG (2001) International AIDS research in anthropology: Taking a critical perspective on the crisis. *Annual Review of Anthropology* 30: 335–361

Shisana O & Simbayi L (2002) *Nelson Mandela HSRC study of HIV/AIDS: South African national HIV prevalence, behavioural risks and mass media. Household survey*. Cape Town: Human Sciences Research Council

Sontag S (1991) *Illness as a metaphor/AIDS and its metaphors*. Harmondsworth: Penguin

Spurlin WJ (2006) *Imperialism within the margins: Queer representation and the politics of culture in southern Africa*. New York: Palgrave Macmillan

Treichler PA (1999) *How to have theory in an epidemic: Cultural chronicles of AIDS*. Durham, NC/London: Duke University Press

UNAIDS (2008) *Report on the global AIDS epidemic*. Geneva: UNAIDS

UNESCO (2008) *Culture, HIV & AIDS: An annotated bibliography* (Prepared for UNESCO by the Social Science Research Council). New York: Social Science Research Council

Van Zyl M & Steyn M (Eds) (2005) *Performing queer: Shaping sexualities 1994–2004* (Vol. 1). Cape Town: Kwela

Waldy C (1996) *AIDS and the body politic: Biomedicine and sexual difference*. London & New York: Routledge

Walker L, Cornell M & Reid G (2004) *Waiting to happen: HIV/AIDS in South Africa – The bigger picture*. Cape Town: Double Storey

Watney S (1997) *Policing desire: Pornography, AIDS and the media* (2nd edition). London: Cassell

Watney S (2000) *Imagine hope: AIDS and gay identity*. London & New York: Routledge

Whiteside A & Sunter C (2000) *AIDS: The challenge for South Africa*. Cape Town: Human & Rousseau/Tafelberg

Williamson C & Martin DP (2005) Origin, diversity and spread of HIV-1. In SS Abdool Karim & Q Abdool Karim (Eds) *HIV/AIDS in South Africa*. Cape Town: Cambridge University Press

Wilton T (1997) *EnGendering AIDS*. London: Sage

# THEORY, METHODOLOGY, CONTEXT

What I would like to insist on is that we have to go back to the ontological and philosophical debate. There are a lot of things to be explored at the philosophical, symbolic level, spiritual level, even language. Language is full of expressions that show different constructions of male-to-male sexuality or woman-to-woman sexuality. There are multiple identities and if we don't know the identities, if we don't work with the multiple identities, we will be sending a message that will not be received. People only receive the message when they think that you are talking to them. You will only reach them when it is clear that you know them, you know each other. You are in a position of empathy, and empathy most of the time is excluded from scientific research. Empathy could help us to understand the other and redesign all the programmes, messages and politics. If you say African societies are homophobic, I say okay, one side only, one level. If you go deep, you will find a completely different story. How can you use what is deep in order to challenge what actually exists in order to arrive at comprehensive HIV/AIDS strategies? We should use a holistic approach towards MSM as a marginalised group and make our research part of the process of social and political transformation. Societies are not rigid, are not fixed. Societies move, they have to evolve. New agendas will push for transformation when they take into consideration everything I said before. *Cheikh I Niang, conference delegate*

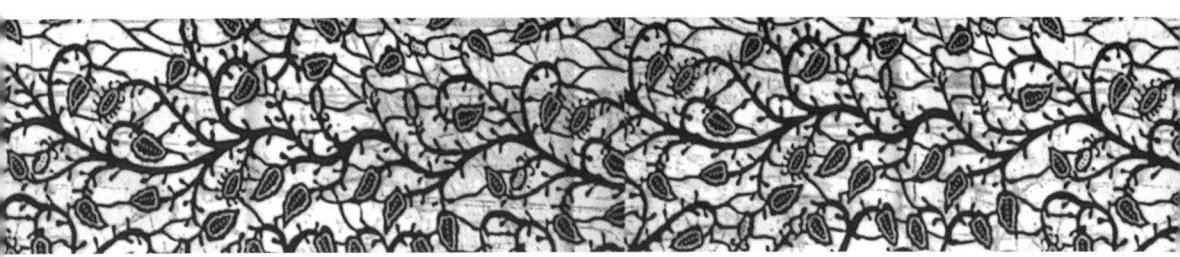

I often remind myself as a researcher of what I think is a very important truism, and that is, how you analyse a problem is going to determine how you choose to intervene in a problem. So if you look at a problem in purely behavioural terms, then you probably are going to intervene in the problem in purely behavioural terms. *Robert Sember, conference delegate*

CHAPTER ONE

# Researching same-sex sexuality and HIV prevention

Peter Aggleton

Some 60 years ago, the Universal Declaration of Human Rights affirmed that all human beings are equal in dignity, in rights and in freedoms, without distinction of any kind. Among the rights delineated in the Declaration are rights to life, liberty and security, to health, education and work, to freedom of opinion and expression, and to freedom of thought, conscience and religion.[1] Subsequent instruments, such as the International Covenant on Economic, Social and Cultural Rights, expanded the field to include reference to a wide range of economic and social rights.[2]

More recently, there have been growing struggles to delineate and achieve sexual rights or the 'rights of all persons to have control over and decide freely and responsibly on matters related to their sexuality…free of coercion, discrimination and violence' (WHO 2004: 3). While this remains a hotly contested field, especially by the 'unholy alliance' of fundamentalist Islam, the Roman Catholic Church and the former government of the United States of America (Pazello 2005), movement has been made, stimulated in part by the Brazilian government's Resolution on Human Rights and Sexual Orientation to the Commission on Human Rights in 2003,[3] and the actions of individual governments, including South Africa, to extend partnership/marriage rights to all citizens.

Within this context, the Yogyakarta Principles on the Application of International Human Rights Law in relation to sexual orientation and gender identity signal a way forward in their commitment to ensuring that the application of existing human rights entitlements should take account of the situations and experiences of people of diverse sexual orientations and gender identities. The Principles affirm the obligation of states to address a broad range of human rights standards and their application to issues of sexual orientation and gender identity. They also highlight the responsibilities of the UN human rights system, national human rights institutions, the media, non-governmental organisations (NGOs) and funders to ensure that the rights of people of diverse sexual orientations and gender identities are protected and upheld.[4]

In relation to HIV, the picture is both more clouded and more clear. Paragraph 64 of the UN Declaration of Commitment on HIV/AIDS, for example, which was adopted by all UN Member States in 2001, emphasised the importance of 'addressing the needs of those at the greatest risk of, and most vulnerable to, new infection as indicated by such factors as…sexual practices, (UN General Assembly Special Session 2001). But the Declaration refrained from naming groups such as gay and other homosexually active men who, on grounds of sexuality, were most vulnerable in the face of the epidemic.

The above commitment was reiterated by UN Member States and by civil society in the Political Declaration on HIV/AIDS, at the High-Level Meeting on HIV/AIDS held in 2006.[5] This Declaration underlined the need for full and active participation of vulnerable groups, and the need to eliminate all forms of discrimination against them, while respecting privacy and confidentiality. But once again, while offering clarity with respect to the channelling of resources towards those most vulnerable within the context of the epidemic, specifically vulnerable forms of sexuality and sexual expression remain unnamed.

## What do we mean by sexuality?

But what exactly do we mean by sexuality? Many different definitions can be found in the literature. The World Association for Sexology (1999), for example, sees sexuality as 'an integral part of the personality of every human being [whose] full development depends upon the satisfaction of basic human needs such as desire for contact, intimacy, emotional expression, pleasure, tenderness and love.'

The World Health Organisation's current working definition of sexuality, on the other hand, views sexuality as:

> …a central aspect of being human throughout life [that] encompasses sex, gender identities and roles, sexual orientation, eroticism, pleasure, intimacy and reproduction. Sexuality is experienced and expressed in thoughts, fantasies, desires, beliefs, attitudes, values, behaviours, practices, roles and relationships. [It] is influenced by the interaction of biological, psychological, social, economic, political, cultural, ethical, legal, historical and religious and spiritual factors. (WHO 2004: 3)

### Sexuality as a set of sensibilities and social practices

Fundamentally, however, sexuality is not so much a 'thing' as a set of sensibilities and social practices that link to issues of identity, and tie into broader social relationships. Ultimately, and in every society, there are many ways of *being sexual*. There may be dominant forms, as well as alternative possibilities. What these different practices are called varies from place to place and from time to time. Some may be understood as the norm; others may be perceived as different.

Sexuality is intrinsically linked to physical acts, yet it is simultaneously conceived in discourse – in words and language. Similar, even identical, acts may have different meanings in different social settings and cultures – being sexual in one context and not sexual in another.

## The ambiguity and situatedness of sexuality

In interactions between people, interpretations of sexuality can vary. Some forms of touch, or talk, may be mutually interpreted as expressions of sexuality. Such meanings are not self-evident or transparent, however, since one person's reading of an interaction as sexual may not be shared by other(s) involved in the communication. Definitions of sexuality are thus dependent on the personal and cultural frames of reference that inform how individuals make sense of their desires. They are also influenced by the relations of power that structure human social interaction. Gender, race, class, age and culture, for example, set limits on what it is possible for some to do. They also privilege some people in their social and sexual negotiations with others.

Why does all this matter, and why is it important to discuss these broader considerations before addressing a research agenda of relevance to same-sex sexualities and HIV with particular reference to developing countries? It is important because sexuality, rather than being a fixed entity, is perhaps best conceived of as something that is constructed both by individuals and by society more generally, in relation to available options and possibilities.

This is particularly important when it comes to understanding same-sex sexualities, since the way in which women's and men's same-sex relationships are often discussed in the West (for example, lesbian/gay, homosexual, bisexual, straight/heterosexual) has limited resonance in many non-Western and in particular African or Asian contexts. In these settings, just as in Europe and North America in the past, such matters, if talked about at all, are often conceived of in respect of local descriptors and vernaculars.

While identities such as 'lesbian' and 'gay' may be subscribed to by some people – particularly those with access to books, travel, television, the internet and other modern means of communication – more often than not, these same identity descriptors are inflected with local meanings. Thus, to be lesbian or gay in modern-day Thailand or in Namibia is not the same as being such in San Francisco. Nor, it should be said, is being gay or lesbian in San Francisco the same as it is in London.

## The importance of gender

Issues of gender are crucial when it comes to understanding same-sex relations. At first sight this may seem strange, since advocacy and activism within the field of sexuality often take place separately from struggles to secure the rights of women, or for greater recognition of the role of dominant masculinities in structuring and limiting men's experiences.

Writers such as Rubin (1984) have highlighted how gender and sexuality systems intersect and interact. Put simply, the one cannot be understood without reference to the other. The heterosexual gender behaviour of many Western men, for example, can only be understood in terms of what it is construed as not being – prissy, effeminate and gay. Likewise, dominant patterns of femininity are often defined through their antitheses – being manly, unladylike or butch. These patterns are true of both rich and poor world contexts, although the sanctions brought to bear for the infringement of local norms may vary.

In the Philippines (Tan 1996) and in Thailand (Ten Brummelhuis 1999), for example, men known as *bakla* and *kathoey* (sometimes described as 'feminised males', being biologically male but socially feminine) both celebrate and challenge prevailing gender norms through their adoption of feminine styles, behaviours and subjectivities – demonstrating in the process something of the malleability of gendered and sexual practices in and across cultures.

Throughout Mexico, central and southern America, *travestis* may dress and to some extent live as women, adapting their clothing, hair and bodies in line with their intent (Parker 1999; Prieur 1998). Some may have prominent roles within their local community as entertainers, hairdressers, beauticians and even politicians. Others may find employment within the sex industry, offering services to men whose masculinity is strengthened, rather than threatened, by playing the nominally 'active' role in their relationship with a feminised male partner (Schifter 1998: Schifter et al. 1996).

In West Africa, feminised men have an important role to play in traditional dance troupes or as *simb* lion dancers. In Burkina Faso, such men have an important role to play in baptisms and marriages (Niang et al. 2004). More recently, research has described the existence of *ibbi* and *yoo* relationships between men in Senegal, the term *ibbi* denoting the receptive partner in anal sex and *yoo* 'he who penetrates'.

But in all of the above contexts there exist countless same-sex attracted men who may, regularly or occasionally, have sex with other men, and who do not construct themselves in a feminised manner. These are the husbands, brothers, sons and fathers who, indistinguishable from the heterosexual majority, live their lives as men, enjoy their lives as men, and whose sexuality, for the large part, remains invisible at home, at work and in the street.

A similar picture prevails for women, although research and scholarship with respect to women's same-sex relationships is, as yet, somewhat less developed. In Taiwan, for example, *T-Po* (Tomboy-femme) identities have been identified among women in same-sex relationships (Chao 2000). In Thailand, *Tom* (as in Tom-boy) and *Dee* (as in Lay-dee) relationships have been documented across a range of settings (Thaweesit 2004). In countries such as Uganda, Kenya, Namibia, Swaziland and South Africa, same-sex relationships of both traditional (for example, woman–woman marriages and mummy–baby relationships) and modern (for example,

Tommy boy and lesbian identities in all of these countries) character have been documented among both young and older women (Morgan & Wieringa 2005).

## Relevance to HIV

But little has been said so far about HIV – overtly at least. This has been deliberate, since to do so without first talking about issues of gender and sexuality, visibility and invisibility, masculinity and femininity, is to do violence to what we need to understand.

All over the world, there exist epidemiological and behavioural studies which construct same-sex attracted people as separate and segregated populations – as different 'species' as it were. In a recent internet posting, for example, it was claimed that HIV-prevention interventions were reaching 96 per cent of men who have sex with men in Bangkok and Chiang Mai, as if the number of men who (regularly or occasionally) have sex with other men were easily measurable in some way.[6]

Worse still, HIV research may relegate to Western or perhaps Northern frames the sophisticatedness and complexity of same-sex relationships as they are lived throughout the developing world, for example with women and men being constructed as 'homosexuals', or as 'gay men' or as 'lesbians', or (more recently) as 'men who have sex with men' and 'women who have sex with women'.

But before continuing, a word of caution and an apology: since the beginning of the epidemic, HIV has been constructed around same-sex sexuality and it often remains difficult for it to be thought of outside the frames of reference that this imposes. Since its early identification among gay men in the USA and other rich countries, HIV has indeed been seen as a disease of gay or 'homosexual' men, a fact which contributes to much (but not all) of the stigma which exists around the disease today – particularly in developing countries.

But HIV is also a disease of absence – with little having been said about the risks that lesbians, bisexual and same-sex attracted women face. Dworkin, for example, has written powerfully about the manner in which the dominant epidemiological categories employed in HIV analysis have quite literally written anything other than heterosexual transmission for women out of the script:

> Under existing classification systems, a woman who always has had long sessions of oral sex with multiple women but has had *one* episode of heterosexual contact is counted as having heterosexual risk. A bisexual female who does not use drugs will be counted as having a heterosexual transmission risk. A bisexual woman who has anal sex with a gay man will be classified as having heterosexual transmission risks. A woman who has sex with women and men, and is the partner of both a female and a male injecting drug user, will be categorized as having heterosexual transmission risks. (Dworkin 2005: 619)

Importantly, the same forces of heteronormativity that are at work here, or the belief that 'adult heterosexuality' is the moral and statistical norm against which all forms of sexual expression should be judged, are those which cause many same-sex attracted women to face avoidable risks in their sexual relations with men. In this respect, it is heartening to see growing attention nationally and internationally to women's same-sex experiences and HIV, particularly in contexts where sexual violence and rape may be used by men against same-sex attracted women to police the boundaries of a normative heterosexuality.

## The importance of masculinity

It is important to recognise that not all men who – regularly or occasionally – have sex with other men are feminised. Some are resolutely masculine in appearance and comportment, and many are indistinguishable from heterosexual men. With respect to identity, some such men may understand themselves as different from the norm in some way. A few may have heard of terms such as 'bisexual' and 'gay', and a very few may identify with them. Perhaps the majority see themselves simply as *men*.

With respect to behaviour, many such men – and many feminised men too – have sex with both women and men, especially in cultures where marriage is socially compulsory, and where heteronormativity is strong.

In this kind of context, it is important to understand both the pervasiveness of male-to-male sexual relations and their invisibility (Aggleton 1996, 1999). Things may happen, but they are not talked about. The family or the community may 'know', but same-sex relations between men are not acknowledged as existing. Sex between men may take place, but it is not seen as 'sex' and rather as 'something that happens' occasionally as fun (as in India where the term *maasti* [mischief], which may be used to describe it, denotes a certain playfulness), and often as 'release', particularly in cultures where the segregation of the sexes is strong (Khan 1996).

This is the context we live with – in both North and South, in Europe and in Africa; and this is the context we need to understand if we are to be constructive in the context of the most serious and life-threatening epidemic the world has known.

## The dangers of similitude

It is often all too easy to take the latest piece of research from the USA, for example, and assume that it has relevance to the other context(s) in which we work. This has happened time and time again with respect to HIV prevention among same-sex attracted men in London, the city in which I work. 'Have you got a "crystal meth." problem in London?', an eminent West Coast professor asked about a year ago. 'What about cultures of barebacking?' asked another. 'What about younger gay men, they are surely at highest risk?'

In the UK, at least, none of these statements are unproblematically correct; it is the specificities of HIV-related vulnerability and risk among homosexually-active men that need to be enquired into – and their situatedness in space and time that is important – not the imagined 'parallels' between behaviours in what are often very different contexts.

In this chapter I prefer to avoid using the term 'men who have sex with men'. In every field, there are terms which were constructed for a particular purpose but have now outlived their usefulness. In my view, the phrase 'men who have sex with men' is one of these. This term was invented in the UK in the late 1980s in an effort to capture within the frame of reference of HIV prevention men who did not see themselves as gay. At that time, prevention workers used the phrase 'gay and other men who have sex with men' to capture something of this diversity.

With the passage of time, however, uses and meanings have changed. Now, it is not uncommon to find men self-identifying as 'men who have sex with men' or even as 'MSM'– a behavioural descriptor is becoming a new identity category. This tendency is particularly acute in South and South East Asia where the impact of MSM projects, such as those undertaken by international NGOs, has been strong. But things can go further than this, with it being reported from several countries that 'MSM groups' exist in which none of the organisers have (or have had) sex with other men! Under the impact of 'MSM organising' globally, this behavioural descriptor is becoming entirely dissociated from its material base in same-sex relations (see Young & Meyer 2005).

## An agenda for action

In the final section of this chapter, I want to turn to some practical issues and, in particular, the delineation of a research agenda of relevance to men's same-sex relations in Africa. Given what has been said so far, it will come as no surprise to learn that the first domain within which enquiry should take place links to how best to understand the problem. It is here that *contextual and interpretative research* has a special role to play.

Research of this kind is likely to stress the importance of appreciating what same-sex roles and practices mean to individuals – both those who practise them and those who do not. It is also likely to direct attention to the effects of contextual factors in influencing when, where and with whom same-sex relations are legitimate. Recent research across Africa has pointed to the prevalence of same-sex relations among men in a rich variety of settings – in religious and spiritual ceremonies, in boarding schools in the military, in prisons, and in mining compounds (Epprecht 2004; O'Murray & Roscoe 1998).

Yet rarely is such behaviour understood within the frames of reference of 'homosexuality', being 'gay', 'same-sex relations' or even 'MSM activity'. More usually, it is not talked about openly – although it may be acknowledged as taking place – or it is made reference to obliquely or via contextually specific frames of reference. As indicated earlier, part of the issue here derives from the fact that 'sex' is often seen as something which by definition takes place between women and men. Other sexual practices may therefore not be seen as explicitly sexual in character, but are construed in other ways.

To this first domain of contextual and interpretative enquiry, however, can be added four other important fields. The categories referred to here have their origins in a recent review of achievements and priorities of relevance to men's same-sex relations and HIV (Sandfort 2006). They are referred to here with due acknowledgement.

## Policy research

Policy research is important, since unless we understand how decisions come to be made about work of relevance to same-sex relations and HIV, it is hard to take action. Of priority, therefore, must be enquiry into the manner in which policy-makers come to understand the HIV epidemic – the individuals and groups who are most affected, the 'needs' that exist (for prevention, treatment and care), and the responsibilities governments have to their citizenry. To date, far too little of this research has been done within any of these fields, although there are some signs that the picture is changing.

Central, too, is policy-focused enquiry into the progressive medicalisation of the epidemic, as biomedical intervention has been given new prominence (for example, around male circumcision, pre-exposure prophylaxis for sex workers, and vaginal microbicides). In this respect, it is important to note that the 2007 International AIDS Society Conference on Pathogenesis, Treatment and Prevention in Sydney had a track called 'biomedical prevention'. Papers within this track made scant reference to the broader-based responses that we know are essential in order to work with men who (regularly or occasionally) have sex with other men.

Moreover, within the biomedical domain itself, how many centres offering post-exposure prophylaxis for HIV in the developing world make their services readily available to men involved in same-sex relations? Why has progress been so slow in the development of (or even discussion about) an effective rectal microbicide? And what protection does male circumcision offer the receptive partner in unprotected anal sex? It seems clear that recent new directions in HIV prevention risk compounding the exclusion and neglect of same-sex attracted men – particularly in resource-poor settings.

## Social research

Social research encompasses several distinct strands of enquiry. First, there is the importance of enquiry into safe and unsafe sex practices in relation to the social position of different groups and in the context of other health behaviours, such as alcohol and substance use. Second, research is needed into men's experiences of same- and opposite-sex intimacy, and the relationship between intimate bonding, sexual expression and sexual risk. Third, it is important – in Southern Africa at least – to better understand community building as it relates to safe-sex practices and offers contexts for prevention.

There are other matters too that need to be addressed within a comprehensive research agenda of relevance to HIV prevention and same-sex attraction. They include research into issues of sexual safety (including harassment, victimisation, exploitation and the rape of both women and men); studies of sexual communication and negotiation (as well as the limits to such practices in different relationships and settings); and enquiry into the nature and practice of HIV serosorting and positive–positive sex – safer-sex practices made possible by the increased availability of new and more effective tests.

Also important is research into the development of sexual subcultures of safety and risk, as well as research into transformations in men's understandings of themselves socially and sexually, under the impact of globalisation, broader struggles for sexual and human rights, and HIV itself. Of central importance in all of this work is seeing sexuality as a socially organised *practice,* rich in social and individual significance, not simply as a behaviour.

Finally, there are issues of stigma and discrimination to consider – both those enacted by individuals, and those which are the consequence of official state repression (Human Rights Watch 2004). Many of these negative reactions have their origins deep within the structures of society – in class, gender and ethnic relations, as well as in the denigration of same-sex practices and relations (Parker & Aggleton 2003). Of special importance in understanding these responses are what Cáceres (2007) has described as three phobias – homophobia, lesbophobia and transphobia – and the forms of irrationality and panic they trigger.

## Epidemiological research

Quality epidemiological research is important if we are to develop stronger and more nuanced understandings of the epidemic. Reference was made earlier to the non-neutrality of many existing epidemiological categories and the partial manner in which they are deployed within the field of public health. But beyond these issues, new forms of epidemiological work are needed – including more representative studies of HIV prevalence and incidence in same-sex attracted populations, better-quality sexual behaviour surveillance, and network epidemiology, to name but a few.

With respect to same-sex sexuality, much existing research is marred by defects, such as biased sampling, which may select groups that are at higher risk or which are otherwise non-representative of the whole. Alternatively or additionally, questions are often not asked about same-sex relations in national or representative surveys (on the assumption that to do so would offend), further compounding ignorance and misunderstanding.

Behavioural surveys are most useful when they identify the prevalence of the riskiest behaviours, such as unprotected anal intercourse with a partner of unknown or opposite serostatus. Counting all forms of unprotected sex in one category – including unprotected oral sex and unprotected anal intercourse with all partners – can make it difficult to determine the real extent of HIV risk behaviours.

### Programme evaluation

Finally, there is the area of programme evaluation. How are the programmes and interventions we make against HIV perceived and evaluated? What works and why, for whom and in what circumstances? In evaluating programmes – be they linked to HIV treatment, prevention or care – regular monitoring and evaluation is needed, with a focus on coverage, quality and effectiveness. Programmes should be assessed for their responsiveness to sexual minority concerns, their equity with respect to 'general population' measures, and their equity across subgroups, for example, with respect to the needs of same-sex attracted women and transgender persons.

In evaluation work it is also important to identify and confront obstacles for programme success, including the need to go beyond HIV so as to embrace sexual health and rights more generally. Small-scale studies and operations research can be valuable in evaluating pilot programmes to reduce inequity across class and other inequalities, and to introduce real comprehensiveness of healthcare services for sexual minorities.

## Conclusion

In the space available, it is not possible to do more than highlight some of the main issues that need to be addressed in researching same-sex sexuality and HIV in the countries of the global South.

Of fundamental importance, however, should be efforts to understand the diversity of both male and female same-sex practices, the contexts in which they occur, and the meanings they carry. For HIV prevention to be successful, we need to move beyond the stereotypes offered by artificially narrow epidemiological and behavioural frames of reference (which would often have us understand the social world in terms of 'species' or 'types' of person – the homosexual, the bisexual, the insertive partner, the receptive partner, the butch lesbian, and the femme) to appreciate the many ways in which women and men *relate* to one another sexually, and transformations in these ways of relating over time.

Research is also needed into the political economy of the epidemic and, in particular, the way in which HIV prevention, treatment and care for same-sex attracted individuals receives neither its fair share of resources nor the political attention it deserves. Finally, there is the need for capacity building among academics, activists and researchers to build the skills necessary to undertake the kinds of studies highlighted here. Good researchers are made, not born, and the gravity of the situation requires commitment and investment on the part of funders, universities and others, to research capacity development.

## Notes

1   See http://www.un.org/Overview/rights.html (Accessed 20 September 2007).
2   See http://www.unhchr.ch/html/menu3/b/a_cescr.htm (Accessed 20 September 2007).
3   See http://www.ilga.org/news_results.asp?FileCategory=44&ZoneID=7&FileID=577 (Accessed 20 September 2007).
4   See http://www.yogyakartaprinciples.org/ (Accessed 20 September 2007).
5   See http://www.un.org/ga/aidsmeeting2006/declaration.htm (Accessed 10 November 2008).
6   See *Update from the Regional Purple Sky Network Meeting in Bangkok* (1) (Accessed 30 August 2007) msm-asia@googlegroups.com.

## References

Aggleton P (Ed.) (1996) *Bisexualities and AIDS: International perspectives.* London: Taylor and Francis

Aggleton P (Ed.) (1999) *Men who sell sex. International perspectives on male prostitution and HIV/AIDS.* London: UCL Press

Cáceres C (2007) *Thoughts on a global research agenda for MSM – HIV and beyond.* Paper presented to a satellite workshop on MSM & HIV at the Toronto International AIDS Conference. Accessed 20 September 2007, http://www.msmandhiv.org

Chao A (2000) Global metaphors and local strategies in the construction of Taiwan's lesbian identities. *Culture, Health and Sexuality* 2(4): 377–390

Dworkin S (2005) Who is epidemiologically fathomable in the HIV/AIDS epidemic? Gender, sexuality, and intersectionality in public health. *Culture, Health and Sexuality* 7(6): 615–623

Epprecht M (2004) *Hungochani: The history of dissident sexuality in southern Africa.* Quebec: McGill-Queen's University Press

Human Rights Watch (2004) *In a time of torture: The assault on justice in Egypt's crackdown on homosexual conduct.* New York: Human Rights Watch

Khan S (1996) Under the blanket: Bisexualities and AIDS in India. In P Aggleton (Ed.) *Bisexualities and AIDS: International perspectives.* London: Taylor and Francis

Morgan R & Wieringa S (Eds) (2005) *Tommy boys, lesbian men and ancestral wives: Female same-sex practices in Africa.* Johannesburg: Jakana Media

Niang C, Moreau A, Bop C, Compaore C & Diagne M (2004) *Targeting vulnerable groups in national HIV/AIDS programs: The case of men who have sex with men in Senegal, Burkina*

*Faso and the Gambia.* Working Paper Series No. 82. Washington, DC: World Bank, Africa Region (Human Development)

O'Murray S & Roscoe W (1998) *Boy wives and female husbands: Studies of African homosexualities.* Basingstoke: Palgrave Macmillan

Parker R (1999) *Beneath the equator: Cultures of desire, male homosexuality and emerging gay communities in Brazil.* New York: Routledge

Parker R & Aggleton P (2003) HIV and AIDS-related stigma and discrimination: A conceptual framework and implications for action. *Social Science and Medicine* 57: 13–24

Pazello M (2005) Sexual rights and trade. *Peace Review* 2–3: 155–162

Prieur A (1998) *Mema's house: On transvestites, queens and machos.* Chicago: Chicago University Press

Rubin G (1984) Thinking sex: Notes for a radical theory of the politics of sexuality. In C Vance (Ed.) *Pleasure and danger: Exploring female sexuality.* New York: Routledge & Kegan Paul

Sandfort T (2006) MSM and HIV/AIDS: Is more research needed? Paper presented to a satellite workshop on MSM & HIV at the XVI International AIDS Conference in Toronto, 13–18 August. Accessed 20 September 2007, http://www.msmandhiv.org

Schifter J (1998) *Lila's House: Male prostitution in Latin America.* Binghampton, New York: Harrington Park Press

Schifter J, Madrigal J & Aggleton P (1996) Bisexual communities and cultures in Costa Rica. In P Aggleton (Ed.) *Bisexualities and AIDS: International perspectives.* London: Taylor and Francis

Tan M (1996) Silahis: Looking for the missing Filipino bisexual male. In P Aggleton (Ed.) *Bisexualities and AIDS: International perspectives.* London: Taylor and Francis

Ten Brummelhuis H (1999) Transformations of transgender: The case of the Thai kathoey. In P Jackson & G Sullivan (Eds) *Lady boys, tom boys, rent boys: Male and female homosexualities in contemporary Thailand.* Binghampton, New York: Harrington Park Press

Thaweesit S (2004) The fluidity of Thai women's gendered and sexual subjectivities. *Culture, Health and Sexuality* 6(3): 205–220

WHO (World Health Organisation) (2004) *Progress in reproductive health research* (No. 67). Geneva: WHO

World Association for Sexology (1999) *Declaration of sexual rights.* Accessed November 2008, http://www.worldsexology.org/about_sexualrights.asp

Young R & Meyer I (2005) The trouble with 'MSM' and 'WSW': Erasure of the sexual-minority person in public health discourse. *American Journal of Public Health* 95(7): 1144–1149

CHAPTER TWO

# Sexuality research in South Africa: The policy context

Robert Sember

## The post-apartheid context

South Africa's shift from apartheid state to secular, liberal democracy is one of the great political feats of the modern period. The jewel at the centre of this transformation is the Constitution of the Republic of South Africa (Act No. 108 of 1996), particularly the Bill of Rights, which is widely considered the most fully realised blueprint for rights-based governance in the world. The anti-apartheid movement was a global phenomenon and the story of South Africa's transition and the promulgation of its Constitution are experienced as personal triumphs by many more than those South Africans who struggled for freedom. The most idealised vision of the new dispensation is that it embraces difference and will create a richly heterogeneous society, free of discrimination and prejudice. This just society will inspire the rest of the African continent and beyond to do the same. Those identities, practices and aspirations that fall within the domain of the sexual, broadly defined, are among the vectors of freedom enshrined in the Constitution. Indeed, it is the expansive articulation of gender rights and the explicit mention of sexual orientation in the non-discrimination clause that are among the real innovations of the document. The vision of gender and sexual rights and freedoms is so central to the Bill of Rights that the extent to which they are realised is a measure of the success of the democracy as a whole.

The confident and unequivocal aspirations espoused in the Constitution are the result of a bloody and bitter history of struggle, and their implementation requires enormous labour. It is impossible in any ultimate sense to build a new society that perfectly mirrors the Constitution, for the past is a necessary presence, an intimate other, to the new. Wendy Isaack, a legal adviser with the Lesbian and Gay Equality Project, sees this paradoxical relationship between past and future as essential to the process of change, for it is by experiencing 'the humiliating legal effect of repressive colonial conceptions of race and gender...the indignity and pain of legally regulated subordination, and the injustice of exclusion and humiliation through law [that] the majority committed this country to particularly generous constitutional protections for all...' (Isaack 2005: 53). Like all narratives of national transformation, her description is both fact and romance: by assigning authorship to 'the majority', she rises above the fractious political process that produced the document, and the long view backward diminishes the hopelessness that was an unavoidable component of the struggle, and helps to redeem some of what was lost with what has been gained.

As Isaack (2005) develops her analysis, she does consider the problematic future suggested by her formulation: how will the Constitution live beyond the experiences of those who produced it and who remain among its most eloquent interpreters? In fact, a vast new archive of experiences has been, and continues to be, constructed in the years since 1994, when the first democratic elections took place, and 1996, when the Constitution was ratified. Many remain downtrodden by inequality and prejudice. Neo-liberal economic policies propose wealth generation as the solution to poverty, shift more and more state responsibilities onto the market, and make technocrats (or millionaires) of political visionaries. Groups who blame either secularism or cultural corruption for South Africa's social ills have also grown more prominent and now advocate alternative trajectories from the one envisioned a decade ago. Their remedy is a return to conservative, Christian morality (the ideological foundation of the apartheid state) or to the revival of essentialist conceptions of traditional African culture imagined to have existed in the pre-colonial period.

Gender and sexual rights are key battlegrounds for these groups which, despite their irreconcilable differences on most matters, find common ground in their intractable opposition to abortion and gay marriage and in their support for the death penalty – the ultimate power a state has to destroy the rights of citizenship.

Gay rights, particularly in relation to marriage, have been a lightning rod for controversy within South Africa and elsewhere on the continent. On close examination, seemingly straightforward cases of homophobia – such as Zimbabwean President Robert Mugabe's judgement that gay men and lesbians are worse than 'dogs and pigs', or former Namibian president Sam Nujoma's judgement that human rights for gay men and lesbians are 'not [part of] our culture'– turn out to be as complex as any other deep-seated prejudice, an amalgam of quasi-scientific postures, naturalised moral codes, historically rooted practices, displays of power, or distractions from political crises. The deconstruction and reformulation of these attitudes requires that one dig deeply into the fundaments of social organisation, to the point where racism, patriarchy and heterosexism knit together into a logic that is the truly dominant organising principle for South African society.

The terms of this logic, such as the concept of 'African culture', or the distinctions between 'masculine' and 'feminine', are not stable. At its most radical the Constitution further destabilises these concepts – it makes them available for debate, struggle and redefinition. Conservative reactions designed to fix these concepts are an inevitable stage in a political formula that Jara summarises as, 'Step 1 – advances; step 2 – reversal; step 3 – struggles; step 4 – maybe final victory! Every day, every week, every month: this is the beat of the story for lesbian and gay equality in South Africa' (Jara 1998: 31). The manner in which this process is shaped by the particular South African context is especially interesting. In fact, it is the stability or instability of the term 'African' that is arguably the one in which we have the greatest stake. The reformulation of this term is perhaps even more ambitious than achieving equality.

'African' is a term that suggests specific configurations of culture and power and particular orderings of race, gender and sexuality. It attempts to situate personal experience geographically and historically and defines the terms by which to conduct the struggle for rights and freedoms. Like the term 'values', 'African' is too often relinquished by progressive activists as inherently conservative and essentialist. If one considers, however, that it marks a particular form of the paradox Isaack (2005) describes – an experience of oppression and suffering that stimulates visions of a liberated future – it can become the focus of debate and creative, political redefinition. One foothold for this debate is the complex historical revisionism used in many post-colonial African states to defend colonial-era sodomy laws as expressly African, which they are, of course, if 'Africa' is considered the sum of its experiences, and these experiences are historically constructed. To not engage in these debates is to risk endorsing homophobia as culturally permissible and immutable. Without this debate, the African context of post-apartheid South Africa becomes fixed. I would rather believe that the struggle for sexual and gender rights is key to the remaking of South Africa.

## The Constitution: writing the non-discrimination clause

The South African Constitution was ratified on 8 May, 1996. It was the first national Constitution to offer protection from discriminations based on an individual's sexual orientation. Clause 9(3) states: 'The state may not unfairly discriminate directly or indirectly against anyone on one or more grounds, including race, gender, sex, pregnancy, marital status, ethnic or social origin, colour, sexual orientation, age, disability, religion, conscience, belief, culture, language, and birth.' While remarkable in its own right, this non-discrimination clause is nested within an ample slate of additional rights. As a collection they provide many tools with which to fashion personal liberties and to ensure that the state protects and advances rather than harms the rights of its citizens.

The array of constitutional rights has enabled individuals, civil society groups, legislators and judges to defend gender and sexual rights against apartheid-era legislation still in force, religious dogma, and cultural, political and other authorities. These rulings have determined, among many other issues, inheritance rights for women, treatment access for persons living with HIV/AIDS, and a slew of rights for same-sex couples, including: the recognition of immigration rights for South African's foreign same-sex partners; granting same-sex partners the same financial rights as heterosexual couples; entitling same-sex couples to the same financial benefits as unmarried, heterosexual couples in a long-term partnership;

acknowledging that children born to same-sex couples by way of artificial insemination are legitimate; and, the right to marry.

Despite the language of the Constitution, none of these rights was granted automatically: individuals or groups must decide to claim them, suffer through the complex and lengthy process of reaching the Constitutional Court and, once there, present a persuasive and constitutionally grounded argument supporting the claim. In many respects this is a continuation of the process of negotiation, coalition building, and philosophical investigation that led to the development of the Constitution itself. The National Coalition for Gay and Lesbian Equality (now known as the Lesbian and Gay Equality Project) was formed in late 1994 with the express goal of ensuring that sexual orientation was retained in the final Constitution's non-discrimination clause. The Coalition included representatives from 32 organisations and was able to unify activist and advocacy groups that had, for decades, been divided along political, racial and gender lines. As a result, they were rather ineffective during the apartheid era. I will speculate, too, that the AIDS epidemic, which had begun a decade earlier in South Africa, with infections concentrated among gay men, provided the experience of a unifying crisis that prepared gay and lesbian groups to work together. In fact, a number of the most prominent movement activists – Simon Nkoli, Zackie Achmat, Edwin Cameron, among others – were living with HIV/AIDS at the time the constitutional negotiations began.

As described in 1998 by Jara, the Coalition's strategy entailed lobbying the Constitutional Assembly with the main aim being to neutralise the African Christian Democratic Party (ACDP), which strongly opposed the clause. Discussion of gay marriage and adoption, as well as military policies concerning homosexuals, was deferred until after the Constitutional Assembly completed its work, for fear that these specific issues would have provoked conservatives within the governing ANC to remove their support for the clause. These early strategic decisions – opposed by many who advocated, among the alternative activist strategies, the development of a mass social movement in favour of gay and lesbian rights – are similar to those made by other civil society groups. This process of government–civil society collaboration continues to the present. While effective in relation to some issues, it has also led to the co-option of various groups or individuals, some of whom have literally moved into government, so creating a leadership gap in many sections of civil society, and has weakened the ability of other groups to use more aggressive strategies to shape policy. The most painful example of the complicated position activists find themselves in as a result of their cooperative relationship with government involves the government's AIDS policies, which have fallen terribly short of what is required to address the crisis. While vehemently opposed to the government's policies in this area, activists have supported the re-election of the ANC because of its progressive policies in relation to gender and sexual rights, poverty reduction and labour rights. A signal of the remarkable shift in ideological balance in the country during the Constitutional Assembly period is the fact that women's and gay and lesbian groups concentrated their efforts on educating and persuading Constitutional Assembly members, while the ACDP took to the streets with thousands of supporters to march against the 'secular state' and for a 'Christian Bill of Rights'.

By April 1996, the month before the Constitution was adopted, every political party, with the exception of the ACDP, had stated their support for including protections of gay men and lesbians in the non-discrimination clause. The cooperative strategy for the post-Constitution period of judicial, legislative and administrative work on gender and sexual rights was confirmed the following year, when delegates to the ANC's 50th National Conference voted for a resolution that explicitly supported the following rights for lesbian and gay workers: access to worker benefits such as housing, medical aid and bereavement leave; recognition of gay and lesbian families; marriage, custody, immigration and adoption rights; the inclusion of gay and lesbian youth in all programmes, policies and laws; protections for these youth from discrimination at school, home, in the media and on the streets; and equalising the age of consent. The ANC government has addressed each of these commitments legislatively or administratively over the past few years, with varying levels of follow-through and success. The elaboration of these rights and policies has not occurred as the result of a uniform strategy. Instead, civil society and government have adopted a variety of judicial, parliamentary and administrative strategies in order to progress toward the translation of the non-discrimination clause into real changes in the lives of the citizens of this country. What follows is an overview of some of the strategies and accomplishments in these three domains.

## Judicial strategies

The posture of the justices in the Constitutional Court's first decade has been, in the words of Gevisser, 'activist and evangelical: they want to be of the people, with the people, and in the people' (2000: 511). This description could also be applied to justices in many of the lower courts who have cleared the path through their rulings and opinions for the Constitutional Court to act. The judiciary's rulings in cases of gender and sexual rights have almost always been ardently progressive with a clear indication in each successive case that they are willing to give more than they have been asked for, thereby helping to shape the overall judicial strategies used by civil society groups and government. In cases concerning gay and lesbian rights, they have acknowledged emphatically that lesbians and gay men are a permanent minority in society, have experienced discrimination, and have a right to appeal to the Constitution for the protection of basic rights. The judiciary has interpreted prejudice and discrimination as symptoms of the fact that gay men and lesbians are seen as being without inherent dignity and not worthy of human respect.

## Decriminalisation

These positions emerged very clearly in various courts' decisions in 1997 and 1998 regarding South Africa's sodomy laws, which were based on those the British colonial regime put in place throughout its empire. The apartheid government had refined the colonial law so that it specifically criminalised homosexuality. Thus, while the English Common Law crime of sodomy prohibited anal intercourse between men and women, as well as between men, South Africa redefined the law so that it applied only to anal and oral sex between men.

No differentiation was made between public and private sex and consensual and non-consensual sex between men. Following police raids of gay parties, a 1968 statute also made it a crime for men to engage in any sort of erotic contact in situations where three or more people were present and to manufacture or use dildos or other erotic devices. This 'anti-dildo' provision was seen to be targeting lesbians who are mentioned explicitly in age of consent legislation. Between 1978 and 1993 convictions for sodomy between consenting adults over 20 years of age ran at a rate of 100 to 200 per year with penalties ranging from 2–6 months imprisonment or fines.

In ruling on the 1997 case *State v Gordon Kampher*,[1] the High Court of the Western Cape was the first to declare that there was no rational basis for criminalising same-sex sodomy. Interestingly, this decision referenced and criticised the *Bowers v Hardwick*[2] case in which the US Supreme Court had denied same-sex partners the right to privacy in upholding a sodomy conviction in the state of Georgia.

This would not be the only time a South African court would criticise anti-gay judgments in other countries as a way of affirming the unique rights-based approach of the South African Constitution. In May 1998, responding to an application by the National Coalition for Gay and Lesbian Equality and the South African Human Rights Commission (one of six state entities established under the terms of the Constitution to advance specific rights), Johannesburg High Court Judge Jonathan Heher struck down as unconstitutional the common law crimes of sodomy and sections of the Sexual Offences Act (No. 23 of 1957). Regarding the burdens these laws had placed on gay men and lesbians, he observed that they represented 'religious intolerance, ignorance, superstition, bigotry, fear of what is different from or alien to everyday experience and the millstone of history'.[3]

In December 1999, the Constitutional Court confirmed this decision in its ruling in *National Coalition for Gay and Lesbian Equality v Minister of Justice*. The Court found that these laws breached rights to equality, dignity and privacy. Judge Ackermann wrote the opinion for the majority and stated that the laws undermined self-esteem, caused psychological harm and legitimated violence and blackmail against lesbian, gay, bisexual and transgender people.

## Benefits

With same-sex sexual relations decriminalised, the judiciary turned its attention almost completely to extending domestic benefits to same-sex couples. The pinnacle of this particular area of concern is same-sex marriage, which registered as an issue in the earliest cases concerning the constitutionality of sexual orientation, specific exclusions and accommodations. In his ruling in early 1998 in a case concerning the refusal of the South African Police Services medical aid to extend health coverage to the partner of a lesbian employee, Judge Roux of the Pretoria High Court stated that heterosexual and same-sex relationships deserved equal respect. Later that same year, the Pension Funds Adjudicator, John Murphy, ordered a pension fund to pay death benefits to a deceased man's same-sex partner. Picking up on Judge Roux's statement, Murphy explained that same-sex unions should enjoy the same status, rights and benefits as a heterosexual union when it comes to the allocation of benefits. The Constitutional Court addressed this issue in its 2002 ruling in favour of Judge Kathy Satchwell, stating that her lesbian partner should have the same benefits as the partners of other married, heterosexual judges.[4]

## Immigration rights

Following its success in having sodomy legislation declared unconstitutional, the National Coalition for Gay and Lesbian Equality, six lesbian couples, and the Commission on Gender Equality (another of the constitutionally established state entities mandated to help advance democracy) filed an application in March 1998 with the Cape High Court, seeking to declare the Aliens Control Act (No. 96 of 1991) unconstitutional because it denied immigration rights to bi-national same-sex couples. In early 1999 the Cape High Court found that the legislation unfairly discriminated against gay and lesbian couples by denying them the same rights as married couples. It gave the government 12 months to amend the Aliens Control Act. On 2 December 1999, the Constitutional Court supported the ruling in *National Coalition for Gay and Lesbian Equality v Minister of Home Affairs*, and used it as an opportunity to affirm that same-sex life partnerships and families are equivalent to those established by heterosexuals.

## Adoption

The apartheid government's Child Care Act (No. 74 of 1983) permitted unmarried or divorced persons to adopt children, but made no provision for two unmarried persons to jointly adopt a child. In August 1995 the Johannesburg Child Welfare Society sanctioned a lesbian adoption. The same year, however, the child commissioner blocked the adoption of an HIV-positive child by a gay couple, who were told they would not make appropriate parents. In September 1996, with a new commissioner in place, the adoption was granted. The only way to prevent this sort of administrative equivocation is to change the law, and the most effective strategy for doing that is to establish a constitutional basis for new laws. This opportunity presented itself when lesbian judges Anne-Marie de Vos and Suzanne du Toit, who had been together for 13 years, filed suit after Du Toit was prevented from adopting Vos's two children. In September 2002, the Constitutional Court confirmed that same-sex couples have the right to adopt children. Writing for the majority, Judge Lewis Skweyiya noted that 'family life as contemplated in the Constitution can be lived in different ways', and that 'excluding partners in same sex life partnerships from adopting children jointly where they would otherwise be suitable to do so is in conflict with the principle enshrined in section 28(2) of the Constitution'.[5]

## Marriage

The accumulation of rulings equating same-sex partners and families with heterosexual partnerships and families provided a firm foundation upon which to build cases supporting same-sex marriage. When Marie Fourie and Cecelia Bonthuys sought the right to marry, they initiated the process of judicial review that finally enabled the court to rule explicitly in this matter. In its review of the case in 2004, the Supreme Court of Appeal declared that under the Constitution, the common law concept of marriage must be changed to include partners of the same gender. Judge Edwin Cameron suggested in his judgment in *Fourie and Another v Minister of Home Affairs and Others* that the definition of marriage be altered to read 'marriage is the union of two persons to the exclusion of all others for life'.[6] In 2005 the Constitutional Court took up the case of *Minister of Home Affairs and Others v Fourie and Bonthuys and Others*, which concerned the marriage rights of same-sex couples. The Court found the common law definition of marriage inconsistent with the Constitution and invalid because it does not permit same-sex couples to enjoy the status, benefits and responsibilities it accords to heterosexual couples.

## Legislative strategies

Judicial decisions concerning same-sex partnerships seldom in and of themselves change the everyday conditions of gay and lesbian South Africans. At best they guide and strengthen the government's own initiatives regarding these issues. Given the ANC's progressive platform concerning gay and lesbian rights, judicial developments have, for the most part, been in harmony with those of the government. The legislative process, however, is one of consultation, debate and compromise and must accommodate opinions beyond those of the courts. This is clearly illustrated by the development of the Same-sex Marriage Bill following the 2005 directive from the Constitutional Court that gave the government one year to remedy the unconstitutionality of laws concerning marriage.

Concerned that the extent of opposition to same-sex marriage would make it difficult to pass legislation, the government initially explored the option of creating civil unions rather than changing the definition of marriage, which is the same strategy used in many other parts of the world. In August 2006, Cabinet approved for submission to Parliament alternative draft bills. One would create civil unions for same-sex couples only, while the other would establish the institution of civil unions for both same-sex and heterosexual couples. In its instructions to government, the Constitutional Court did not provide the explicit suggestion offered by Judge Edwin Cameron on how to redefine marriage but, clearly anticipating this manoeuvre, it did caution against any 'separate but equal' solution, which is how the apartheid government had at various points attempted to resolve issues of racial discrimination. Such a remedy would almost certainly not meet the test of constitutionality, the Court cautioned. The State Law Advisors, who review draft legislation for form and constitutionality, echoed this concern and recommended a direct amendment of the Marriage Act (No. 25 of 1961). The South African Law Reform Commission issued a similar caution.

Government had to contend with opposition to same-sex marriage legislation on many fronts, including among the general public. On 16 September 2006, thousands of people protested against gay marriage in a number of cities across the country and ministers from the ACDP promised to introduce a constitutional amendment banning same-sex marriage. At public hearings the following week on the Civil Unions Bill opinions were polarised. In some cases, some of the hearings had to be moved because officials were denied access to facilities in certain locations. Opponents of gay marriage pressed for a hold on the Constitutional Court's ruling so that a constitutional amendment could be presented, while gay rights groups criticised the proposed Bill because it would create a separate class of citizens and would not fulfil the mandate of the Constitutional Court. In the days following these hearings, the government acknowledged that the definition of marriage in the Marriage Act was indeed unconstitutional.

The Marriage Alliance, a group advocating for a constitutional amendment that would preserve the 'traditional' definition of marriage, held a public protest in Pretoria on 7 October 2006 and marched to the Union Buildings, where representatives deposited a memorandum stating their demands. Two days later the ANC voted to support the Civil Unions Bill, ensuring that it would have sufficient votes to pass the legislation. In a last minute change to the Bill, the government permitted the 'voluntary union of two persons, which is solemnized and registered by either a marriage or a civil union'. The Bill was passed by the National Assembly on 14 November 2006, the National Council of Provinces on 28 November, and signed into law on 30 November, just a day before same-sex marriage would have been legalised by court order. This made South Africa the fifth country in the world to legalise same-sex marriage. Thus, the government had avoided amending the Marriage Act while still permitting marriage for same-sex couples. In statements following the signing of the Bill, government representatives acknowledged that a fuller marriage law would need to be formulated to harmonise the different pieces of marriage legislation.

Gay and lesbian rights activists both applauded and criticised the Bill. Among their objections was government's failure to amend the Marriage Act, as this reinforced the notion that there was a need to separate same-sex couples from heterosexual couples when it comes to marriage. They also observed that the provision allowing marriage officers to refuse to marry same-sex couples on the grounds of conscience, may be unconstitutional. Under this provision the Catholic, Baptist, Anglican and Presbyterian churches notified government that they would not perform same-sex marriages. Acknowledging the divisive nature of the debate over the Bill, the Joint Working Group, a national network of lesbian, gay, bisexual and transgender organisations, urged government to launch a series of public education campaigns designed to increase acceptance of rights for gay men and lesbians.

While the Civil Unions Bill was the most controversial legislation concerning same-sex rights, it had been preceded by a series of laws designed to fulfil the equal rights and non-discrimination clauses of the Constitution. For example, the Labour Relations Act (No. 66 of 1995) prohibits unfair workplace discrimination based on sexual orientation. In 2000 the government passed the Promotion of Equality and Prevention of Unfair Discrimination Bill, which contains 17 grounds on which no person may be discriminated against, including sexual orientation, age, culture, pregnancy, marital status, conscience, social standing and language. The Bill also bans hate speech. And in 2003, in an amendment to the Sexual Offences and Related Matters Bill, government harmonised the age of consent. A 1968 law raised the age of consent for same-sex behaviour from 16 to 19 years of age. This created an additional statutory offence to the sodomy laws for any same-sex activity between a man 20 years and older and a male sexual partner who was 19 years or younger. The penalty for such an offence was up to six years imprisonment.

## Administrative strategies

In addition to its legislative initiative, the government also has the power, authority and responsibility to advance constitutionally projected rights through its administrative branch. This includes changing policies in the various branches of government to ensure that they are in line with the Constitution as well as providing services in a manner that does not frustrate the rights of citizens. For example, the 1996 White Paper on Social Welfare stipulated that all services should promote non-discrimination, tolerance, mutual respect, diversity, and the inclusion of all groups in society, including gay men and lesbians. The definition of family implicitly recognised same-sex families and same-sex headed households, which enabled welfare officials to process adoptions by lesbians and gay men. However, with explicit legislation governing this, its implementation is subject to the whims of particular officials. There are also infrastructure limitations and failures to translate legislation into explicit administrative policies, as is the case with the re-issuing of identity documents for transsexual men and women. The law concerning sex change was amended in 2003, but it remains difficult to get the Department of Home Affairs to process applications for new documents.

Among the most significant administrative changes initiated by the state is the promotion of non-discrimination policies with the police and the military. Following the passing of the Labour Relations Act which prohibits unfair workplace discrimination based on sexual orientation, the South African Police Service issued a new policy directive on gay and lesbian police officers in which it affirmed the right to equality in any appointment, promotion or transfer. It also noted that discrimination on the basis of sexual orientation would not be tolerated.

Under apartheid, the police services and the military were used to enforce discriminatory apartheid policies. The treatment of gay men and lesbians was notorious. Over the past few years, the aVersion Project has investigated human rights abuses perpetrated by the South African military against gay men during the apartheid era. Gay men and lesbians were not allowed to join the permanent force in the military and conscripted gay soldiers were often hospitalised and subjected to aversion therapy, including shock therapy, hormonal treatment and even sex-change operations and chemical castrations (Canaday 2002). As early as 1996, while the final Constitution was still being debated, the military initiated a comprehensive review of its policies at the urging of the National Coalition for Gay and Lesbian Equality, which had allied itself with the trade union movement and lobbied for workers' rights within the defence force. The consortium also lobbied for the lifting of the ban on gay and lesbian personnel, which had occurred two years before the repeal of the sodomy laws. In response to this lobbying, the Ministry of Defence issued a White Paper in which it made specific provision that the South African National Defence Force would not discriminate against any of its members on the grounds of sexual orientation.

## Beyond rights

With well over 10 years of judicial and legislative developments in place in the democratic South Africa, it is possible to appreciate the extraordinary influence the Constitution has had on the South African state. Among the signal accomplishments of the judiciary is the Constitutional Court's decision in *State v Makwanyane* in which it unanimously declared the death penalty unconstitutional. This was clear confirmation that the racist South African police state had given way to a new rights-based dispensation in which the state's total power over the bodies of its citizens – the very essence of the apartheid state – was curtailed. This single decision consolidated the constitutional protection of rights to bodily integrity, dignity and life, each of which is essential to fundamental freedoms. Legislation of comparable stature in the history of the post-apartheid Parliament is the Choice of Termination of Pregnancy Bill, legislation which reflects the basic principle of autonomy and confirms the transformation in conditions for women following the end of apartheid. During apartheid women's control over their bodies was severely curtailed.

In the midst of these courageous and revolutionary decisions and laws are ones that mark significant points of vulnerability, places where one is reminded that even the most robust of rights-based systems cannot take their accomplishments for granted. The Constitutional Court's 2002 decision in *State v Jordan*, which questioned the constitutionality of laws criminalising sex work, is perplexing. The justices unanimously determined that these laws did not infringe on the rights to human dignity and economic activity, and that a limit to the right to privacy was 'justifiable' in this instance. In a separate decision, justices O'Regan and Sacks argued that because the law considers the patrons of sex workers to be accomplices rather than equally culpable, it 'reinforces the sexual double standards prevalent in our society'. '[This] difference in social stigma,' they continue, 'tracks a pattern of applying different standards to the sexuality of men and women...thereby fostering gender inequality.'[7] The implied remedy in this argument is the increased criminalisation of sex work. In light of this argument, I become concerned that the progressive expansion of privacy and domestic rights for same-sex couples is palatable precisely because it domesticates sexuality, sees it as essential to the person, always intimate and, dare I say, sacred. Following her 2004 review of the state of sexuality in South Africa, Posel observes that, 'The constitution created the spaces for moral and cultural alternatives in the midst of – rather than displacing – the taboos of old' (2004: 60). I would suggest that, in addition to this basic conservative context, the conventional ontological definition of sexuality remains closed.

The South African government's response to the AIDS epidemic has been its greatest betrayal of its constitutional obligations to sexual rights and sexual health. Another curious example of its contradictory stance on sexual rights is evident in the positions it has taken in various UN forums. The generous promise of the post-apartheid era was clearly evident in the South African delegation's suggestion at preparatory meetings in 1995 for the UN World Conference on Women, that the words 'sexual orientation' be included in a paragraph addressing discrimination. Later that year, in her address to the delegates at the Fourth World Conference on Women in Beijing, the South African lesbian activist Bev Ditsie (1995) called for the inclusion of sexual orientation in the draft Platform for Action. Although this did not occur, South Africa presented itself as unequivocally devoted to international sexual rights, including the rights of gay men and lesbians. However, the actions of the South African representatives at the August 2007 meeting of the UN Economic and Social Council (Ecosoc) were a painful betrayal of this apparent commitment. Two gay rights organisations, one Swedish, the other Canadian, petitioned Ecosoc for accreditation, which would permit them to have 'consultative status' at the UN in January 2008 (approximately 2 000 civil society organisations have this accreditation). Ecosoc's NGO subcommittee, whose members include Egypt, Pakistan and the Sudan, rejected the applications.

South Africa joined with representatives from Belarus, China, Pakistan, Russia, Saudi Arabia, Somalia and the Sudan, countries that deny rights to gay men and lesbians, to oppose the applications, and abstained on the actual vote. Thankfully, these countries were in the minority, so their position did not hold.

Kirchick (2007) suggests that this shift in position in little more than 10 years is evidence of a growing anti-Western sentiment within the South African government. 'As the most economically developed and politically stable country on the African continent,' Kirchick observes, 'South Africa envisions itself as the chief advocate for the underdeveloped world in the courts of Western Europe and North America' (2007: 1). He goes on to lament the fact that this trend undermines the progressive influence South Africa could have in the UN on states in both the global North, such as the United States, and the global South, with respect to sexual rights. South Africa has just taken a two-year seat on the Security Council and could use its heightened status 'to make the case for, at the very least, tolerance for gay rights in countries where homosexuality is illegal…with its anti-imperialist bona fides [South Africa] could speak about these issues far more effectively to the developing world than any gay activist in the US or western Europe' (Kirchick 2007: 1).

If the representative function of government is defined as the simple reflection of the opinions of its population, the government's apparent shift to the right brings it more in line with the country's majority with respect to sexuality. A global survey of moral attitudes conducted by the US-based Pew Research Center for the People and the Press (2003) revealed that when South Africans were asked whether homosexuality should be accepted by society, 63 per cent responded 'no' with 33 per cent agreeing that homosexuality should be accepted. Similar results were obtained by the Human Sciences Research Council in its survey of South Africans' social attitudes and moral values (Rule & Mncwango 2006). Of the almost 5 000 adults aged 16 years and older included in the survey, 81 per cent of Africans consider same-sex relations as 'always wrong', and 64 per cent of coloured people, 70 per cent of white people and 76 per cent of Indians hold this opinion. In some rural areas, such as those in the Eastern Cape, 90 per cent of those polled considered homosexuality to be 'always wrong'. The majority of those polled also supported capital punishment, condemned premarital sex and opposed abortion. I caution against an over-determined response to these statistics; they need to be assessed in relation to a variety of contradictory trends, such as the fact that the ANC, the author of the most progressive legislation, has received the overwhelming majority of the votes in all elections and that everyday behaviour, specifically the widespread practice of extramarital sex, suggests opinions quite different from those reported here. Careful analysis of these contradictions is required and is likely to reveal a substratum of political thinking and action on the part of South Africans that cannot be reduced to pre-defined responses to closed-ended survey questions. Nevertheless, as Gevisser observed during the highly contentious process leading up to the passing of the Choice of Termination of Pregnancy Bill, 'the further away from the moment of liberation we get, the easier it will be for religious conservatives to mobilize South Africans around THEIR agendas…'[8]

South Africa's democratic structures demand that in order for principles to be truly secured, they must be entrenched at all levels of society. As progressive principles are realised in policy and jurisprudence, they need to be translated into terms that affect the everyday circumstances of the country's citizens, including the generation of children who have not experienced the oppression and analysis of that oppression that Isaack (2005) considers the foundation for the country's Constitution. For many, the status of a rights-based citizenship is eclipsed by the struggles of poverty. Equality of rights is simply impossible in a grossly unequal society. These hardships represent a continuation of the hardships of prejudice and inequality in place during apartheid, but there is no analysis of or mobilisation against these conditions comparable to what existed during the apartheid era. The most compelling structure of experience for many in South Africa today is not dignity and individual freedom, but the apparently unbreakable bond between racial inequality and suffering. How instrumental can a human rights-based analysis of these experiences be in helping to shift this experience?

The disjuncture between advancement in policy and experience is what Isaack (2005) terms 'mere formal equality'. She notes that the acknowledgement by the courts and Parliament of the right to be free from discrimination has not substantively changed the lives of most black lesbians and black gay men. Racism and class still stifle freedoms and deny people access to services and recourse. This is an echo of the painful division between sexual activism and the broader context of apartheid inequality that fractured gay and lesbian rights movements under apartheid. The several gay rights organisations formed at the time the ruling National Party expanded the sodomy laws in 1976 (also the year the Soweto uprising began and the anti-apartheid struggle entered its final, most bloody and ultimately victorious phase) were divided along racial lines and larger political questions. The Gay Association of South Africa was a mostly white, male organisation that did not declare its opposition to apartheid, whereas the Rand Gay Organisation was multi-racial and considered itself part of the anti-apartheid struggle, an acknowledgement that in South Africa one always has multiple identities. That is, one is never just gay, or black, or a woman. Coalitional rather than identity politics is the logical strategy by which to advance social change. The fact is, as Isaack notes, 'in practice lesbian and gay men, specifically black lesbians and gay men, continue to be failed by the education system, losing their jobs, being denied access to public housing, having their needs ignored by the medical profession and being unfairly treated by the legal system' (2005: 55).

One contemporary struggle that does offer a comprehensive and collaborative platform for the advancement of a broader social agenda than is permitted by a population or identity-exclusive agenda, is the struggle around the AIDS crisis. Social movements concerned with addressing the epidemic have used the authority of the constitutional process while also tacitly acknowledging its limitations. The constitutional discourse on rights and citizenship provides a vocabulary of citizenship that has enfranchised many. But rights in themselves are not a panacea for the complex historical and contemporary inequalities that shape the AIDS epidemic and a host of other prejudices. Magnifying and colouring all of this, of course, is the inertia of social forces conditioned by the racist, sexist and patriarchal regimes of religion, morality and traditionalism.

## The politics of research

Given the remarkable advances in securing sexual and gender rights within the judicial, legislative and, to a lesser extent, administrative branches of the state, what should be the focus of future research in this area? This question arises from the fact that rights conferred are of little use unless materialised in everyday practices. In South Africa, 'everyday practices' are defined by multiple state and non-state forces and respond to political, economic and cultural forces from far beyond the borders of the country. South African society is generally socially conservative and remains divided by sharp racial, gender and income inequalities. Given this context, it is necessary that rights be claimed, performed, defended, habituated and vigilantly monitored. In other words, the realisation of sexual and gender rights requires fundamental social transformation, a process that must be governed by the principle that specific rights cannot be pursued in isolation from other rights.

Sexuality and gender research is informed by, and has the capacity to influence, every level of South African society. As a subset of the country's multinational social research enterprise, such research may either directly or indirectly draw resources, discourses and methods from the South African state, other governments, development programmes, and a vast network of philanthropies. Many, if not most, of the country's public and private sector institutions are either engaged in or are the focus of social science research. As is the case with the country's public health system, some institutions are both the source *and* focus of research. If sexuality and gender concerns were to be integrated into these research processes, they would rapidly become visible to a vast array of social institutions. The ANC government has made research an essential component of the administration of the country by insisting that all government programmes are monitored/measured. Data for government programme evaluation are drawn from the state's own research initiatives (such as the census) as well as from research conducted by countless other groups. Thus, research is a venue for the interaction of government and civil society, and among the issues to be debated in this venue is how 'citizenship' is translated into ideological and practical methods, and what the particular terms of analysis will be that will determine the terms by which governmental and non-governmental forces intervene in society.

I am concerned that these terms of analysis will be drawn uncritically from long-established research conventions in place within South Africa and in research institutes elsewhere in the world, and which now define and direct a great portion of the social research taking place in the country. Research is neither value-neutral nor ideologically pure. Method is political and the manner in which questions are framed and answered transmits ideologies and conditions consciousness, as was evident in an interaction I recently had with South African demographers concerning the absence of same-sex sexuality and gender diversity questions on national surveys. I argued that an AIDS epidemic as large as the one among the gay population in the 1980s does not simply end. In light of this, the almost complete silence among South African social scientists and public health professionals in response to same-sex sexual risk and the prevalence of HIV/AIDS among men who have sex with men, appears deliberate. A concerted effort is required to deny that the AIDS epidemic does not involve same-sex sexual activity.

Their response was that South Africa is an 'Africanist' context and they simply cannot ask such questions; it is too taboo. They also claimed that asking such questions would so outrage respondents that it would harm the research process as a whole. Following this public debate, a number of the women demographers approached me and spoke of the similar justifications used to exclude questions concerning women's sexuality. It was clear to them that the problem is not the respondents, but the patriarchal and conservative attitudes of the survey designers and directors. Whether and how those surveyed will respond to questions about same-sex attraction, behaviour, desire or fantasy, or questions about women's desires, sexual fantasies and behaviours, is an empirical question. Without investigation, the opinion of the populace is a blank slate, available for the projection of prejudices rooted not in the population but in those in authority.

Clearly, one of the greatest threats to the advancement of sexual and reproductive rights is the notion that such freedoms are 'un-African'. The fact is that the majority of South Africans are separated from their rights and movements in favour of their rights by social marginalisation, poverty and persistent racism. Silenced by these circumstances, those in power, including researchers, can practise an insidious ventriloquism that posits the majority as a homogeneous and static bloc, an ahistorical 'Africanist' constituency. Engaged research can help shift the power that sustains the status quo, but it can also further fragment and weaken the terms of progressive analysis by compartmentalising issues – such as sexual rights for gay men and lesbians from those for sex workers. If we accept the position that no one is free until we are all free, it behoves us to see a common purpose in our aspiration for autonomy and bodily integrity and in the aspiration of the men and women who wish to make commerce of pleasure. It is this politics of affiliation and affirmation that is most likely to secure the rights that are particular to our own desires, as different as those may appear from the practices of others. Thus, for those involved in research, discussions of the politics of method should not be ignored or lightly dismissed, for it is in the search for questions, the manner of their articulation and the terms by which they are investigated, that power is constructed and directed.

## Notes

1 *State v Gordon Kampher* (Case No. 232/1997).
2 *Bowers v Hardwick* 478 US 186 (1986). The US Supreme Court directly overruled *Bowers v Hardwick* in *Lawrence v Texas*, 539 US 558 (2003).
3 *The National Coalition for Gay and Lesbian Equality and the South African Human Rights Commission v The Minister of Justice, the Minister of Safety and Security, and the Attorney-General of the Witwatersrand* (Case No. 97/023677). Information accessed at: http://www.qrd.org/qrd/world/legal/ncgle-v-south.africa.
4 *Satchwell v President, Republic of South Africa* 2002 (6) SA1 (CC).
5 *Du Toit and Another v Minister of Welfare and Population Development* 2002 (CCT40/01: pp. 13; 16).
6 *Fourie and Another v Minister of Home Affairs and Others* (Supreme Court of Appeals, Case No. 232/2003).
7 *State v Jordan and Others (Sex Workers Education and Advocacy Task Force and Others as Amici Curiae)* 2002 (CCT31/01: p. 39).
8 Gevisser M (1997) 'The ANC's great divide'. *The Nation*, 17 February 1997.

## References

Bentley K & Brookes H (2005) The great leap sideways: Gender, culture and rights after 10 years of democracy in South Africa. *Agenda – Special Focus (Gender, Culture and Rights)* 1(71): 2–13

Canaday M (2002) *The effect of sodomy laws on lifting the ban on homosexual personnel: Three case studies.* Accessed April 2008, http://repositories.cdlib.org/isber/cssmm/cssmm04

Dirsuweit T (2006) The problem of identities: The lesbian, gay, bisexual, transgender and intersex social movement in South Africa. In R Ballard, A Habib & I Valodia (Eds) *Voices of protest: Social movements in post-apartheid South Africa.* Scottsville: University of KwaZulu-Natal Press

Ditsie PB (1995) Statement delivered on behalf of the International Gay and Lesbian Human Rights Commission at the United Nations Fourth World Conference on Women, 13 September. Accessed December 2008, http://www.hartford-hwp.com/archives/28/014.html

Gevisser M (2000) Mandela's stepchildren: Homosexual identity in post-apartheid South Africa. In P Drucker (Ed.) *Different rainbows.* London: Gay Men's Press

Hassim S (2006b) The challenges of inclusion and transformation: The women's movement in democratic South Africa. In R Ballard, A Habib & I Valodia (Eds) *Voices of protest: Social movements in post-apartheid South Africa.* Scottsville: University of KwaZulu-Natal Press

Isaack W (2005) LGBTI mainstreaming: Inculcating a culture of human rights. *Agenda – Special Focus (Gender, Culture and Rights)* 1(71): 50–57

Jara M (1998) Gay and lesbian rights: Forcing change in South Africa. *Southern African Report* 13(3): 31

Kirchick J (2007) *South Africa's gay betrayal.* Accessed April 2008, http://www.guardian.co.uk/commentisfree/2007/aug/21/southafricasgaybetrayal

Manjoo R (2005) Gender rights within the framework of traditional or cultural norms and rights. *Agenda – Special Focus (Gender, Culture and Rights)* 1(71): 80–83

Ndashe S (2005) Human rights, gender and culture – a deliberate confusion? *Agenda – Special Focus (Gender, Culture and Rights)* 1(71): 36–41

Pew Research Center for the People and the Press (2003) *Views of a changing world: The Pew global attitudes project.* Washington, DC: Pew Research Center for the People and the Press

Posel D (2004) Getting the nation talking about sex: Reflections on the discursive constitution of sexuality in South Africa since 1994. *Agenda – Empowering Women for Gender Equity* 62: 53–63

Potgieter C-A (2005) Gender, culture and rights: Challenges and approaches of three Chapter 9 institutions. *Agenda – Special Focus (Gender, Culture and Rights)* 115: 154–160

Rule S & Mncwango B (2006) Rights or wrongs? An exploration of moral values. In U Pillay, B Roberts & S Rule (Eds) *South African social attitudes: Changing times, diverse voices.* Cape Town: HSRC Press

Terreblanche S (2002) *A history of inequality in South Africa, 1652–2002.* Scottsville University of KwaZulu-Natal Press

Whiteside A (2001) AIDS and poverty: The links. *AIDS Analysis Africa* 12(2): 1, 5

CHAPTER THREE

# Same-sex sexuality and health: Psychosocial scientific research in South Africa

Juan Nel

Sexuality is a core value and central to self, identity, culture and nation (Pigg & Adams 2005). Issues of sexuality and gender touch upon some of the most intimate and personal aspects of human existence. They carry much cultural weight and are therefore vulnerable to exploitation for political reasons (HRW 2003). In many cultures and communities, sexuality is a highly value-laden terrain and most societies attempt to control the sexual behaviour of their members in some way (Goodwatch 2005). The realm of sexuality is thus recognised as a powerful domain, both of general social prejudice and stigmatisation and, more specifically, of the pathologising of minority groups or 'deviant' categories of people (Hook 2002).

Large parts of the African continent have been devastated by the effects of sexual problems and suffering brought about by, among other things, a lack of sexual rights and education and, sadly, limited access to professional sexual healthcare. South Africa is no exception in this regard. While having one of the most progressive constitutions in the world, which includes freedom of sexual orientation in its Bill of Rights, South Africa has one of the highest incidences of HIV and AIDS infections and of sexual assault in the world.

In this chapter, international developments within sexology regarding sexual orientation and, to a lesser extent, gender identity, are outlined and 'gay-affirmative' approaches explained. Against this international backdrop, the social and legal position of and healthcare provision for sexual minorities in South Africa are indicated. Current psychosocial scientific research in South Africa is also referred to.

## Perspectives from medicine and the social sciences

Sexology, the study of sexuality, is an interdisciplinary field of scientific enquiry and an area of specialisation. A sexologist requires highly specialised knowledge, skills and attitudes. Medical specialists, psychologists and other health service providers, social and other scientists, academics and sex educators, health policy-makers, sexual health activists and sexual health product marketers, all contribute to the understanding of sexuality and the promotion of sexual health and rights. Sexology is placed within notions of population management, human rights, disease prevention, risk reduction, family planning, child survival and material health, each with an implicit set of moral assumptions about the purposes of sexual relations and human nature (Pigg & Adams 2005).

Internationally, research on sexuality issues is mainly done in the humanities and social sciences, most notably within the departments of history, literature, ethnology, sociology, and social anthropology. The field is rather small, but growing (Samelius & Wägberg 2005). The values, beliefs and stereotypes of the researcher are central in studying lesbian women and gay men. These values will directly influence the way in which problems are defined, formulated and evaluated and the types of intervention offered. There are tensions between an understanding of sexuality as universal and a sexuality that is context-specific in meaning, practice and outcome (Pigg & Adams 2005). In scientific discourse, with claims of neutrality and objectivity, sex and sexuality are universalised in the name of health and well-being. Patriarchal Westernised ways of defining sexual orientation and gender identity make the assumption that biological sex forms the basis for people's identity and determines their sexual expression, which is essentially fixed (Pigg & Adams 2005). The medical model is interested in objective knowledge that is unaffected by the subject's/knower's values and meanings. Both subject and knower are seen as solitary objects, stripped of the contextual particularities of sex, race and culture (Unisa 2006). The assumption is thus that an expert can 'diagnose' objectively and linearly apply a solution. 'Clinical technologies' include psychological treatment modalities (such as psychotherapy, psychiatry and their systems of diagnosis) at the interface of client/patient/community and the mental health professional (Hook 2002).

Not so long ago, same-sex sexual orientation was seen as psychopathology within biomedicine and treated as a mental disorder. Same-sex sexuality was declassified as a disorder by the American Psychiatric Association in 1973 (Shidlo & Schroeder 2002), and in 1975 the American Psychological Association (APA) passed a resolution supporting this action (APA 1998), encouraging professionals to work against the prevailing idea that same-sex sexuality was 'perverse' (Goldfried 2001). The American National Association of Social Workers brought out its first policy statement related to same-sex sexuality in 1977, emphasising that its position of non-discrimination and affording equal status to all, regardless of sexual orientation, served the mental health and welfare interests not only of affected individuals, but of society as a whole (Tully 2000). However, the 'expert' opinion of same-sex sexuality as undesirable, and research aimed at 'converting' same-sex sexual behaviour to that of the mainstream, persisted until the late 1970s (Sandfort & De Keizer 2001). As of the early 1970s, the term 'homosexual' was increasingly rejected as pathologising and replaced with the term 'gay' by same-sex minorities, activists and affirmative healthcare practitioners. 'Ego-dystonic homosexuality', an incomprehensible and unpopular diagnosis, was excluded from the revision of the *Diagnostic and Statistical Manual of Mental Disorders* (DSM) III in 1987 (Gonsiorek 1988). While the American Psychiatric Association's DSM classification system declassified homosexuality as pathology in

1973, the World Health Organization followed suit in 1990, and the *International Classification of Diseases* (ICD) delisted homosexuality in 1999 (MACGLH 2002). Now 'officially' seen as a sexual variation rather than a problem, same-sex sexual orientation itself is no longer seen as a condition to be treated.

Not all scientific disciplines that study sexuality are equally affirming in their approach to the needs and issues of individuals from sexual minorities. In particular, tensions exist between medico-psychosocial sciences and other academic disciplines, which has major implications for loss of currency of the social sciences in favour of literary studies and other disciplines. It may be argued that psychology does not enjoy prominence in the field of sexology. For some, psychology is neither enough of a pure science nor medical enough; and for others it's not progressive or affirming enough. Internationally, recent studies indicate that awareness and understanding of the psychological issues faced by lesbian, gay, bisexual, transgender and intersex (LGBTI) individuals are limited. Reflective of prevailing heterosexist attitudes, the majority of psychology textbooks still inadequately address lesbian- and gay-related issues in human development, relationships and other such areas (Steffens & Eschmann 2001).

Scientific enquiry to establish causality is an enduring feature of conventional psychology. The same applies with regard to same-sex sexual orientation. Ongoing debates highlight 'nature' on the one hand and 'nurture' on the other, or suggest a combination of both. Predetermination and predisposition, as well as inherent qualities such as the biochemical prenatal influences of hormones and nutrition, feature in theories of causality supportive of nature as cause. Theories supportive of nurture as cause, for example psychoanalysis, emphasise disrupted development (Carl 1990). Social learning theory purports that same-sex sexual orientation is not a pervasive psychiatric disorder, but a set of behaviours learned through social reinforcement, observation of persons and events without direct reinforcement, and/or incidental association of events during critical periods (Feinberg 1987 cited in Carl 1990).

Treatment of lesbians and gay men based on the medical model had limited results when 'heterosexual shift' was the goal (Coleman 1982). In fact, since 1990, reparative therapy has been strongly discouraged by the APA and others, due to poor prognosis, the ethics involved in trying to change a trait that is not a disorder and that is vital to a person's identity, and because such a practice can do more harm than good (APA 1998). However, the disaffirming and oppressive attitude of same-sex sexual orientation as undesirable still persists in many 'expert' circles. Same-sex sexual orientation, feelings and urges are acknowledged by some, but rejected as problematic by many others. Despite practice guidelines for psychologists indicating poor prognosis and advising working towards acceptance of sexual orientation, there are professionals who still attempt conversion therapy (Cochran 2001).

Internationally, activism within the LGBTI community attaches a very high premium to the notions of inclusion and representation. This approach is reflected in, for instance, the principles on which the Federation of Gay Games (the LGBTI equivalent of the Olympic Games) are built, namely participation, inclusion and personal best. Use of the abbreviation LGBTI in reference to sexual minorities, not only on the basis of alternative sexual orientation, but also gender non-conformity and biological variance, is another indication of this inclusive stance. Not only is such a position a corrective measure in response to lifelong experiences of marginalisation, exclusion and disqualification (on the basis of competitiveness), but it is also politically informed by the need for solidarity among minorities in the face of discrimination at the hands of a vast majority.

In contrast with the mentioned activist position, specificity is, however, highly valued in academic endeavours and scientific practice. The abbreviation LGBTI minimises theoretical distinctions drawn between biological variance, gender, and sexual orientation, which may not be feasible in psychosocial academic and research endeavours, nor in psychosocial intervention programmes. Such blurring of distinctions also has very real consequences for scientific classification.

The evolution of the social and legal position of same-sex orientation from sick to just another aspect of human diversity is important to emphasise. 'Gender identity disorder' (GID), also known as 'gender dysphoria', and previously referred to as 'transsexuality', is, however, still firmly considered psychopathology and included as a diagnostic category in the DSM IV-R (American Psychiatric Association 1994). The ICD-10 similarly lists 'transsexualism' and GID as sexual deviations and disorders of psychosexual identity (MACGLH 2002). Many progressive and LGBTI-affirmative therapists, however, do not consider transsexuality to be a mental illness, and believe there is no need for psychotherapeutic treatment for transsexuality *per se*.

## Affirmative perspectives on sexual orientation and gender identity

Viewed from a rights-based approach, the goals of sexology include the eradication of ignorance and prejudice and the promotion of sexual and reproductive health rights. The rights-based approach is a conceptual framework for understanding the process of human development that is normatively based on international human rights standards and operationally directed to promoting and protecting universal human rights (WHO 2002).

Regardless of sexual orientation or gender identity, all people have the right to: recognition; legal protection against discrimination; social rights that include marriage and adoption; participation in decision-making; social and cultural rights, including visibility and freedom of speech; access to education, healthcare and sexual health services; inclusion in statistics and research; and initiating and registering new organisations and arranging meetings and events (Samelius & Wägberg 2005).

Health is a fundamental human right, therefore sexual health must also be considered a basic human right. The sexual rights of all persons must be respected, protected and fulfilled. Such rights serve to protect everyone regarding their choices and decisions about their sexuality and reproductive health, and especially those who are deemed vulnerable to abuse and sexual and other health problems. Sexual rights embrace certain human rights already recognised in national laws, international human rights documents and other consensus documents. Sexual rights include access to healthcare services, information regarding sexuality, sexuality education, respect for bodily integrity (security in and control over one's body), choice of sexual partner, deciding to be sexually active or not (self-determination), consensual sexual relations, entering into marriage only with full and free consent of both partners, deciding whether or not to have children, and pursuing a satisfying, safe and pleasurable sexual life (WAS 1999).

Sex and sexuality (not only in relation to HIV or pathology, but also with regard to wellness and rights) ought to be included more fully on the agenda – socially, in policy processes, and in research. Sexual health requires a positive, respectful approach to sexuality, free of coercion, discrimination and violence. Programmes, policies and laws conducive to sexual well-being and that do not discriminate against anyone, are required for sexual health to be attained and maintained. Sexual health requires access to private and confidential information, education and care on matters of sexuality. Most notably, sexuality education through information, skills building and values clarification will enable people to make choices about their sexuality and take charge of their sexual lives (WAS 1999).

Internationally, research findings suggest that sexual minorities are susceptible to discrimination and victimisation (APA 1998; Nel 2007), psychological ill-health (Cochran 2001; Eliason 1996), decision-maker deprioritisation (Tully 2000), and healthcare provider neglect (Rich 2006; Steffens & Eschmann 2001). They are 'vulnerable' to, 'marginalised' or 'at risk' not only of being verbally and physically victimised, but also of contracting HIV and other sexually transmitted infections (STIs). Several factors may increase the risks faced by sexual minorities, including their own (sexual) behaviour, occupation, stigma, internalised oppression, marginalisation, sexual orientation and gender expressions. Their susceptibility to institutional and societal discrimination implies a high incidence of not being selected for an opportunity or employment. Minorities are thus in effect 'cut down to size', 'put down', disaffirmed (the feeding ground for internalised oppression) or disqualified (oppressed), which substantially limits their prospects of entry into or advancement in employment, so limiting their opportunities for growth, development and progression.

Differences do exist and ought to be recognised. A diversity mindset (respect for difference regarding people's sexuality and other aspects of their lives) should apply.

Healthcare providers for sexual minorities require diversity awareness, especially regarding gender identity and sexual orientation. Exposure to their issues and needs and adequate information on LGBTI concepts, realities, practices and lifestyles will enable helpful responses and affirmative healthcare.

Several European Union member states, such as the Netherlands, Denmark and Sweden, have shown long-term commitment to the international struggle for LGBTI equality and human rights, and South Africa can benefit from findings of related psychosocial research endeavours. Internationally, the Netherlands is renowned for its progressive social and political attitudes, and its views on sexual matters.

The Dutch have arguably led the way in the European struggle for LGBTI equality (Sandfort 1998). Dutch society has also made significant contributions in recent years to assist in the development of LGBTI-affirmative health services and intervention programmes in South Africa. Events and processes in Dutch history relevant to the development of their expertise in affirming healthcare provision are thus of interest to South Africa.

Regardless of the fact that the Netherlands is internationally considered most accepting of same-sex sexuality, LGBTI-specific healthcare provision remains vital, and lesbian and gay emancipation is incomplete (Ministerie van Volksgezondheid, Welzijn en Sport 2001; Sandfort 1998; Schippers 1998). Segregation is a precondition for integration (Sandfort 1998). Identity, health, solidarity and continued need for social change, count among ongoing concerns (Stienstra 1991 cited in Veenker 1998). Challenging and addressing the image of same-sex sexuality and its subculture held by society in general will have to remain a continuous concern of the gay movement (Schippers 1998).

## Sexual orientation

The USA is prominent in the development of gay-affirmative healthcare policy and practice. In 2000, the APA became the first psychological association to formally adopt LGB-affirmative psychotherapeutic guidelines (APA 2000). In 2001, Division 44 of the APA co-hosted the first international meeting on sexual orientation and mental health, held in San Francisco, USA. Sponsored by several national and international psychological associations, the meeting, which aimed to establish global perspectives on practice and policy, was attended by people from 20 countries. Division 44 of the APA continues to provide administrative and financial support to the International Network on Sexual Orientation-Related Matters and Gender Identity Concerns in Psychology (INET), founded at this meeting. The Psychological Society of South Africa has been represented on INET since 2007.[1]

The gay-affirmative approach is a 'political-ideological' approach that significantly resembles the feminist approach to therapy in that it gives attention to, and takes into account, the specific, the 'own' interest. Gay-affirmative therapy is a specialised treatment modality with implications for attitude and attention to specific themes integrated into conventional methods to conduct therapeutic conversation and group process facilitation. A basic premise of a gay-affirmative stance is that homosexuality is a normal variation in human sexuality and not psychopathological. The gay-affirmative therapy model assumes that, similar to heterosexuals, lesbian women and gay men incorporate learned negative attitudes and beliefs about same-sex sexuality in the process of growing up – a complicated process of stereotyping and image formation (Schippers 1997). This approach is sometimes also referred to as the 'lesbian- and gay-affirmative' approach, as internationally reference to 'LGBTI-affirmative' is not commonplace. Although criticism against the gay-affirmative therapy approach includes the dearth of rigorous research findings on the effectiveness thereof (Cochran 2001), this approach is highly valued by LGBTI-affirmative healthcare practitioners, communities and persons.

'Good practice' when dealing with LGBTI clients includes neither avoiding sexual orientation issues nor focusing solely on this factor when the client does not see it as pertinent to their problem. Inappropriate practice includes assuming that a client is heterosexual, indicating that a gay or lesbian identity is bad or inferior, and a lack of knowledge on issues of concern to LGBTI clients (APA 2000; Liddle 1996). For 'political' reasons (to gain societal and decision-maker acceptance), understanding causality may be important. However, therapeutic responses to concerns regarding causality include being open to 'nature' and also 'nurture' arguments, or a combination of both but, more importantly, challenging the significance of establishing the 'causes'. Fact is, we not only don't know what exactly causes same-sex sexual orientation, but the causes of heterosexual sexual orientation are also unknown. Therefore, as same-sex sexual orientation is a variant and not abnormal, the 'cause' is, in fact, irrelevant.

Furthermore, it is important that the therapist does not assume that the rules and solutions applicable in heterosexual relationships can always be applied in same-sex relationships. A primary goal in therapy must often consist of restructuring the couple relationship and legitimising the right of the couple to be a couple. In addition, the solutions applied must be appropriate to the situation and not based entirely on the therapist's experience with heterosexual couples.

## Gender identity

Feminist thinking and its interest in gender and power emerged in the 1970s. Feminist analyses of the gender biases have informed scientific work on nature and normative masculinity and femininity (Pigg & Adams 2005). Feminism, largely seen as developing and giving equal status to the role of women, also increased the awareness that the dominant positions held by men in certain respects also applied to gay men, and that use of the term 'gay' in reference to both women and men with a same-sex orientation in fact rendered lesbians invisible. Many of the key contributions to the study of lesbian women, however, came from outside the social sciences (Nardi & Schneider 1998). Contemporary gender research focuses on how femininities and masculinities are constructed as unequal dichotomies regarding power and material resources. The work to address anti-gay violence is playing a crucial role in challenging dominant constructions of masculinity.

'Queer' became a key concern from the late 1980s. Queer theory separates the natural relation between sexed bodies, gender and desire. Developed through activism and social science enquiry, sexuality and erotic desire can be conceptualised independently of gender and outside the heterosexual matrix (Pigg & Adams 2005). Queer theory enables us to question Western and scientific naturalist assumptions. Social constructionism emphasises historical change and context. It considers sexuality to exist within economic, social and political structures and within the systems of meaning and representation they sustain. All sexualities are thus local (Pigg & Adams 2005).

Most people (inclusive of trans people) feel that having a recognised gender identity accords with their sense of self. Dreger (2006), together with others, however, challenges the notion that everyone has a true, core, single, unchanging gender identity: just as sex anatomies don't come in only two types that never change, neither do genders. A libertarian view of legal gender/sex identity advocates that, instead of the state adjudicating who is who in terms of sex and gender, people ought to have their own say about what their genders are, regardless of their anatomies (Dreger 2006).

Transsexuals have, more often than not, been misunderstood and misdiagnosed by their caregivers, who have frequently allowed their own personal prejudices to adversely affect their judgement (WPATH 2001). In recognition of the scarcity of so-called qualified gender specialists, standards of care (SOC) for GID were established by the World Professional Association for Transgender Health (WPATH),[2] with the assistance of professionals in both the medical and psychological sciences. The SOC specify the minimum requirements for proper care and protection of both the person with GID and the professionals who provide treatment. The SOC articulate WPATH's professional consensus regarding the psychiatric, psychological, medical and surgical management of GID. Included are requirements for determining a client's acceptability for hormone therapy and gender reassignment surgery (GRS). The SOC specify the treatment goal of psychotherapy, endocrine and surgical therapy for persons with GID as lasting personal comfort with their gendered self in order to enhance their overall psychological well-being and self-fulfilment (WPATH 2001).

Intersex persons are extremely marginalised and almost totally invisible in society, yet mostly regarded as abnormal (Samelius & Wägberg 2005). The standard protocol in the treatment of intersex children is GRS to alter the genitals of the person and, in so doing, ascribe them to one of the two recognised biological sexes – male or female.

Internationally, a small but growing intersex movement is lobbying against this practice, which they consider discriminatory, disrespectful and, at times, responsible for inflicting physical and psychological harm (Samelius & Wägberg 2005).

## South African perspectives on same-sex sexuality

Apartheid South Africa is notorious for having been a particularly repressive society (Nel 2005; Seedat et al. 2001). Until the early 1990s, also with regard to sexuality, strong emphasis was placed on restriction, with several laws regulating sexual behaviour, such as the prohibition of sex across the colour line, the criminalisation of sex between men until as recently as 1996, and the laws against all forms of pornography (Nel 2005; Potgieter 1997). Sex work is still illegal.

Freedom of political association, of speech, as well as of sexual expression is new. Sexuality-related issues elicit strong (negative) emotional responses, including feelings of guilt and shame, and are considered 'private' and 'personal' and 'not to be discussed'. The sexual behaviours of others are viewed in strict and rigid terms of 'rightness' or 'wrongness', and those behaviours departing from the norm are severely criticised. For these reasons, sexuality has more often than not been veiled in secrecy. However, following decades of Calvinist rule, the post-1994 multi-billion rand South African sex industry (including upmarket entertainment venues, strip clubs, several chains of sex shops, house parties and sex work) suggests that a sexual revolution has occurred.[3]

Yet, heterosexism remains characteristic of contemporary South African culture (Hattingh 1994; Miller & Romanelli 1991). Heterosexism refers to the assumption or belief that everyone is and should be heterosexual and that the other sexual orientations are unhealthy, unnatural and a threat. In everyday life this manifests as the assumption that everyone is heterosexual, until proven otherwise. In other words, there is a lack of awareness and thus an omission of homosexuality as a viable alternative to heterosexuality. Heterosexist assumptions and attitudes are pervasive in the media, religious teachings and practices, legal discourses, education and healthcare. Neglect or deliberate exclusion of LGBTI persons in gender analyses and policy discussions reflects the pervasiveness of heterosexism (Samelius & Wägberg 2005). Silencing implies a taboo and undesirability, and perpetuates prejudice (Eliason 1996).

The South African LGBTI community also has to contend with homoprejudice and transphobia (Du Plessis 1999; Hattingh 1994). Not too long ago – and some will argue still today – being lesbian or gay in South Africa was considered a 'sickness', a 'sin', 'criminal', or un-African. Theoretically, being homoprejudiced is today considered sick, or even criminal, if expressed either verbally or physically, yet religious condemnation, harassment in the workplace, open harassment, public homoprejudiced statements, and violence towards LGBTI people are still rife. Internalised homoprejudice is prevalent in many LGBTI persons (Isaacs & McKendrick 1992; Nel 2007).

Internationally, the rise of an activist gay liberation movement as a critical force in establishing the validity of a gay identity is recognised (Isaacs & McKendrick 1992). In several ways, it is not feasible to compare South African LGBTI persons and communities to those found in metropolitan cities of developed countries such as the UK, the Netherlands, Australia and the USA. Firstly, in South Africa there are no so-called 'gay ghettos', such as those found in New York or San Francisco, nor are there any locations with a major concentration of predominantly LGBTI businesses, such as in London, Sydney and Amsterdam.

LGBTI identities in South Africa differ significantly along the designated 'racial' categories of African, coloured, Indian and white. Given our history of apartheid and patriarchy, the most visible and vocal subsection of the LGBTI 'community', until recently, was white and predominantly male, many of whom are well positioned in the workplace and affluent in comparison to other sectors of society. They are, however, not a true reflection of the community as a whole: the vast majority of LGBTI individuals in South Africa are black, unemployed, poor and have low literacy levels (Reid & Dirsuweit 2002). Being economically disadvantaged and disempowered, they thus share the general profile of South African society.

Due to the multiplicity of their minority status in terms of gender, sexual orientation, socio-economic status, and race, under-resourced black lesbians are assumed to be the most vulnerable subsection of the community (Reid & Dirsuweit 2002). As a result of their historic invisibility, the associated difficulties with gaining access to them, and also their deprioritisation, this subsection is also severely under-researched. Recent research findings indicate disproportionately high levels of risk of victimisation among this group, including so-called corrective rape (Polders 2006; Reid & Dirsuweit 2002; Rich 2006; Wells 2006). Also, their levels of HIV infection are significantly higher than what has become known internationally with regard to the risk associated with lesbian sexual practices (Polders 2006; Rich 2006; Wells 2006). Whether their HIV prevalence and the aforementioned vulnerability to corrective rape victimisation are linked is yet to be determined.

To date, most local LGBTI-related research, albeit limited, is focused on resourced white gay men. Internationally most comparable, this subsection of the South African LGBTI community is generally considered to be the beneficiary of the power associated with being male, white and resourced within a patriarchal society. Being the most privileged, the assumption is made that they are also the least vulnerable or the least at risk of victimisation and distress. This general assumption, however, appears faulty when considering recent research findings (Nel & Joubert 1997; Polders 2006; Rich 2006; Wells 2006).

Similar to the identity construction of LGBTI persons in Europe and northern America, among white South Africans sexual orientation is considered a basis for identity. In rural and poorer African and coloured communities, however, sexual practices do not necessarily constitute an identity-forming practice for all people.

In these contexts, sexual identities are more often based on sexual activities along traditional gender roles prescribed for men and women, without fixed boundaries. In practice, this may translate into someone considering himself a gay man, yet referring to his sexual partner as a straight man, and clearly stating that he will not have sex with another gay man (Reid 2007). Similar to elsewhere in Africa, the receptive role during sex greatly determines gender presentation (often overtly effeminate), self-identification (as gay), and sexual attraction (to masculine, insertive, self-identified heterosexual men only) in men who have sex with men (MSM) (Samelius & Wägberg 2005).

As in Euro–America, and for very much the same reasons, use of the abbreviation LGBTI in reference to sexual minorities is common practice in South African activist circles. Implications for psychosocial studies and interventions of this naming practice, which in fact minimises or disregards scientific distinctions between biological variance, gender and sexual orientation, have not yet been sufficiently considered. Use of this abbreviation is, however, not a true reflection of representation or inclusion in decision-making. In fact, participation of bisexual, trans and intersex persons in the so-called LGBTI sector or movement is very limited. As a consequence, knowledge of bisexual-, transgender- and especially intersex-related issues is very limited.

## Sexual healthcare provision

In South Africa, the field of sexology is poorly developed, and specialised healthcare, including sex therapy, is available only to a select few, and almost exclusively at private healthcare facilities in urban centres. Until recently, very limited funds and support were made available in South Africa for research and education on sexuality issues. Human sexuality, and most certainly the issue of sexual orientation, has been neglected in the research, practices and theoretical concerns of healthcare professionals. These professionals seldom receive formal training in matters related to sexual health and well-being. A limited number of medical professionals, psychologists and therapists can consider themselves as sexologists. Very few have adequate multidisciplinary knowledge of, and skills in, sexuality-related issues, and most have no recognised formal qualification.

Viagra, as oral treatment for erectile dysfunction, changed the lack of funding for sexuality research in South Africa. Pfizer, the pharmaceutical company that produces Viagra, has prioritised the provision of credible information and education on sexual health issues from a multidisciplinary perspective to the general public, the media and healthcare professionals. The subsequent availability of alternative treatments (such as Cialis and Levitra) for erectile dysfunction further strengthened sexology in South Africa.

In South Africa, HIV and AIDS have contributed significantly to the public healthcare system becoming more overstretched, with state hospitals bearing the brunt as they accommodate people suffering from HIV/AIDS-related illnesses.[4] The endemic prevalence of HIV/AIDS, but also rape and women and child abuse (De la Rey & Eagle 1997), may be partly related to the lack of sexuality education and inadequate understandings of gender issues. Until the mid-1990s, very little emphasis was placed on sexual rights, and it is only recently that public campaigns and debates on sexuality issues and the responsibilities that go with freedom have been introduced. Despite strong recommendations in this regard, sex education and gender awareness are yet to be comprehensively introduced in schools (OUT 2006).

South Africa, as a Member State of the UN, has committed itself to work towards the achievement of the Millennium Development Goals, of which at least four have direct bearing on sexual and reproductive health. Being a signatory of the International Agreement reached at the Fourth World Conference on Women held in Beijing in 1995, South Africa subscribes to the rights contained in the Sexual Health Charter and is therefore obliged to ensure that the sexual rights of all persons are respected and protected. Furthermore, several sexual and reproductive rights are included as human rights in the South African Constitution, such as the right to expression of sexual orientation without interference from others, equality and equity for all, and freedom to make choices free from gender-based discrimination, freedom from sexual violence or coercion, and the right to privacy (Gender Manual Consortium 1999).

South Africa is, however, far from translating these 'paper rights' into practice. High levels of poverty and unemployment provide the bedrock for HIV/AIDS. The relentless HIV pandemic and the very high levels of rape, domestic violence, incest and teenage pregnancies, suggest that many people are not able to claim their sexual and reproductive rights (Gender Manual Consortium 1999). The unconvincing responses of the public health sector to the HIV/AIDS pandemic have raised grave concerns. LGBTI issues are virtually non-existent in the Department of Health, and also in HIV prevention and care. Similarly, reports on HIV transmission do not differentiate between male-to-male and male-to-female modes of transmission (Samelius & Wägberg 2005). Non-gay defined MSM and women who have sex with women (WSW) are deprioritised in services provided by both the state and civil society organisations. As indicated, government-initiated HIV prevention and treatment programmes and interventions insufficiently recognise diversity of sexual expressions, behaviours and needs, and generally only target the mainstream. LGBTI-specific organisations, on the other hand, specify resource limitations as an excuse. The paucity of referenced accounts of bisexual life in South Africa, and the under-representation of bisexual concerns in lesbian and gay organisations in general, is striking. Their greater invisibility, but also preconceived ideas of bisexual persons as fence-sitters who are fearful of disclosure of their sexual orientation, have been suggested as possible reasons (Nicholas, Daniels & Hurwitz 2001 cited in Francoeur 2001). Because bisexual persons may be more integrated into mainstream culture and can 'pass' as being heterosexual, they may not be as marginalised as lesbian and gay persons.

As part of its mandate to share its expertise internationally, the Dutch Schorer Foundation entered into a three-year collaborative agreement with OUT LGBT Well-being (OUT) in Gauteng, South Africa, in 2001, which was subsequently extended by a further two years (Ministerie van Volksgezondheid, Welzijn en Sport 2001). Funded by the Humanist Institute for Co-operation with Developing Countries, the mandate was primarily to assist in the development of a range of LGBTI-affirmative healthcare practices with a focus on HIV prevention, lesbian programmes and materials development. In 2006, the Dutch Ministry of Foreign Affairs allocated substantial funding to the Schorer Foundation for an HIV/STI prevention programme for sexual minorities in, among other places, southern Africa. This programme emphasises prevention activities, capacity enhancement, mainstreaming, and advocacy, emancipation and dissemination. Partner organisations in four southern African countries, namely South Africa, Botswana, Namibia and Zimbabwe, participate in this four-year programme (2007–2010). South African partner organisations are OUT (Gauteng), the Triangle Project (Cape Town) and the Durban Lesbian & Gay Community & Health Centre.[5]

The South African Constitution (Act No. 108 of 1996) guarantees non-discrimination regardless of, among other things, race, sex or sexual orientation. Furthermore, the Preamble states: 'South Africa belongs to all who live in it, united in our diversity.' Yet in many communities, and for countless individuals, service provider neglect, deprioritisation, marginalisation, exclusion, discrimination and even victimisation are everyday occurrences. Experiences of treatment as a second- or even third-class citizen are even more commonplace for those who differ from the 'norm'.

Current practice in mainstream healthcare in South Africa and by deduction also in the rest of Africa is, more often than not, to render services with an assumption of sameness, rather than with respect for difference or diversity. It goes without saying that everyone has the right to be treated as equal and to healthcare services that adhere to the minimum standards. However, because of the diverse peoples who inhabit the land, it is erroneous and inappropriate to think that 'one size fits all'. On the rare occasion when sexuality issues are addressed in professional contexts or in public forums in South Africa, it is often from a heterosexist (Potgieter 1997) and, until recently, also a patriarchal perspective (De la Rey & Eagle 1997).

Despite South Africa's claim to be a 'rainbow nation' and committed to non-discrimination, human rights awareness, change management and diversity sensitisation (including around sexual orientation) are seldom included in the curricula of healthcare and other relevant service providers. Too often healthcare providers ascribe to the prevailing norms in South African society. Attitudes towards social marginality are reflected by the tendency to blame one or other problematised sector of society for prevailing social problems, such as HIV and criminality. When those who get to judge the sexual orientation or gender presentations of others are in positions of power, such as psychologists, politicians and religious leaders, the effects of their disapproval can be devastating in terms of the associated neglect, deprioritisation, marginalisation, exclusion, discrimination and victimisation.

Sexual orientation is the one ground for non-discrimination contained in the Constitution that a vast majority of healthcare providers are either ignorant of or experience difficulties in appropriately and skillfully addressing within their services. Reasons for such difficulties may include discomfort, unfamiliarity, a lack of understanding or skills, the low priority attached to sexual orientation-related matters, or downright prejudice and unwillingness.

While the LGBTI sector in South Africa renders (sexual) health and psychosocial services, recognition is seldom given to LGBTI clients/patients or their rights and needs in the mainstream (including government and civil society initiatives). No LGBTI-specific healthcare service is provided by government. Increasingly, clients demand the services of LGBTI-affirming therapists, and although the number of therapists who advertise their services in the LGBTI media has significantly increased in recent years, not many therapists in South Africa, especially outside the major city centres, qualify as LGBTI-affirmative. Transgender-related treatment programmes and services, albeit only a few and in major cities, are available for pre- and post-operatives.

The first specifically transgender organisation on the continent, Gender DynamiX, located in Cape Town, South Africa, was only launched in 2005. While transgender rights are now protected, and it is possible to legally change gender on birth certificates and in identity documents (Samelius & Wägberg 2005), bureaucratic procedures and the ignorance and prejudice of state officials render many of these rights useless.

## Psychological research and teaching practices

The formal training of psychologists and psychology professionals is currently not sufficiently inclusive of the issues and needs of sexual minorities. University prescribed textbooks may inadvertently or otherwise reinforce prevailing negative attitudes by linking LGBTI persons directly to HIV/AIDS or psychopathology. Not consciously counteracting notions of same-sex sexuality as psychopathology or as criminal behaviour is inexcusable.

A Teaching Psychology in South Africa conference held at the University of the Free State in 2007 included a round-table discussion on counteracting heterosexism and homoprejudice in the curriculum, facilitated by the author of this chapter. Discussions, which included representatives of the universities of Fort Hare, Free State, Johannesburg, Zululand and the University of South Africa, called for greater provision within the curriculum for diversity, and recognition for the fluidity of sexual orientation, gender and biology. Representatives acknowledged that sexual orientation- and gender identity-related content is often restricted to subfields such as social and abnormal psychology. Inclusion of related content in case studies, examples and discussions in all subfields of psychology will contribute to the required desensitisation and recognition of same-sex sexuality as normal variance.

Representatives considered the inherent conservatism (inclusive of patriarchy) in South Africa and resistance, also within the profession, to addressing themes of sexuality and gender as considerable challenges. Related terminology (such as sex, gender, sexual orientation, gender identification, sexual behaviour, LGBTI, MSM, WSW, homosexuality versus same-sex sexuality) is often confusing, poorly understood and controversial (conventional classification has contributed to labelling and stereotypes) and requires careful 'unpacking' and complexification, rather than linear descriptions (the fluidity needs to be acknowledged).

A search of South African journals indicates the paucity in local research on sexual orientation and gay-affirmative therapy. No article dealing with this subject is found in an electronic search of the Index of South African Periodicals and South African Studies databases. The author, often having served as external examiner for master's dissertations in psychology at several South African universities, is aware of the following patterns in current research into sexual minorities:

- Topics contribute to psychological knowledge and are suitable for research at a master's level, however, while South African research on lesbian and gay-related issues is severely lacking, some very relevant local research findings and texts are seldom cited.
- The vast majority of findings and literature cited are of American sources, without students necessarily always contextualising them as such when reporting the findings. Not contextualising the findings of the literature study, geographically and with regard to demographics, may be misleading and even irresponsible. More caution ought to be taken not to apply these studies as if they are necessarily equally valid for South Africa. Also, key concepts such as 'homophobia', 'heterosexism' and 'internalised homophobia' are mostly insufficiently defined or applied in a faulty way.
- With regards to research methodology, insufficient indications are given of how it was ascertained that participants were lesbian/gay. Insufficient demographic information is provided with regard to issues such as race, age and socio-economic status of the participants, leaving the reader to assume that they are all white, middle class and part of the gay subculture or 'gay community'.
- In analyses and conclusions, identity politics is insufficiently recognised – the differences between those adopting the so-called gay identity (and subculture, for that matter) versus those who have sex with others of the same sex, but cannot associate with being gay or lesbian, and most certainly do not identify with what the 'gay subculture' has come to signify.
- Limited reference is made to cultural variants in the use of terminology, whether to refer to the self or to describe same-sex attraction in others. Differences in the development of a gay identity, including the process of 'coming out', not only between the developed world and the developing world, but also between the

first world and third world segments of South African society, are insufficiently highlighted.
- Local researchers often reflect an insufficient grasp of the South African 'gay community' and/or recognition of the role played by 'gay subculture'. Insufficient emphasis is placed on the significance of gender within this phenomenon as well as within the feminist construct of 'patriarchy'.
- Finally, there is a tendency to generalise the findings to the South African 'gay community' and, in so doing, the significance for South Africa of variables such as race and socio-economic status are not recognised.

## Conclusion

In this chapter, declassification of same-sex sexual orientation as psychopathology in Euro-American psychiatry and psychology was emphasised, and international developments affirming same-sex sexuality as variance were introduced. The potential for secondary victimisation at the hands of healthcare providers and often unhelpful and disempowering interactions between them and sexual minority clients and communities in South Africa were also indicated. LGBTI persons are at risk and vulnerable to stigmatisation, discrimination and victimisation. They therefore require mainstreaming of their issues and needs, but also LGBTI-specific services and legal protections. For this reason, lesbian- and gay-affirmative practices and clear guidelines are urgently required in South Africa with regard to the use of reparative therapies and the normalising of same-sex sexuality.

## Notes

1  The author of this chapter in fact serves as a representative.
2  WPATH was formerly known as HBIGDA – the Harry Benjamin International Gender Dysphoria Association.
3  H Geldenhuys, Inside South Africa's sex boom: Post-apartheid sexual revolution breeds over multi-billion Rand industry, *Sunday Times*, 24 December 2006.
4  B Boyle, Fight crime, Africa tells SA, *Sunday Times*, 3 December 2006.
5  F Strijthagen, *Programme to fitness: MFS information*, email correspondence, 14 December 2006.

## References

American Psychiatric Association (1994) *Diagnostic and statistical manual of mental disorders* (IV). Washington, DC: American Psychiatric Association

APA (American Psychological Association) (1998) *Hate crimes today: An age-old foe in modern dress.* Accessed on 4 August 2004, http://www.apa.org/monitor/jan98/hate.html

APA (2000) Guidelines for psychotherapy with lesbian, gay and bisexual clients. *American Psychologist* 55(12): 1440–1451

Carl D (1990) *Counselling same-sex couples.* New York: W.W. Norton & Company

Cochran SD (2001) Emerging issues in research in lesbians' and gay men's mental health: Does sexual orientation really matter? *American Psychologist* 56(11): 932–947

Coleman E (1982) Developmental stages of the coming out process. *Journal of Homosexuality* 7(2/3): 1–9

De la Rey C & Eagle G (1997) Gender and mental health policy development. In D Foster, M Freeman & Y Pillay (Eds) *Mental health policy issues for South Africa*. Cape Town: Medical Association of South Africa

Dreger A (2006) *Really changing sex bioethics forum: Diverse commentary on issues in bioethics.* Accessed 9 November 2006, http://www.bioethicsforum.org/New-York-City-plan-to-change-gender.asp

Du Plessis J (1999) *Oor gaywees*. Cape Town: Tafelberg Publishers

Eliason MJ (1996) *Institutional barriers to health care for lesbian, gay and bisexual persons*. New York: National League for Nursing Press

Francoeur RT (Ed.) (2001) *The international encyclopedia of sexuality. Volume I – IV, 1997–2001*. New York: Continuum Publishing Company. Accessed on 24 November 2006, http://www2.hu-berlin.de/sexology/IES/index.html

Gender Manual Consortium (1999) *Making women's rights real: A resource manual on women, gender, human rights and the law*. Cape Town: Gender Manual Consortium

Goldfried MR (2001) Integrating gay, lesbian and bisexual issues into mainstream psychology. *American Psychologist* 56(11): 977–988

Gonsiorek JC (1988) Current and future directions in gay and lesbian affirmative mental health practice. In M Shernoff & WA Scott (Eds) *The sourcebook on lesbian/gay healthcare* (2nd edition). New York: National Lesbian/Gay Health Foundation

Goodwatch R (2005) Sex therapy: Historical evolution, current practice, Part 1. *Anzjft* 26(3): 155–164

Graziano KJ (2004) Oppression and resiliency in a post-apartheid South Africa: Unheard voices of black gay men and lesbians. *Cultural Diversity and Ethnic Minority Psychology* 10(3): 302–316

Hattingh C (1994) The experience of gays and lesbians who are covert at work. Honours dissertation, Grahamstown, Rhodes University

Hook D (2002) Introduction: A 'social psychology' of psychopathology. In D Hook & G Eagle (Eds) *Psychopathology and social prejudice*. Cape Town: University of Cape Town Press

HRW (Human Rights Watch) (2003) *More than a name. State-sponsored homophobia and its consequences in southern Africa*. New York: Human Rights Watch

Isaacs G & McKendrick B (1992) *Male homosexuality in South Africa: Identity formation, culture and crisis*. Cape Town: Oxford University Press

Liddle BJ (1996) Therapist sexual orientation, gender, and counseling practices as they relate to ratings of helpfulness by gay and lesbian clients. *Journal of Counseling Psychology* 43(4): 394–401

MACGH (Ministerial Advisory Committee on Gay and Lesbian Health) (2002) Gay, lesbian, bisexual, transgender and intersex community consultations: Stage one. Introductory paper to accompany issue papers on major health issues affecting GLBTI Victorians, Australia. Accessed 13 February 2002, http://www.dhs.vic.gov.au/phd/macglh/ index.htm

Miller DJ & Romanelli RE (1991) From religion: Heterosexism and the golden rule. *Journal of Gay and Lesbian Psychotherapy* 1(4): 45–48

Ministerie van Volksgezondheid, Welzijn en Sport (2001) *Paars over roze: Nota homo-emancipatiebeleid.* Den Haag: Directie Sociaal Beleid

Nardi PM & Schneider BE (Eds) (1998) *Social perspectives in lesbian and gay studies: A reader.* London: Routledge

Nel JA (2005) Moving from rhetoric to creating the reality: Empowering South Africa's lesbian and gay community. In M van Zyl & M Steyn (Eds) *Performing queer: Shaping sexualities 1994–2004 (Vol. 1).* Cape Town: Kwela Books

Nel JA (2007) Towards the 'Good society': Healthcare provision for victims of hate crime from periphery to centre stage. PhD thesis, University of South Africa

Nel JA & Joubert KD (1997) Coming out of the closet: A gay experience. *Unisa Psychologia* 24(1): 17–31

OUT (OUT LGBT Well-being) (2006) School violence and safety: Addressing issues of sexual orientation and gender identity. Submission to the South African Human Rights Council. Pretoria: OUT LGBT Well-being

Pigg SL & Adams V (2005) Introduction: The moral object of sex. In V Adams & SL Pigg (Eds) *Sex in development, science, sexualiy and morality.* Durham: Duke University Press

Polders LA (2006) Factors affecting vulnerability to depression among gay men and lesbian women. MA dissertation, University of South Africa

Potgieter C (1997) From apartheid to Mandela's Constitution: Black South African lesbians in the nineties. In B Greene (Ed.) *Ethnic and cultural diversity among lesbians and gay men.* Thousand Oaks: Sage Publications

Reid G (2007) Sexual orientation and gender: Making identities. Presentation at OUT LGBT Well-Being Study Group, Pretoria

Reid G & Dirsuweit T (2002) Understanding systemic violence. *Urban Forum* 31(3): 99–126

Rich E (2006) Overall research findings on levels of empowerment among LGBT people in Western Cape, South Africa. Report, University of South Africa

Samelius L & Wägberg E (2005) *Sexual orientation and gender identity issues in development.* Stockholm: Swedish International Development Co-operation Agency Health Division

Sandfort T (1998) Nog lang niet klaar. De permanente noodzaak van een lesbische en homobeweging. In J Veenker (Ed.) *Roze tijden: Kansen en risico's voor de lesbische en homobeweging.* Amsterdam: Schorer Boeken

Sandfort T & De Keizer M (2001) Sexual problems in gay men: An overview of empirical research. *Annual Review of Sex Research* 12: 93–120

Schippers J (1997) *Liever manner: Theorie en praktijk van de hulpverlening aan homoseksuele mannen.* Amsterdam: Thesis Publishers

Schippers J (1998) Sodoms eicellen. Biologische opvattingen over homoseksualiteit bij mannen. In J Veenker (Ed.) *Roze tijden: Kansen en risico's voor de lesbische en homobeweging.* Amsterdam: Schorer Boeken

Seedat M, Duncan N & Lazarus S (Eds) (2001) *Community psychology. Theory, method and practice*. Oxford: Oxford University Press

Shidlo A & Schroeder M (2002) Changing sexual orientation: A consumers' report. *Professional Psychology: Research and Practice* 33(3): 249–259

Steffens MC & Eschmann B (2001) Fighting psychologists' negative attitudes and prejudices towards lesbians, gay men and bisexuals. In MC Steffens & U Biechele (Eds) *Annual review of lesbian, gay and bisexual issues in European psychology* (Vol. 1). Trier: ALGBP

Tully CT (2000) *Lesbians, gays and the empowering perspective*. New York: Columbia University Press

Unisa (University of South Africa) (2006) *Community psychology: Re-imagining community*. Study guide PYC205 of the Department of Psychology. Pretoria: University of South Africa

Veenker J (Ed.) (1998) *Roze tijden: Kansen en risico's voor de lesbische en homobeweging*. Amsterdam: Schorer Boeken

WAS (World Association for Sexual Health) (1999) *Universal declaration of sexual rights*. Accessed on 27 February 2007, http://www.worldsexology.org/about_sexualrights.asp

Wells H (2006) Levels of empowerment among lesbian, gay, bisexual and transgender (LGBT) people in KwaZulu-Natal, South Africa. Report commissioned by OUT LGBT Well-being, Pretoria

WHO (World Health Organization) (2002) *Sexual health working definitions*. Accessed 27 February 2007, http://www.who.int/reproductive-health/gender/sexual_health.html

WPATH (World Professional Association for Transgender Health) (2001) *Standards of care for gender identity disorders* (Version 6). Accessed 16 February 2007, www.wpath.org/Documents2/socv6.pdf

CHAPTER FOUR

# Homosexual and bisexual labels: The need for clear conceptualisations, operationalisations and appropriate methodological designs

Theo Sandfort and Brian Dodge

The title of this chapter is somewhat ambitious. Fully addressing the various issues mentioned would require a much longer chapter. Fortunately, what we want to discuss is not new. Several people have written intelligibly about this topic (see Asthana & Oostvogels 2001; Boyce 2007; Caceres & Rosasco 1999; Muñoz-Laboy 2004; Parker & Caceres 1999).

Our aim is to critically assess the labels that we use to identify men who engage in sexual behaviour with other men, and to challenge the underlying assumptions. We will conclude with recommendations for future research.

## 'Gay' and 'bisexual' labels in cross-cultural contexts

The idea for this chapter came up while reading a study about what was called 'men who have sex with men' (MSM) (Allman et al. 2007). The study was carried out in Nigeria. In the description of the sample, the authors mentioned that a third of respondents identified themselves as 'gay' and two-thirds of respondents identified themselves as 'bisexual'.

It is not our intention to criticise this particular study, because almost all studies about the so-called MSM population report these kinds of percentages. Besides, the study is very informative. But these percentages make one wonder: how did these answers come about? And what do they actually mean?

Let us first explain that the data were collected in focus groups, and the focus group discussions were conducted in English. Even though English is the official language in the country where the study was done, many other languages are commonly spoken, including Yoruba and Igbo. The researchers explained that while the focus groups were conducted in English, informal translation between English and these two indigenous languages constantly occurred between group members while the focus group discussions were in progress.

We might assume that the researchers used the words 'gay' and 'bisexual' when they asked the participating men about their sexual identity. Did they actually use the term 'sexual identity' as well? We do not know this.

But what about the participants? It is very likely that several if not most knew the words 'gay' and 'bisexual'. But what about 'sexual identity'? Participants might have known these words, but how likely is it that these words had identical meaning for the researchers and the participants? What happened with the translation of these words into Yoruba and Igbo? Assuming that the words 'gay', 'bisexual' and 'sexual identity' do not exist in these languages, what kind of local concepts were used to replace these words, what is left from the meaning that we usually attach to these words, and what got lost in translating the local terms back into English? We do not have answers to these questions, but our conviction is that the correspondence is limited.

Let us illustrate this with an example from a study by the South African anthropologist Graeme Reid (2006). He observed a series of workshops organised in Ermelo, a town in the north of South Africa. The workshops were organised by and aimed at 'homosexual men and lesbians' (words used by the researcher himself).

The word 'gay' was indeed used by the participants at the workshops; however, it did not have the same meaning as it has in industrialised societies. Reid writes, 'being gay in these environs is almost invariably synonymous with being effeminate or, in local parlance, a "lady" or *sis-Buti*' (Reid 2006: 139). Cross-dressing is a substantial part of what is being defined as gay in this community. Cross-dressing actually seems to promote acceptance of these men's homosexuality. While we assume 'gay' men to have sex with each other, this is definitively not the case in Ermelo: here gay men do not have sex with each other. The idea itself seemed hilarious to the participants: to them, two 'ladies' having sex with each other is akin to lesbianism.

So whom do these gay men in Ermelo have sex with? They have sex with so-called '*Injongas*' and 'gents'. An *Injonga* is a man who is 'attracted to and involved with other men, but who maintains a male social and sexual role in a same-sex relationship' (Reid 2006: 139). 'Gents' are straight men who are, as the local people call it, 'somewhat bended'. These men are straight, but are known or suspected to be available as sexual partners for homosexual men. These straight men's defence for what, from a Western perspective, is homosexual involvement, is that they do not have sex with men but with ladies.

The situation becomes even more complex when we also look at gender. While Western gay men (homosexual men who identify as gay) have few, if any, doubts about the maleness of their sex, gay men in Ermelo see themselves as belonging to a third gender category, separate from men and women. One of Reid's informants said: 'In my family it is my mother and we are six [children]. I would say that at home there were three boys and two girls. Then it is me, who is gay' (Reid 2006: 140).

The experiences of these South African MSM are likely to be completely unrelated to the experiences of the MSM in the Nigerian focus groups. This is sufficient reason to doubt that we understand what it means when researchers report about the gay and bisexual identities of the study's participants. These reservations go beyond the words 'gay', 'lesbian' and 'sexual identity'. They also apply to concepts such as 'sexual attraction' and to the meanings men attribute to sexual activities.

The diffuse meanings of homosexual and bisexual identities in an African context might seem obvious. But we started to wonder: do we not have the same problems when we are dealing with Western countries?

## Concepts of 'gay' and 'bisexual' also limited in the West

Quite early in the HIV/AIDS epidemic, research (re)discovered that not only men who identify as gay had sex with men. This became clear when we stopped asking about orientation and identities, and focused on behaviour. One of the first major studies to do so was outlined in the paper *Homosexually and nonhomosexually identified men who have sex with men: A behavioral comparison* (Doll et al. 1992). This discovery sparked an interest in bisexuality, both as behaviour and cultural practice, resulting in new research and critical publications (see Aggleton 1996; Tielman et al. 1991). This interest was driven by the idea that bisexually behaving men might form a bridge from the gay population to what was called the general population.

Research into bisexuality made it clear that in industrialised countries too, the meanings of labels such as 'gay' and 'bisexual' are not uncomplicated. We would like to illustrate this with a study we recently completed at the HIV Center (Dodge et al. 2008; Sandfort et al. 2007). The goal of the study was to understand the HIV risk behaviour of black men in New York who have sex with men and with women. All 30 men who were interviewed had had sexual interactions with both men and women in the year preceding the interviews. We also discussed with the men how they perceived and labelled their own sexuality. And their accounts are revealing.

While most of these men, in line with their actual behaviour, saw themselves as bisexual, two men said they see themselves as exclusively gay. Many men used more than one label, including 'straight'. A third of the men were very explicit about their preference not to use any labels. When probed, these men came up with several somewhat elusive labels, such as 'freak', 'bi-curious', 'free', 'open' and 'just me'.

We discussed with the men why they used specific labels. Their reasoning was rather varied. Some men said the label reflected their behaviour. For others, the label reflected their feelings, sometimes regardless of the fact that their relationship status did not match their feelings. But there were other reasons as well. Some men said they preferred the label 'bisexual' because it was less stigmatising than 'gay'. For some men the label 'bisexual' also had a strategic meaning; these men said that it helped them to accept homosexual feelings and practices and that 'bisexual' instead of 'gay' made it easier to sell homosexual behaviour to others. The men who did not want to use labels used arguments such as: 'Labels are limiting', 'I don't want to be categorised', and 'people are more than their sexuality'.

We would like to highlight something a 25-year-old man said:

> Gerald: Are you gay, are you straight? You know. I would say it depends on who you're with.
>
> Interviewer: Depends on who you're with. Do you ever use 'bisexual', 'straight', 'gay'?
>
> Gerald: I've used bisexual. And I've used straight. And I've used gay... Because it's like, you know, if you have sex with a girl, then you're straight. And if you have sex with a guy, then you're gay.

This quote destabilises our notion of sexual orientation. This man does not seem to have a stable orientation. The label that he uses depends on whether he is sexually involved with a man or a woman. These findings suggest to us that notions of bisexual and gay sexual identities are also not as self-evident in the Western industrialised world.

While thinking about these issues, we also started to wonder about social-scientific research that was done in the Western world under the label 'gay and lesbian studies' before AIDS started to dominate the research agenda.

## Pre-AIDS research presented a limited perspective on homosexuality

Looking back, it seemed that there was a moment in history when self-identification as gay or straight meant a lot and it was pretty obvious what it meant: men were either gay or straight and men knew exactly which category they belonged to.

Researchers were aware that there were MSM who did not label themselves as gay or homosexual. These men were thought to constitute a minority however, and there were even labels to describe their behaviour: 'situational homosexuality' and 'pseudo homosexuality'.

To be really homosexual, a man had to feel attracted to men and this sexual attraction was supposed to be an integral part of his self-identification. 'True' homosexuals had a fixed sexual identity, clearly specified as the final outcome of the models about homosexual identity formation. Research used to have a very essentialist understanding of sexuality. One way to understand the dominance of this perspective is the political role that a lot of research used to play: gay and lesbian studies were an important ingredient of identity politics.

So for our research we recruited men using the concept of 'gay' or 'homosexual'. Of course, most of these studies used convenience instead of probability samples.

We wonder now, though, who was being left out by the recruitment procedures we used and how that has affected our understanding of male same-sex sexuality. The inclusion of sexual behaviour data and measures of sexual attraction in large scale probability samples made clear that our perspective was biased (Sandfort 1997, 2007). One such comparison made clear that a convenience sample usually captures men:

- with higher levels of education;
- who tend to live in urban areas;
- who are more likely to be in an intimate relationship;
- who are less likely to be, or to have been, legally married to a woman; and
- who are less likely to have children.

The health status of gay men in the convenience sample was on average better than that of homosexual men in the probability sample (Sandfort & Bos 1998).

This example shows that there is tension between the researcher's terminology, especially as used for the recruitment of participants, and the population he or she is interested in.

## The concept of MSM is only partially helpful

To circumvent the problems of sexual identity, researchers started using the concept of 'men who have sex with men'. This concept became popular at the end of the 1980s. It was intended to describe men who engage in same-sex sexual practices. Nothing more and nothing less. The homosexual behaviour of these men could be exclusive or they could be involved in sexual interactions with women as well. The homosexual behaviour of these men could be permanent, temporary and situational. It could be practised in the context of a gay identity, any other identity, or without a clearly defined identity.

The concept of MSM has been criticised (see Dowsett et al. 2004). In their critiques, the concept was attributed more meaning than it was intended to have. However, the concept has started to live a life of its own. The funny thing is that, although the concept was invented by researchers, men involved in same-sex sexuality started to use MSM as a label for themselves. For some men, MSM became a category that they identified with. This even happened in countries where English is not the official language and the acronym MSM is meaningless. It should be clear, though, that whenever researchers use the label MSM, we do not know anything yet about the men involved: how they see themselves; what their homosexual practices mean to them, or to the men they are sexually involved with; and how their practices are seen in the culture in which they live.

This leaves us with two major conclusions: (1) When we ask men about their sexual self-identification, we do not know what their answers mean unless we also assess what the answers mean to the men themselves; and (2) Circumventing the issue of self-identification by adopting the label 'men who have sex with men' is meaningless if we do not also assess what the behaviour means to these men.

## Recommendations

Instead of using existing sexual identity categories or adopting the all-encompassing MSM label, researchers of same-sex sexuality may consider the following set of recommendations:

- Researchers should pay explicit attention to how their recruitment methods include some MSM and exclude others, and try to develop strategies that fully capture the population of interest.
- Researchers should be clear about the labels that they use: are these labels 'scientific' labels, imposed on the research participants' accounts, or are these labels used by the participants themselves?
- Whatever labels participants use for their sexual behaviour, attraction or orientation, the meaning of that label should not be taken for granted. Even if researchers and participants use the same label, it does not automatically follow that the meaning that researchers and participants attach to these labels is identical.
- In order to effectively reach and involve men who engage in sexual behaviour with other men, it is essential to understand the meaning of that particular behaviour for these men: how do they understand that behaviour as part of who they are? How do they see their sexual practices and themselves as sexual actors in the context of their social environment? And how do other people see them?

## Acknowledgements

A version of this chapter was presented at the AIDS Impact Conference, Marseille, France, 1–4 July 2007. The preparation of this chapter was supported by NIMH center grant P30-MH43520 to the HIV Center for Clinical and Behavioral Studies (PI Dr Anke A Ehrhardt). The authors thank Henny Bos, Gary Dowsett and colleagues at Columbia University for sharing their thoughts on issues discussed in this chapter.

## References

Aggleton P (Ed.) (1996) *Bisexualities and AIDS. International perspectives.* London: Taylor & Francis

Allman D, Adebajo S, Myers T, Odumuye O & Ogunsola S (2007) Challenges for the sexual health and social acceptance of men who have sex with men in Nigeria. *Culture, Health and Sexuality* 9(2): 153–168

Asthana S & Oostvogels R (2001) The social construction of male 'homosexuality' in India: Implications for HIV transmission and prevention. *Social Science & Medicine* 52(5): 707–721

Boyce P (2007) 'Conceiving *Kothis*': Men who have sex with men in India and the cultural subject of HIV prevention. *Medical Anthropology* 26(2): 175–203

Cáceres CF & Rosasco AM (1999) The margin has many sides: Diversity among gay and homosexually active men in Lima. *Culture, Health and Sexuality* 1(3): 261–275

Dodge B, Jeffries IV W & Sandfort TGM (2008) Beyond the down low: New findings on sexual risk and disclosure among at-risk black men who have sex with both men and women (MSMW). *Archives of Sexual Behavior* 37(5): 683–696

Doll LS, Johnson ES, Petersen LR, Ward JW, White CR & the Blood Donor Study Group (1992) Homosexually and nonhomosexually identified men who have sex with men: A behavioral comparison. *Journal of Sex Research* 29: 1–14

Dowsett G (2007) The way forward: Knowledge development. *Pukhaar, the Journal of the NAZ Foundation International* 56: 26–27

Dowsett G, Grierson J & McNally S (2004) MSM – a catch-all term that may not catch enough: Rethinking MSM epidemiology and prevention in Asia following a review of MSM research in four countries. Poster presented at the XV International Conference, Bangkok, 11–16 July

Muñoz-Laboy M (2004) Beyond 'MSM': Sexual desire among bisexually-active Latino men in New York City. *Sexualities* 7(1): 55–80

Parker R & Cáceres C (1999) Alternative sexualities and changing sexual cultures among Latin American men. *Culture, Health and Sexuality* 1(3): 201–206

Reid G (2006) How to become a 'real gay': Identity and terminology in Ermelo, Mpumalanga. *Agenda. Empowering Women for Gender Equity* 67(13): 137–145

Sandfort T (1997) Sampling male homosexuality. In J Bancroft (Ed.) *Researching sexual behavior: Methodological issues*. Bloomington, Indiana: Indiana University Press

Sandfort T (2007) *Same-sex sexuality, HIV/AIDS and population surveys*. Paper presented at the International conference Gender, Same-sex Sexuality and HIV/AIDS in South Africa, Pretoria, South Africa, 9–11 May

Sandfort T & Bos H (1998) *Sexual preference and work. This is what makes the difference.* Zoetermeer: ABVAKABO FNV

Sandfort T, Dodge B, Fontaine YM, Jeffries IV WL & Udoh I (2007) *Sexual self-identifications and perceptions of the down low in black bisexual men*. New York: Grand Rounds, HIV Center for Clinical and Behavioral Studies

Tielman RAP, Carballo M & Hendriks AC (Eds)(1991) *Bisexuality & HIV/AIDS. A global perspective*. Buffalo, New York: Prometheus

## CHAPTER FIVE

# Gender, same-sex sexuality and HIV/AIDS in South Africa: Practical research challenges and solutions

Pierre Brouard

I was approached to explore the topic of gender, same-sex sexuality and HIV/AIDS in South Africa from the perspective of the work done by the Centre for the Study of AIDS (CSA) at the University of Pretoria (UP), where I am employed as the deputy director. It is therefore appropriate to begin with a review of the work of the CSA.

The CSA was established in 1999. It is responsible firstly for ensuring that the UP as a whole is able to plan for, and cope with, the impact that HIV and AIDS will have on the institution and the tertiary education sector; secondly, to prepare students personally and professionally to engage with HIV and AIDS in their families, workplaces and communities; thirdly, to critique and debate critical areas of HIV and AIDS; and fourthly, to initiate research, policy and programme development on prevention and care regarding HIV and AIDS.

As the CSA has evolved, it has reached out to communities to develop a better understanding of how they operate and of the impact of HIV and AIDS at local level. It runs projects which explore innovative education methodologies and has developed a significant grasp of the social determinants of behaviour. The CSA has become known for its critical stance on issues around HIV testing and treatment, arguing that the biomedical model has been inadequate in promoting the uptake of diagnostic and treatment services. In recent years, the CSA, with the Centre for Human Rights at UP,[1] has focused on the role of human rights and stigma in the pandemic (Viljoen 2005) and has developed tools to understand and impact on stigma.

From a research perspective, the CSA has a variety of approaches. It has conducted purely desktop research, published as its annual *AIDS Review*, which explores topical issues in the HIV/AIDS epidemic in South Africa. While publications may be based on literature reviews and interviews with key informants, they are essentially attempts to speculate and develop new theory and ideas. Although there is a strong emphasis in the world of social issues such as HIV on research which is 'practical' and 'applied', it is the view of the CSA that there is also room for research which is purely intellectual, as this is appropriate for academic-based institutions and also because pure research has value in and of itself.

Of course, as an institution working in and with communities severely affected by HIV and AIDS, some of the CSA's research is aimed at supporting and illuminating the focus of its community-based projects; this may be in the form of evaluation of project activities or understanding forms of stigma, leading to stigma-mitigation activities. Other research is aimed at improving services. An example of this is a forthcoming piece of research conducted at the UP campus aimed at exploring attitudes to HIV and HIV testing; this research will help to improve and streamline the HIV testing and treatment service currently available to students on the campus. The CSA is also often invited to be part of research consortia; such collaborative research comes with its own tensions and advantages.

From this range of research experience, the CSA is in a useful position to comment on practical challenges in conducting research and how these may be addressed, even if only partially. In addition, while the CSA has not done much research around same-sex practices and practitioners, understandings of sex and sexuality inform its work, and I personally have collaborated in same-sex focused research. Thus, a combination of organisational and personal experience infuses this chapter.

## Identity and practice

Several contributors to this volume have identified a crucial tension around whether labels such as MSM (men who have sex with men) and WSW (women who have sex with women) are useful. Do they focus on practices at the expense of the identities which individuals choose to shape and configure their world? Are these terms an invention of the West, attempting to reduce complex behaviours to epidemiological sound bites and oversimplifying HIV/AIDS programme objectives and indicators? Has an unintended consequence been the emergence of an MSM identity label ('I am an MSM') which needs to be unpacked and explored more fully? Perhaps, in our attempts to understand same-sex practice, we have avoided complex identity politics, understanding that identity labels such as 'gay' and 'lesbian' may be Western constructs, of little value and use in an African context. But it is also true to say that identity labels are useful: the words people use to identify themselves are a window into how they view their practice. Practice does not occur in a vacuum; it is shaped by social, cultural, economic and political contexts and so there is a complex and fluid interrelationship between identity and practice. Some of these tensions have been noted by writers such as Lorway, who writes in a Namibian study, 'What emerges in my analyses is a picture of sexuality that *cannot* be viewed as a fixed set of predictable roles or behaviours that can be readily mapped onto the parameters of Western sexual identity categories of lesbian, gay, bisexual, transgender and heterosexual' (Lorway 2007: 3).

So it is crucial always to ask people we work with what they wish to be called and how they describe what they do sexually. I am reminded of the words of a transgender activist, Robert Hamblin, who has resisted labels and simply says of himself, 'I am just a kind of a person.' So a willingness to be surprised and challenged by research participants is a fundamental principle of all research.

## Some research challenges

### The research question

Who defines the research question may have an impact on the integrity and usefulness of the findings, as well as on the willingness of communities and individuals to participate freely and openly. Many organisations in the world of HIV and AIDS, and in a context of donor-driven imperatives, are tempted to conduct research which meets needs of donors, managers or academics, but which may not be viewed by participants as useful and valuable. In addition, research may have a political and moral imperative, setting out to confirm a particular agenda. An example of this may be research conducted by a faith-based organisation to 'prove' that abstinence-only education for young people can prevent new HIV infections. All research should, of course, meet appropriate ethical standards, but other agendas can creep in.

It may be useful in some situations to develop research questions in collaboration with affected communities. This may require a process of engaging with and listening to these communities in a way which allows for research questions to emerge. Sometimes it may be relevant to build consensus over time as a more 'pressing' or 'useful' research question can emerge after initial concerns and needs are worked through. Many communities do not 'see' lesbian or gay people and would thus never identify homosexuality, or the effect of HIV on same-sex practising people, as a topic worthy of research and focus (Johnson 2007).

Research fatigue can creep into the terrain and it is crucial that researchers endeavour to ask questions that are fresh and relevant for target communities. It is also important to go beyond the obvious when asking research questions – too much research replicates what is already known and builds cynicism in communities if their genuine concerns are not addressed.

Sometimes, in working with communities and individuals affected by HIV and AIDS, there is a misunderstanding about what research is. It is often seen as 'intellectual', divorced from the 'real' world, or something that only highly trained people can do. While in no way diminishing the importance of well-trained researchers – because much of what passes for research fails to meet appropriate standards – it can also be helpful to develop in communities and in community-based projects a sense of curiosity about the world around them. Skilled discussions with communities can reveal a myriad of research questions that were there, just never articulated.

And finally, there is a sense that research is an 'elitist' exercise, that enough research has been done in HIV and AIDS, and that our imperative now is to intervene programmatically or with new laws and policies. This is a flawed view: epidemics change, contexts and terrains shift, communities and individuals adapt, practices adjust and it is critical to keep researching, keep understanding and keep being reflective and reflexive in the work we do.

## The research site

Where we conduct our research is of vital importance. Sometimes research sites are chosen for their convenience and while this is not wrong, it can lead to laziness and a certain predictability of the results. If possible, research sites should also be chosen for their ability to generate new and useful findings which can lead to interventions that are helpful. However, depending on the research methodology, obscure research sites can prevent generalisability. So, all research sites should in some senses be seen as unique, and results generalised with caution.

In some cases, communities are over-researched, leading to 'research experts' who become practised in the art of being a research respondent. They may give responses which they believe will please researchers, or which minimise creativity and spontaneity. All efforts should be made to avoid such situations so that research findings are fresh and usable. All researchers need to focus on 'outliers', examples of points of view which are different and unpredicted, casting a new light on assumptions and simple, reductionist explanations of complex phenomena.

In the CSA's experience, it can be useful to set up a research advisory committee, a group made up of researchers, key local actors and target-group representatives, where many of the issues mentioned above can be addressed and avoided. This group can also be part of a process of reflecting on and interpreting the results of research, adding depth and power to the analytical process.

## The research methodology and methods

Both quantitative and qualitative methodologies have their strengths and weaknesses. Guiding principles should be: the purpose of the research, the nature of the target group, and the issue under consideration. For hard-to-reach populations, large-scale quantitative studies may not be possible, yet such studies may be powerful lobbying and advocacy tools. A case in point is the research conducted under the umbrella of the Joint Working Group in South Africa, a collective of lesbian, gay, bisexual, transgender and intersex (LGBTI)-focused organisations. Their research on experiences of homophobia, well-being and HIV has received significant media coverage, creating the possibility for changes in laws and policies. Yet large-scale studies may miss nuances, and given the identity/practice challenge outlined at the outset of this chapter, it is crucial that qualitative work be done to tease out the complexities in the lives of same-sex practising people in South Africa. Both approaches can complement each other and it is the view of the CSA that both are useful.

Whatever methodology is opted for, a range of methods may allow for 'triangulation', with each method illuminating a different segment of the whole and offering more complete evidence for an emerging theme. So, focus groups, individual interviews (particularly life history interviews) and observation may all contribute to a more sophisticated understanding of complex phenomena. A good example of this is the work of Graeme Reid (2006), who has done innovative research exploring black same-sex sexuality in small towns, using interviews, group discussions and participant observation. Interestingly, the blurring of subject/object allowed for a richness of data which may otherwise have been lost.

Focus groups are an extremely useful and common tool in qualitative work, perhaps used too uncritically at times. They can generate an enormous amount of information, sometimes almost too much to usefully analyse, but there can be a breadth which other methods do not achieve. However, they do sometimes fail to achieve the same depth as individual interviews, dominant members may shape the discourse and these groups can arrive at an artificial consensus, especially in gender-mixed groups, even if the 'mixed' nature of the group produces interesting dynamics. If the group is run by facilitators who come from the same community that is being researched, this can present an 'insider advantage' in that nuances can be elicited and superficial answers challenged. However, there is also the danger that assumptions can creep in and a facilitator who is a 'naïve' outsider may bring unique possibilities. Nevertheless, focus groups are still the most powerful way of obtaining information 'in situ'.

Another pressing issue in research is whether researchers come to the field with a theoretical position which frames and contextualises the enquiry. This is often very useful, providing substance and rigour to data collection and analysis. In other instances theory may be absent, unhelpful or restrictive, in which case the grounded-theory approach is very powerful. Here, theory emerges from the data and the process of the research, constantly being adapted, reflected on, and moulded by what is found and observed. Again, the terrain of same-sex practice and identity lends itself to this approach, in many cases because there is just insufficient theory to draw on. The last 60 years or so have brought about so many changes in visibility and rights for homosexual people, and phenomena such as AIDS have brought fresh and unique challenges. In such cases, new theories have to be developed. It has proved useful for the CSA to revisit research communities and present findings and re-examine them with the community – this can avoid stereotypical or formulaic interpretations of results.

## Finding and recruiting participants

The literature on recruiting participants for research is replete with methods, including new ones such as respondent-driven sampling (Heckathorn 1997), which allow one to access hard-to-reach populations, such as people living with HIV or AIDS (PLHA) or people involved in same-sex practices. In the end, there are limitations to all methods, and interpretation of results should bear this in mind. Often key informants provide entry points to communities; it is always useful to interrogate who such informants are and why they are assisting researchers. In the CSA's experience, while key persons are useful and important, some 'gatekeepers' may in fact have their own agenda (Platzer & James 1997). Working closely with such gatekeepers can minimise their conscious agendas or unconscious motivations. When we have worked with key persons who hold positions of power and influence (such as traditional leaders and healers), and who may be concerned with holding onto this power or who have a strong sense of entitlement to extra levels of privilege and respect, sensitivity and tact are paramount. Again, this speaks to the issue of who owns and drives the research – the greater the investment in the target community, the greater the possibility that a useful spread of participants may be found. In some instances there is a multitude of local actors with different points of view and it is advisable to attempt to reflect all voices and not simply to settle for the easiest route to obtain participants.

Many research projects use incentives to recruit participants, particularly in situations where communities are poor and where travelling to and from the research site may take time and money. In this case the CSA has found it helpful to use stipends to cover basic costs. It is always worth interrogating whether this confounds the sampling process, especially where representivity is the goal. In some instances we have found that people compete to be in focus groups.

A final word of caution may be relevant here: when recruiting HIV-positive participants, a technique often used is to approach existing support groups, some of which may be under the banner of larger, sometimes national organisations. It is always necessary to explore whether such participants may reflect the 'political' position of their organisation, rather than their own point of view. Will this adequately reflect the voices of PLHA who are not in the support group network or culture? Stigma around HIV, and indeed same-sex practice, may prevent certain voices from being heard.

## Managing the research process

In conducting the research, researchers need to be mindful of challenges which can emerge during the process: has something happened in the local, regional or national context which may affect participants (for example, an experience of discrimination or harm to a person living with HIV); do participants truly understand what they are consenting to, especially if what they say may prove to be unpopular with someone higher up in their organisation; can researchers maintain proper confidentiality around who participated in the research; is the language that researchers use appropriate to the participants if the researchers do not come from that community – and what might get 'lost in translation'; has the identity of the researcher been factored into understanding how participants respond to certain questions; and, ultimately, are we getting a true reflection of what people think and feel?

## Feedback

The CSA has found that going back to communities to talk about the research process and findings is a powerful process: it keeps the researchers focused; evens out the power relations to some extent; empowers participants and communities to own and interpret the findings; and promotes the notion of 'what do we do now with these findings?' We found feedback to participants, communities and researchers to be critical for the integrity of the research and to promote good relations with the community. Not only did it create 'buy in' for further interventions in the community, but it also led to other research possibilities and programmatic interventions. However, a word of caution is necessary: be careful about what you promise, as not keeping promises leads to distrust and cynicism.

In some cases, and where possible, research participants have been involved in opportunities where the research findings are presented in other forums and they have spoken of their own experiences as participants. This has made the presentations more 'real' and brought immediacy to the findings, has helped to build capacity and research savvy in participants, and has allowed for advocacy to happen – especially around PLHA concerns.

## Using the research

Research is often political and can have an impact on individuals and communities after the researchers have left. Mistrust can develop, relationships can break down, and it may be difficult to do subsequent work. In the light of this, the CSA has found that it is important to use the research findings with care and caution, to limit generalisations, to respect the integrity and privacy of participants, and to encourage other researchers to challenge, duplicate or build on their own work.

# Conclusions

Research is always a complex and multifaceted exercise, as it should be if justice is to be done to complex phenomena. This is particularly so when conducting research into same-sex practices, which have been illegal until recently in South Africa and which are still subject to much stigma and discrimination. This chapter has outlined a number of pitfalls and some strategies to address these research challenges. Key to more thoughtful research is a willingness to be reflexive, flexible, respectful, ethical and consultative, while at the same time remaining committed to high standards, unrelenting curiosity and healthy wariness.

## Note

1. More information on the Centre, its activities and publications can be found at www.csa.za.org.

## References

Heckathorn D (1997) Respondent-driven sampling: A new approach to the study of hidden populations. *Social Problems* 44(2): 174–199

Johnson CA (2007) *Off the map: How HIV/AIDS programming is failing same-sex practising people in Africa.* New York: International Gay and Lesbian Human Rights Commission

Lorway R (2007) Breaking a public health silence: HIV risk and male-male sexual practices in the Windhoek urban area. In S La Font & D Hubbard (Eds) *Unravelling taboos: Gender and sexuality in Namibia.* Windhoek: Ford Foundation

Platzer H & James T (1997) Methodological issues in conducting sensitive research on lesbian and gay men's experience of nursing care. *Journal of Advanced Nursing* 25(3): 626–633

Reid G (2006) How to become a 'real gay': Identity and terminology in Ermelo, Mpumalanga. *Agenda. Empowering Women for Gender Equity* 67(13): 137–145

Viljoen F (2005) Disclosing in an age of AIDS: Confidentiality and community in conflict? In F Viljoen (Ed.) *Righting stigma: Exploring a rights-based approach to addressing stigma.* Pretoria: University of Pretoria

CHAPTER SIX

# From social silence to social science: HIV research among township men who have sex with men in South Africa

Tim Lane

Although it has long been recognised that men who have sex with men (MSM) are at high risk for HIV infection, the published scientific literature on same-sex sexuality and HIV in South Africa is sparse. A June 2007 PubMed database search, using the standard MeSH (medical subject headings) terms 'homosexuality' and 'South Africa' returned 60 items. Of these, nine are concerned with same-sex sexuality in history and anthropology (only one of which makes a specific mention of HIV/AIDS); three with the treatment of homosexuality under apartheid, with no mention of HIV/AIDS; three with the recent controversies involving blood donation by gay men; seven related to the epidemiology of HIV/AIDS in South Africa (four of which describe the shift in South Africa's epidemic from 'male homosexual' to 'heterosexual' in the 1990s); and three case reports of HIV/AIDS among gay men in the 1980s.

What is apparent from this literature is how the research community came to define South Africa's HIV epidemic as heterosexual in the years around South Africa's transition to democracy. The first reported cases of AIDS in South Africa appeared in white, gay-identified men in 1982 (Puren 2002), and for most of the 1980s, white MSM were believed to be disproportionately affected by South Africa's developing HIV epidemic. In 1986, surveillance data from two sexually transmitted infection (STI) clinics in Durban and Cape Town estimated prevalence among MSM in those two cities at 8 and 11 per cent respectively (UNAIDS/WHO 2004). The epidemic was characterised by Western 'type 1'(HIV I) pattern infections, and the medical community presumed that the epidemic in South Africa was an offshoot of the North American and Western European epidemics, where sex between men was the predominant route of transmission.

However, by the mid-1980s cases of African 'type 2' (HIV II) pattern infection were observed among heterosexual black South Africans.[1] By 1989 medical researchers hypothesised that these two epidemics would co-occur in South Africa, and that the African pattern would soon overtake the Western pattern as the dominant type of HIV infection in South Africa (Schoub et al. 1989). Antenatal clinic data from the early 1990s bore out this prediction. In 1997, two papers asserted that South

Africa was experiencing two 'independent' HIV epidemics: one among (white) MSM, characterised by declining incidence, and one among (black) heterosexuals, characterised by increasing incidence (Maartens et al. 1997; Van Harmelen et al. 1997). The interpretation of this science became highly politicised in South Africa in the run-up to the Thirteenth International AIDS Conference, held in Durban in July 2000, when President Mbeki attempted to articulate his understanding of how heterosexually transmitted AIDS in Africa was distinct from the experience of 'homosexually transmitted' AIDS in the West (Van der Vliet 2001: 172).

In the ensuing controversy, the scientific community produced volumes of evidence about heterosexual and mother-to-child HIV transmission that supported their claim that South Africa was facing an AIDS crisis more severe than any the world had yet seen (Van der Vliet 2001). This seems to have had the effect of solidifying the African HIV epidemic as 'heterosexual' in both academic and public discourse.

Certainly, the magnitude of the problem of heterosexual transmission of HIV in South Africa explains why it has received an enormous amount of attention from academics and civil society organisations, as well as why the South African government has spent so much energy engaging with the problem in the way it has. South Africa is not alone among African nations in the scant attention it has paid to the problem of HIV infection among same-sex practising men in a generalised HIV epidemic. But the possibility that black South African MSM might be a vulnerable group in South Africa's growing 'African' HIV epidemic seems not to have been considered at the time the demographics of the South African epidemic began to shift. Black MSM did not figure prominently in the HIV literature of the 1980s. In ethnographies of the 1990s that discussed the emergence of township gay communities, the HIV epidemic was a backdrop to analyses of emerging gay identities (Donham 1998; Gevisser 1995), but township gay men themselves seem not to have wanted to discuss HIV with researchers or reflect much on it themselves (McLean & Ngcobo 1995).

The reticence of township MSM to discuss the impact of HIV on their lives is at last fading away. As researchers, we are presented with an opportunity to move from social silence to social science on MSM sexualities and HIV. The lessons learned about HIV transmission and risk from a quarter century of epidemiological and behavioural science research will be important as we begin to put South Africa's MSM population back on the HIV research agenda. But the effort should be truly interdisciplinary, paying careful attention to issues of identity and sexuality both in understanding risk behaviour, and in structuring research itself. In this chapter, I offer some preliminary thoughts about the questions that this interdisciplinary research should begin to answer, and lay out some of the logistical and ethical challenges that conducting HIV research with South Africa's MSM population may present.

## MSM as a vulnerable population in South Africa

The *HIV & AIDS and STI National Strategic Plan for South Africa 2007–2011* (DoH 2007) – known as the National Strategic Plan or NSP – recognises MSM as a vulnerable population group, noting that 'there is very little currently known about the HIV epidemic amongst MSM in the country', and that 'MSM who practise receptive anal intercourse have an elevated risk for HIV infection'. It also realises that 'MSM behaviours and sexualities are wide-ranging and include bisexuality, and the HIV epidemic amongst MSM and the heterosexual HIV epidemic are thus interconnected' (DoH 2007: 38).

That the issues of MSM vulnerability and the relationship of HIV transmission among MSM to South Africa's generalised epidemic are being addressed in the NSP is a positive development. However, the lack of specific research on MSM leads the NSP to an unfortunate characterisation of male same-sex sexuality: it notes only that sex between men is 'more likely to occur in particular institutional settings, such as prisons, often underpinned by coercion and violence' (DoH 2007: 38). While it is certainly true that sexual transmission of HIV between men in prisons is a problem, much, and probably most, sex between men is consensual and takes place in non-institutionalised settings. Furthermore, although Goal 16.3 of the NSP is to 'ensure a supportive legal environment for the provision of HIV and AIDS services to marginalized groups', and proposes to 'develop and distribute information materials on rights to HIV prevention, treatment and support that responds to the special needs of...MSM, gay, and lesbian people', among other groups (DoH 2007: 119), it does not indicate how it will measure progress towards this goal. Nor does the NSP's call for improved HIV surveillance suggest specific methods of conducting HIV surveillance among MSM (DoH 2007).

As far as MSM are concerned, the NSP should be viewed as a call to researchers to fill the information gaps that exist in the challenges that South African MSM face in the HIV epidemic. This requires understanding the socio-economic and cultural diversity of South African MSM communities. In cities like Johannesburg and Pretoria, for example, there are communities of gay-identified men that would be recognisable to inhabitants of similar gay communities in San Francisco, London or Sydney. But do similar gay communities exist in township communities like Soweto or Mamelodi? Do MSM in these townships exist in similar social and sexual HIV risk environments? The socio-economic gap that exists between the well-resourced communities like Johannesburg's northern suburbs and the less well-resourced areas that make up Soweto, suggest the need for a more specific focus on township environments. Moreover, in an epidemic where HIV transmission has been characterised as 'heterosexual' for so long, it is important to understand the specific structural, social and individual contexts of township MSM's HIV risk behaviours in order to respond meaningfully and appropriately to the challenges these MSM face.

Some of these factors have been explored in an emerging body of MSM HIV research in sub-Saharan Africa more generally, as outlined below. Countries where this research has taken place include Botswana, Ghana, Kenya, Mali, Nigeria, Senegal, Uganda and Zambia. In all of these countries, homosexuality is illegal and same-sex practising people suffer the effects of varying degrees of stigma and discrimination. Although South Africa has decriminalised same-sex sexuality and outlawed discrimination on the basis of sexual orientation, stigma against same-sex sexual identities and practices remains high, and experiences of de facto discrimination are common, particularly in township communities. Therefore, many of the external structural and social factors that contribute to the vulnerability of township MSM in South Africa are likely to be similar to those that have been identified by researchers elsewhere in the sub-Saharan African region.

Structural factors that influence MSM vulnerability include poor access to HIV prevention services in the public health sector, including voluntary counselling and testing (VCT) (Onyango-Ouma et al. 2005; Washington & Semugoma 2006). In addition, African MSM experience structural barriers to accessing HIV prevention information and materials, including condoms and latex-compatible lubrication (Onyango-Ouma et al. 2005). It is important to determine whether and how these structural barriers operate for MSM in South Africa in light of the NSP's aim to meet the HIV prevention needs of same-sex practising people.

Where structural barriers exist, these are quite likely to be related to some of the social factors that contribute to MSM's HIV vulnerability in their communities. For example, it should not be surprising to find that an environment in which access to MSM-specific HIV prevention information and materials is poor, is also one where many MSM perceive that anal sex between men is less risky than vaginal sex with women, and where there are weak peer norms supporting condom use (Zulu et al. 2006). Discrimination in healthcare services could lead to MSM delaying or avoiding treatment for STIs (Broqua 2006), and this may contribute to HIV incidence among MSM. Models from Kenya suggest an annual incidence rate of 4.5 per cent among MSM, who may account for 21 per cent of all new HIV infections in that country (Gouws et al. 2006). Fear of discrimination may also lead some MSM to avoid testing for HIV. A fear of discrimination in healthcare services is likely to be indicative of a larger community context in which stigma and homophobia are rampant (Broqua 2006; Geibel et al. 2006; Onyango-Ouma et al. 2005; Skodval et al. 2006; Washington & Semugoma 2006).

The ways in which structural and social factors interact with individual behaviours, beliefs or psychological states that influence risk for HIV infection should be a central focus of future research. The individual risk factors that researchers have explored in African MSM populations include: multiple concurrent partnerships, including sex with both women and men (Geibel et al. 2006; Skodval et al. 2006; Wade et al. 2005; Zulu et al. 2006); group sexual activity (Geibel et al. 2006); substance use, particularly alcohol (Ehlers et al. 2001); peer norms that do not support condom use (Zulu et al. 2006); the erroneous perception that anal sex with men is 'safer' than vaginal sex with women (Zulu et al. 2006); and psychological distress and depression (Ehlers et al. 2001).

Identifying the structural, social and individual components of vulnerability is vital to developing interventions. However, research still needs to explore how MSM relate to each other sexually; that is, we need to better understand sexuality itself. Although HIV is largely an STI, sexuality has remained peripheral to much of the epidemiological and psychological research on HIV that has taken place in Africa to date. My reference to 'same-sex practising' men or my use of the acronym MSM connotes a category of sexual behaviours and the biological sex of those who practise them, but not necessarily the social and sexual identities that make their behaviours meaningful to themselves and each other. Understanding how same-sex practising men relate to each other socially and sexually is crucial to understanding the dynamics of HIV risk and transmission. As Gagnon and Parker wrote, it requires shifting the field of enquiry from the sexual actions of specific bodies to the cultural and social contexts in which sexuality occurs (Gagnon & Parker 1995), and coming to terms with how local cultures of desire organise the same-sex practices and HIV risks of township MSM.

## Identity, sexuality and MSM

In contrast to the lack of scientific literature on HIV among MSM in South Africa, there has been some investigation of same-sex sexuality, particularly among black South African men. It is not surprising that this scholarship has focused largely on the two all-male environments that were instrumental in the construction and maintenance of apartheid: the mining industry's migrant labour compounds, and prisons.

Historians have written about 'mine marriages' between men in early and mid-twentieth century mining compounds, but have generally attributed the phenomenon of masculine men coupling with men who displayed or adopted feminine identities to the absence of biological women in these institutions, and not to the presence of authentic same-sex desires (Harries 1994; Moodie 1994). When some scholars permitted the possibility of these desires, there was disagreement that same-sex activities in either of these institutions was evidence of nascent modern homosexual identities (Achmat 1993; Niehaus 2002).

Indeed, what preoccupied most scholars of same-sex sexuality in South Africa during the 1990s was not HIV, but the question of whether and how modern 'gay' identity traversed the historical and cultural distance from its Anglo–European origins to take root in non-institutionalised settings in South Africa's townships. Some emphasise external, transnational forces in the emergence of township 'gay' identity during the anti-apartheid struggles of the 1980s and 1990s (Niehaus 2002).

The fact that exiled and gay anti-apartheid activists travelled along global networks that linked Johannesburg and Cape Town with cities like London, New York and San Francisco, allowed for the transportation of ideas about gay social and sexual identity to South Africa; black activists brought these ideas the further step from urban gay neighbourhoods like Johannesburg's Hillbrow to townships like Soweto (Gevisser 1995). On the other hand, this view of history may underestimate the role played by social changes internal to South Africa. For example, Donham (1998) suggests it was only because women were allowed to migrate to cities and live with their male partners in or near labour compounds after the 1960s, that it became possible for both partners in a same-sex 'mine marriage' to identify as males, and potentially as 'gay'.

Understanding the identities that MSM claim is important to behavioural and epidemiological research on HIV. Questions of identity are central to understanding how township MSM organise their social and sexual lives. Returning to a question posed earlier: assuming there is a 'gay community' in Soweto or Mamelodi, what kind of social and sexual life does being part of the 'gay community' entail? And, for the purposes of HIV research, does HIV risk behaviour that takes place among members of this community represent the HIV risks of all MSM?

Using the acronym MSM to describe a population of same-sex practising men does have many limitations and complications where questions of identity are concerned, particularly if it is used uncritically to denote a particular identity, type of sexual behaviour, and form of same-sex desire (Young & Meyer 2005). As researchers, we cannot simply transport our research assumptions about MSM from societies in the global North, where 'MSM' and 'gay' have largely been conflated and used synonymously, to describe a single target population. Nonetheless, the acronym MSM and the behaviours it attempts to categorise remain useful to defining a target population of same-sex practising men in which HIV risk and transmission must be better understood. It is critical for researchers to listen to how individuals within this target population describe themselves and their experiences, and we need to probe sensitively and carefully around the meanings of identity terms for clues to how sexuality is organised and HIV risk experienced. Recognising that there may be a number of different identities claimed by individuals whom we might categorise as MSM, the proper questions of research become not only 'what do they call themselves?' but 'who desires whom?' and 'how do they enact their desires?'

## Logistical and ethical challenges of MSM HIV research

Although research has only begun to understand the social and sexual lives of township MSM, it is well established from research on heterosexual HIV transmission in South Africa that residents of township communities face many social and economic challenges that increase their vulnerability to HIV. Township MSM are not likely to be different in this regard. Clearly, research that establishes accurate population-based estimates of risk behaviour and HIV prevalence is an important step in developing a long-term HIV prevention strategy and programme for township MSM. What may be less clear is how to gather it. MSM in South African townships are both hidden and stigmatised. This fact presents two major challenges to HIV research that must be overcome: developing a sampling methodology, and addressing the medical and psychosocial needs of HIV-positive MSM.

Although no published study has quantified levels of stigma against same-sex practising men in South African townships, it is safe to assume that it is high. MSM who are open about their identity and desires report experiencing stigma and discrimination from others in their communities, including healthcare workers (Lane et al. 2008). Those MSM who are not open may therefore be keeping their identities and behaviours well hidden from their friends, families and healthcare providers for fear of the social consequences. But MSM do make themselves visible to each other in the social situations and venues that they have claimed for themselves. In other parts of the world where MSM are stigmatised, researchers have used social venues, including gay bars, pubs and clubs, as research sites (Choi et al. 2003; Colby 2003). These venues do exist in South African townships. Will it be possible to use similar sites in Gauteng townships for MSM research?

In 2006, the Perinatal HIV Research Unit of the University of the Witwatersrand in Johannesburg and the University of California's San Francisco Center for AIDS Prevention Studies conducted exploratory research to determine how to sample MSM for future behavioural and epidemiological studies. We conducted structured observations at 23 bars, taverns and shebeens in Soweto and Mamelodi that MSM identified as 'gay friendly' establishments. We evaluated venues based on our observations of the following criteria: the venue itself, including its location, structure, cleanliness and lighting; the people in attendance, including whether women were present; whether MSM were easily identified among attendees; the amount of alcohol and other drug consumption; and how individuals interacted with each other, including non-sexual and sexual interactions between men and women, as well as between men. We concluded that, in general, these were not sites that could accommodate research activities.

The primary obstacle to using drinking establishments as research sites is that they are public spaces, lacking the privacy necessary to protect participant confidentiality. The presence of women, many of whom may be female partners of some MSM, could complicate recruitment. Even if private space to carry the dissemination of study information, screening and recruitment could be arranged on these premises, many men may not want other patrons to see them participating in MSM HIV research because of the stigma attached both to HIV and to MSM identity and behaviour. Furthermore, the fact that alcohol is consumed on the premises – generally in large quantities – and that some drug use (for example, marijuana) may be tolerated, means that any MSM successfully recruited in these venues may not be able to offer fully informed consent to participate in research conducted on the premises, or at a convenient off-premises location. Finally, the fact that these venues really come alive only late at night on the weekend makes study recruitment at peak hours logistically difficult at best, and dangerous at worst.

Despite these obstacles, MSM in Soweto are highly motivated to participate in research, suggesting that a peer-driven, chain-referral sampling strategy is more feasible. One promising option for recruiting a diverse MSM sample for the purposes of estimating HIV prevalence is respondent-driven sampling (RDS). The RDS method has been used with a variety of hidden and stigmatised populations around the world, including commercial sex workers, injection drug users, and MSM. In RDS, participants are recruited into a study sample by peers whom they know and trust. Theoretically, RDS proceeds from the same assumptions as simple snowball sampling: that individual members of the target population know best how and where to recruit others, and that individuals tend to recruit others similar to them ('like recruits like', known as *homophily*). Where RDS differs from snowball sampling is that it limits the number of participants any one individual may recruit. In practice, this limit has been set at three recruits per person. This reduces homophily in the sample by preventing individuals with larger social networks from dominating the composition of the sample, and is meant to allow for population estimation through statistical adjustments that compensate for the fact that the sample was not recruited randomly (Heckathorn 1997, 2002; Magnani et al. 2005).

In the case of South African township MSM, this is crucial. Using snowball sampling, for example, we may start recruitment with those MSM who are most visible – gay-identified men who are 'out' about their sexual identity. It is possible that participants may recruit a few non-gay identified MSM with whom they are acquainted, but placing no limits on peer recruitment would make it highly likely that more visible, gay-identified men would continue to recruit an overwhelmingly 'out' gay-identified sample. In the end, the sample is likely to be too homogeneous to allow for generalising predictors of risk behaviour or estimates of HIV prevalence to the population of MSM in the community. But the RDS limit of three peer recruits makes it more probable that when the more hidden, non-gay identified MSM enter the sample, their efforts to recruit others like themselves will not be overwhelmed by larger, more visible networks of gay-identified men. The resulting sample MSM may more accurately reflect the diversity of sexual identities in the MSM population, which in turn makes generalised measures of risk behaviour or HIV prevalence more plausible.

It is also possible that RDS will provide better privacy protection for those MSM who are not 'out' and who, for whatever reason, may need to keep their identities and behaviours hidden. Recruiters in an RDS study will not be professional research staff operating conspicuously in a drinking establishment or other public place, but rather individual MSM who have already participated in the study and who recruit others from within their social networks, operating 'under the radar' as necessary. MSM would recruit other MSM by means of 'coupons' designed by the study and given to potential participants by their peer recruiters. Actual study enrolment takes place only when an individual decides to contact the research team at the research site, presents the coupon, is screened for eligibility, and consents to enrolment.

Aside from recruitment, conducting a study that asks MSM to test for HIV may pose a challenge to researchers. Although many MSM may be eager to participate in social and behavioural research, the stakes are much higher when we ask participants to test for HIV. It is therefore important to conduct preliminary research to understand MSM's prior testing behaviour and experiences, and to use research as an opportunity to begin to address unmet needs. Discrimination against MSM by healthcare workers and the generally high levels of HIV-related stigma in South African township communities may be operating as a powerful disincentive to learning one's HIV status. It is highly likely that many MSM who participate in an HIV prevalence study will be testing for HIV for the first time. It is therefore incumbent on researchers to provide VCT services in research projects that demonstrate to MSM that it is possible to receive HIV VCT in a non-stigmatising environment, and that they are, in fact, entitled to such services as South African citizens. Furthermore, perhaps a quarter or more of MSM participants who consent to VCT through research will receive a positive result. It will be important to assess whether the medical and psychosocial needs of HIV-positive MSM can be met through available public sector services. The HIV testing experiences and needs of MSM may vary by community, but researchers must ensure that these needs can be met in other ways if we are to assess HIV prevalence for MSM in an ethical manner.

Understanding and overcoming the difficulties inherent in working with South Africa's township MSM populations for HIV research is a challenge the research community must meet. Recommendations for proceeding with this research in South Africa include:

- Build trust with MSM: HIV researchers and South African MSM are, for the most part, strangers to each other. In South Africa's largest major urban centres we can work in partnership with lesbian, gay, bisexual and transgender (LGBT) community-based organisations that already have strong programmes of community building, human rights advocacy, and HIV education and prevention for same-sex practising people. In areas that lack formal LGBT organisations, it is possible to work with knowledgeable community members to meet local MSM individuals, groups and stakeholders who can help build a working relationship with wider MSM networks.
- Adopt an integrated, interdisciplinary approach to research: with a population about which so little is known, ethnography is a crucial first step to understanding the social and sexual lives of MSM on their own terms. It will bring the more hidden aspects of MSM community life to light, and allow for culturally sensitive adaptation of quantitative measures. In addition, knowing how MSM self-identify their sexuality, as well as how and where they interact

with each other sexually, will guide the selection of appropriate sampling frameworks for survey work.
- Frame research protocols around community needs: engaging South African MSM in research immediately makes clear that many MSM lack access to HIV prevention information and materials. Study-related outreach to MSM should at a minimum provide information about condoms, lubricants, non-stigmatising HIV testing services, and treatment literacy and access. MSM should be involved in the development of research strategies and protocols when possible.

MSM in South Africa's townships have finally broken their silence about their sexual identities and their HIV prevention and treatment needs. It is up to researchers to listen carefully and sensitively, and work together with these communities to ensure that the suffering inflicted by the HIV epidemic does not continue to make the Constitution's promise of non-discrimination on the basis of sexual orientation ring hollow.

## Note

1   In this chapter, the term 'black' when applied to people refers to South Africans of African ancestry.

## References

Achmat Z (1993) 'Apostles of civilized vice': 'Immoral practices' and 'unnatural vice' in South African prisons and compounds, 1890–1920. *Social Dynamics* 19(2): 92–110

Broqua C (2006) *Men who have sex with men and behaviours adopted to counter the risk of HIV infection in Bamako (Mali)*. Paper presented at the 16th International AIDS Conference, Toronto, 13–18 August

Choi KH, Liu H, Guo Y, Han L, Mandel JS & Rutherford GW (2003) Emerging HIV-1 epidemic in China in men who have sex with men. *Lancet* 361(9375): 2125–2126

Colby DJ (2003) HIV knowledge and risk factors among men who have sex with men in Ho Chi Minh City. *Journal of Acquired Immune Deficiency Syndromes* 32(1): 80–85

DoH (Department of Health) (2007) *HIV & AIDS and STI National Strategic Plan for South Africa 2007–2011*. Pretoria: DoH

Donham D (1998) Freeing South Africa: The 'modernization' of male-male sexuality in Soweto. *Cultural Anthropology* 13(1): 3–21

Ehlers VJ, Zuyderduin A & Oosthuizen MJ (2001) The well-being of gays, lesbians and bisexuals in Botswana. *Journal of Advanced Nursing* 35(6): 848–856

Gagnon JH & Parker RG (1995) Conceiving sexuality. In RG Parker & JH Gagnon (Eds) *Conceiving sexuality*. New York: Routledge

Geibel S, Birungi H & Onyango-Ouma W (2006) *Factors associated with reported STI symptoms among MSM in Nairobi, Kenya*. 16th International AIDS Conference, Toronto, 13–18 August

Gevisser M (1995) A different fight for freedom: A history of South African lesbian and gay organisation from the 1950s to 1990s. In M Gevisser & E Cameron (Eds) *Defiant desire: Gay and lesbian lives in South Africa*. New York: Routledge

Gouws E, Brown T, Stover J & White PJ (2006) Short term estimates of adult HIV incidence by mode of transmission: Kenya and Thailand as examples. *Sexually Transmitted Infections* 82(3): 51–55

Harries P (1994) *Work, culture, and identity: Migrant laborers in Mozambique and South Africa, c. 1860–1910*. Portsmouth: Heinemann

Heckathorn D (1997) Respondent-driven sampling: A new approach to the study of hidden populations. *Social Problems* 44(2): 174–199

Heckathorn D (2002) Respondent-driven sampling II: Deriving valid population estimates from chain-referral samples of hidden populations. *Social Problems* 49(1): 11–34

Lane T, Kegeles AM, McIntyre J, Mogale T & Struthers H (2008) 'They see you as a different thing': The experiences of men who have sex with men with healthcare workers in South African township communities. *Sexually Transmitted Infections* 84(6): 430–433

Maartens G, Byrne C, O'Keefe & Wood R (1997) Independent epidemics of heterosexual and homosexual HIV infection in South Africa – survival differences. *Quarterly Journal of Medicine* 90(7): 449–454

Magnani R, Heckathorn DD, Sabin K & Saidel T (2005) Review of sampling hard-to-reach and hidden populations for HIV surveillance. *AIDS* 19(2): S67–72

McLean H & Ngcobo L (1995) *Abangibhamayo Bathi Ngimnandi* (Those who fuck me say I'm tasty): Gay sexuality in Reef townships. In M Gevisser & E Cameron (Eds) *Defiant desire: Gay and lesbian lives in South Africa*. New York: Routledge

Moodie T (1994) *Going for gold*. Berkeley & Los Angeles: University of California Press

Niehaus I (2002) Renegotiating masculinity in the South African lowveld: Narratives of male-male sex in labour compounds and in prisons. *African Studies* 61(1): 77–97

Onyango-Ouma W, Birungi H & Geibel S (2005) *Understanding the HIV/STI risks and prevention needs of men who have sex with men in Nairobi, Kenya*. Washington, DC: Population Council

Puren AJ (2002) The HIV-1 epidemic in South Africa. *Oral Diseases* 8 (Sup. 2): 27–31

Schoub B, Martin D et al. (1989) Development of the AIDS epidemic in South Africa. Paper presented at the 5th International AIDS Conference, Montreal, 5–9 June

Skovdal M, Mwangi E & Meegan M (2006) An investigation of the impact of migration among men who have sex with men in Kenya. Paper presented at the 16th International AIDS Conference, Toronto, 13–18 August

UNAIDS/WHO (Joint United Nations programme on HIV/AIDS/World Health Organization) (2004) *Epidemiological fact sheets on HIV/AIDS and sexually transmitted infections – South Africa*. UNAIDS/WHO

Van der Vliet V (2001) AIDS: Losing 'the new struggle'. *Daedalus* 130(1): 151–184

Van Harmelen J, Lambrick M, Rybicki M, Williamson AL, Williamson C & Wood R (1997) An association between HIV-1 subtypes and mode of transmission in Cape Town, South Africa. *AIDS* 11(1): 81–87

Wade AS, Diallo PAN, Diop AK, Gueye K, Kane CT, Largarde E, Mboup S & Ndoye I (2005) HIV infection and sexually transmitted infections among men who have sex with men in Senegal. *AIDS* 19(18): 2133–2140

Washington T & Semugoma P (2006) *Social justice through social work: Identifying barriers to HIV prevention in Uganda.* Paper presented at the 16th International AIDS Conference, Toronto, 13–18 August

Young RM & Meyer IH (2005) The trouble with 'MSM' and 'WSW': Erasure of the sexual-minority person in public health discourse. *American Journal of Public Health* 95(7): 1144–1149

Zulu K, Bulawo N & Zulu W (2006) Understanding HIV risk behavior among men who have sex with men in Zambia. Paper presented at the 16th International AIDS Conference, Toronto, 13–18 August

# HISTORY, MEMORY, ARCHIVE

Research is itself a cultural process, it is a political process, it has its institutions, it has its power systems, it has its protocols, and it has its language. It is as complicated, as fraught, as contradictory a sort of social world as any other. And part of what we are doing here strategically is a kind of 'sociology of science' in relation to the political issues of the marginalised. What I found very persuasive today was this notion that one achieves visibility through doing research. I made a sort of facetious comment about all methodological problems involved in getting one or two questions about same-sex behaviour onto national surveys, and whether the knowledge that gets generated is going to be useful. In fact, what might be more important is that the questions are there in the survey, that they actually exist within that particular scientific realm. That is a political accomplishment – that we actually register within the institution of science. And that is part of the sociology or the politics of the scientific process. *Robert Sember, conference delegate*

In our research and prevention, we should not only focus on behaviour. Behaviours don't occur in a vacuum, they occur in a social context. Ideas circulate in the social sphere and I think it is important to look at the labels people use. I am thinking about research Graeme Reid has done in townships outside Ermelo, where you define yourself as a 'lady' or a 'gent' and the ladies are the 'bottoms', the gents are the 'tops'. And the tops often are involved with women and marriages as well. Those labels define your behaviour and your roles and your identity, what you do sexually and how you negotiate this. So I think it is worth looking at labels and language too. *Pierre Brouard, conference delegate*

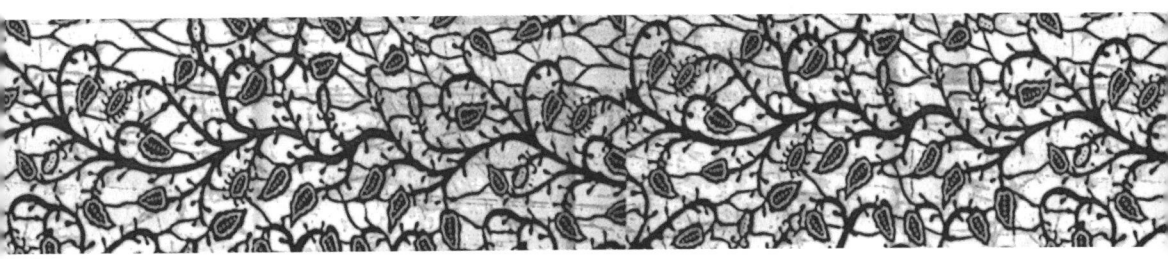

In my community, which is a Deaf community, there's a high level of illiteracy. We hardly have workshops on HIV and AIDS, which is a huge problem. We have a lot of young Deaf people who are dying, and half of them (or more) don't even know why they are dying. Lots and lots of them are dying out there…Another problem is that within the Deaf community because of the low literacy level, they think being positive means something good. So they tend to be excited when they are told that they are positive. We need to go to the community and educate people about what it means to be HIV positive because really they don't know, and when they go to these healthcare clinics, the doctors or health workers use huge technical words which do not reach people on the grassroots level. *John Meletse, conference delegate*

CHAPTER SEVEN

# Gay AIDS activism in South Africa prior to 1994

Mandisa Mbali

For most of the 1980s, the vast majority of AIDS cases were seen by epidemiologists as being concentrated in the white 'homosexual population'. This chapter addresses some of the key issues in the history of AIDS activism, such as which social movements and political networks AIDS activists emerged from, and how these movements and networks politically strategised around AIDS; how the politics of gender and sexuality shaped AIDS activism over time; and why South African AIDS activism was non-radical for most of its existence.

The first section argues that the early history of AIDS activism by lesbian and gay activists in South Africa can only be understood against the backdrop of the diverse and evolving identities, social practices and organisations which have been constructed around same-sex sexuality over time. It discusses how the non-militant nature of gay organisations in the 1980s partially explains the social support orientation of early gay AIDS activism.

The chapter's second section addresses more directly how AIDS entered into the gay and lesbian social and organisational world. It makes the case for a social constructionist problematisation of early AIDS epidemiology. In particular, it brings into question the underlying assumption of many early studies that homosexuality was an almost exclusively white phenomenon in its first few years in South Africa. This section argues that social support for those gay men living with AIDS, and information dissemination for those deemed to be at risk, remained the focus of early gay AIDS activism.

The third section goes on to argue that the biggest single barrier to more explicitly political gay AIDS organising in the 1980s was the jailing of key anti-apartheid, gay rights activists such as Ivan Toms and Simon Nkoli. With greater political freedoms from the early 1990s, and the release from jail of anti-apartheid political activists such as Nkoli and Toms, a move towards more political AIDS activism began.

This development dovetailed with the emergence of a new, more militant black-led gay activism, which exploited the freer political climate in the transition era to make the case for gay rights to be recognised in the new South African Constitution, which was under negotiation. This more militant, black-led gay rights activism developed hand in hand with gay AIDS activism: the two struggles were increasingly seen as interrelated and as demanding similar tactics. However, some lesbian activists felt that gendered factors, such as so-called corrective rape, which placed them at risk of HIV infection were under-addressed by this nascent gay and lesbian movement.

Simultaneously, gay rights activists were increasingly drafting rights-based charters to use as opening salvos in carefully co-ordinated campaigns for rights-based responses to diverse sexual orientations and AIDS, as shown in section four of the chapter. While gay activists affiliated with the Organisation of Lesbian and Gay Activists (OLGA) drafted a Gay Rights Charter, Edwin Cameron brought together a number of AIDS activists to draft the AIDS and HIV Charter. This group later formed the AIDS Consortium, a human rights-focused advocacy coalition of AIDS activists. The tactic of openness about status was used by Shaun Mellors to push for wider acceptance of this new charter in AIDS policy-making circles at the National AIDS Convention of South Africa (NACOSA) Conference.

Meanwhile, gay rights activists lobbied and advocated for a sexual orientation clause to be added to the section of the Bill of Rights which outlawed unfair discrimination. These efforts were central to liberating AIDS-related speech and expression in ways which would facilitate freer promotion of safer sex post-1994.

The final section discusses ways in which HIV-positive gay activists became increasingly bold in their choice of platforms to reveal their HIV status to promote gay rights and to put an end to AIDS-related discrimination. Indeed, Gay and Lesbian Organisation of the Witwatersrand (GLOW) activist Linda Ngcobo's funeral actively drew on the iconography of the anti-apartheid political funerals. From the late 1990s onwards, political AIDS funerals would increasingly become a platform from which to lobby for increased access to treatment.

## Changing lesbian and gay identities and non-militant early gay politics

A discussion of the history of gay AIDS activism should begin by situating it in relation to the wider history of gay and lesbian identities and social life because, as Gevisser and Cameron have noted, '...the making of queer societies and an assertion of "queer culture" – is always a precursor to the establishment of a lesbian and gay liberation movement' (Gevisser & Cameron 1994 :4).

This chapter will use this observation as a starting point for its own examination of how gay activists' responses to AIDS have been enmeshed in the political progression of South African 'queer culture', from bar culture, to social support organisations, to political activism.

Firstly, any exegesis of same-sex identities, solidarities and practices in South Africa in relation to AIDS activism must be placed within a historical perspective.

Historians have shown that same-sex sexual practices have taken place in southern Africa for centuries. The stigmatising idea that same-sex sexual practices are an 'un-African' Western import is oft repeated in the region, most vocally by leaders such as Zimbabwean President Robert Mugabe and former Namibian President Sam Nujoma. Marc Epprecht contends that as sex was only understood in terms of acts which resulted in pregnancy in pre-colonial southern African societies, there was a '*de facto* tolerance of sexual difference and individual non-conformity...because "sex" in pre-modern context was not sex the way it is usually construed in modern Western discourse' (Epprecht 2004).

However, an important distinction needs to be made between those individuals who engaged in same-sex sexual practices in the past, and those who *both* engaged in such practices *and* claimed identities such as gay, lesbian, bisexual and/or transgendered, which are based upon an open admission of a preference for sex with persons of the same sex.

In relation to this, it is worth noting that the terms 'gay', 'lesbian', 'heterosexual' and 'bisexual' are seen by many theorists of sexuality as being inherently unstable and always evolving over time. Indeed, there is a significant and ongoing debate over whether sexuality is biologically determined or socially constructed. Social constructionists argue that sexuality is not objectively fixed into three mutually exclusive categories of 'homosexual', 'bisexual' and 'heterosexual' (Foucault 1976). By contrast, those holding essentialist views of sexual orientation argue that '...there are objective, intrinsic, culture-independent facts about what a person's sexual orientation is' (Stein 1990: 5).

In the absence of conclusive research proving the existence of a 'gay gene', social constructionists appear to have the upper hand in this debate for the meantime.[1] Most social constructionists have drawn on the work of Michel Foucault in arguing for the social fashioning of sexual orientation. In his *History of Sexuality*, Foucault (1976) showed how the modern category of 'the homosexual' was produced as a category by medicalisation and other forms of modern power-knowledge (Altman 1993). This means that any political mobilisation based on categories such as 'homosexual', 'bisexual' and 'heterosexual' is bound to be complex and contested.

These wider debates around sexuality chime with Graeme Reid's ethnographic research on same-sex practising Africans living in and around Ermelo in Mpumalanga province, South Africa. Reid (2006) found that gay identities and the ways in which they are expressed generated a great deal of discussion and debate. He discovered that African men who had sex with men, and women who had sex with women, were well integrated into social life in the area and occupied certain niche professions. Gender ambiguity was seen as enhancing traditional healers' healing ability, for example, and some even had their own specific local argot to describe their identities and practices. This mirrors Ronald Louw's (2001) discussion of homosexual talk in the isiZulu language.

Same-sex sexual activity has historically been associated with institutions and spaces which tend to house members of one sex (Epprecht 2004). However, only a minority of those who engage in same-sex sexual practices identify themselves using terms of Western origin such as 'lesbian' or 'gay'. A diverse and growing number of South African terms have been used for persons who engage in same-sex sexuality, both in the past and the present. Some of these terms are derogatory, for instance, 'moffie', 'dyke', '*isitabane*' and '*ungqingili*' are commonly used.[2] These terms are only considered acceptable when they are reclaimed and used as self-descriptors in an empowering way by people engaging in same-sex practices (Louw 2001).

There is also a great diversity of identities adopted by people engaging in same-sex practices and many different self-descriptions of their relationships. As Epprecht argues:

> Africans on their own did initiate the development of new types of same-sex relationships in the modern era including mine marriage, transvestitism, prison sex, female *amachicken* or mother/baby relationships, same-sex prostitution, homosexual romantic love and some specific sexual positions and acts like oral sex. (2004: 224–225)

Moreover, the relationships between female *sangomas* (traditional healers) and their female ancestral wives have provided spaces for expression of female same-sex sexuality (Nkabinde & Morgan 2005). There is also a contemporary butch/femme subculture among urban black women who self-identify as lesbians (Keswa & Wieringa 2005).

This is relevant to gay AIDS activism in that the lesbian and gay organising on which it was based was limited in terms of the numbers it could attract by the fact that not everyone who engaged in same-sex practices identified as lesbian or gay. Moreover, not everyone who identified as lesbian or gay was prepared to do so in a political way to combat homophobia or push for law reform. And among those who did want to conduct advocacy opposing homophobia, fewer still wanted to link their struggle against homophobia to the wider and more popular struggle for national liberation and against racism and apartheid. Indeed, in this vein, there was a debate within the Gay Association of South Africa (GASA), South Africa's first national gay organisation, on the issue of whether the organisation should be 'political', especially in relation to racism and apartheid: a debate which, as we shall see, led to its fragmentation.

GASA was not the first gay organisation in South Africa, however. In the 1960s, the South African police raided a private gay party in Forest Town in Johannesburg. This is sometimes referred to as South Africa's 'Stonewall'[3] as it catalysed the development of the first gay law reform movement in 1968. As Gevisser (1994) has argued, this lobby group was mostly white dominated and was not radical or mass-based. In consequence, while fresh homophobic legislation was prevented, discriminatory amendments were still added to the Immorality Act.[4] As discussed below, these amendments, especially the outlawing of dildos, had an adverse effect on HIV prevention work by and for gay men.

In 1972 an ephemeral South African gay 'liberation' movement was formed at the University of Natal in Durban (Epprecht 2004). Given its fairly radical political orientation, the apartheid state deemed it to be a political threat, so the police rapidly forced its founder to disband the movement, threatening to charge him for inciting people to sodomy, which was then a common law offence (Gevisser 1994).

The first truly national gay and lesbian organisation, GASA, was only formed in January 1982. By the end of that year it had nine branches across the country and linked up with a similar Cape Town-based group called 6010, which became GASA 6010 (Gevisser 1994). The organisation grew rapidly and by May 1983 it had over 1 000 signed up members and affiliated sports clubs, religious societies, support and counselling services and *Link/Skakel* (a gay newspaper which later changed its name to *Exit*, and is still in existence) (Gevisser 1994).

GASA social functions reflected much of the petty racism of the gay social scene from which the organisation emerged. From the mid-1980s black gay people started trying to visit white nightclubs. There were some gay venues where black people were refused entry on the grounds of the colour of their skin (Gevisser 1994; Luirink 2000).

Despite the segregation of gay nightclubs, there was certainly interracial gay sex in South Africa in this period. Luirink (2000) argues that much of this sex was paid for – the richer white man would pay the black man for sex. Luirink's black informants described this as follows, 'The price then was simple: sex. Taken in the middle of the night, hidden in the boot, to the white suburbs. If you were caught the next morning in an area forbidden to blacks, it was assumed you would pretend to be the master's "garden boy"' (Luirink 2000: 122).

As argued in the next section, the mere fact that black gay men who had white same-sex sexual partners became infected with HIV in the period, undermines the dominant epidemiological model that emerged in the 1980s of two epidemics segregated according to race and sexual orientation (Luirink 2000).[5]

In addition, when Simon Nkoli formed a black gay group called the Saturday Group which initially met at GASA's offices in Hillbrow, it was quickly prevented from meeting there by the organisation (Gevisser 1994). While the Saturday Group was primarily social in nature, discussions within the mostly black group began to take on a more radical flavour (Gevisser 1994).

The Saturday Group was short-lived and collapsed when Nkoli was jailed in 1984 with other United Democratic Front activists on trumped up treason charges. While Nkoli became a *cause célèbre* for anti-apartheid, gay rights activists around the world, GASA refused to condemn apartheid or support Nkoli, leading to its expulsion from the International Lesbian and Gay Association (Gevisser 1994). While GASA splintered, several new anti-apartheid, gay organisations were formed, such as GLOW and the mostly white OLGA.

## Enter AIDS

It was into this context of gay and lesbian organisations riven by racial and political divisions that the first South African cases of AIDS were identified in 1982 in white gay men.

For most of the 1980s, early gay AIDS activism, like lesbian and gay activism in general, was non-militant and focused on provision of social support for those diagnosed with AIDS, and information for those who feared they were at risk of infection. Moreover, partially as a consequence of the wider political divisions discussed above, the most visible and effective responses to the AIDS epidemic were regional, and there was little in the way of a coherent national and political gay response for most of the 1980s.

This was especially true in comparison to the relatively militant response by the gay movement in the United States, which became increasingly shrill towards the end of the decade, especially as manifest in the AIDS Coalition to Unleash Power (ACT-UP) (Pegge 1995).

Almost a quarter of a century ago, in late 1982, two South African Airways stewards were diagnosed with AIDS; these were the first two cases in the country (Malan 1986). Almost as soon as the epidemic emerged in South Africa, gay activists were forced to respond as the epidemic was framed in the media as being a 'gay plague', which generated homophobic stigma and discrimination.

Ruben Sher, a white South African immunologist, played a key role in identifying South African AIDS cases. Soon after AIDS was first identified internationally, Sher read about the strange new disease during a trip to the United States. He visited the Center for Disease Control in Atlanta and met inspiring and determined young virologists and immunologists working in the field (Sher interview, 2007). At this stage, the cause of AIDS had not yet been identified. HIV would only be identified as the cause of AIDS in 1983 by scientists in France in 1984 and by those in the United States (Vilmer et al. 1984; Safai et al. 1984).

Soon after Sher's return to the country in late 1982, two young gay men died of unusual chest infections; both had worked for SAA. The newspapers heard about the story and decided to phone Sher to find out what he knew about the men's deaths. Sher 'put two and two together and figured out that they had died of AIDS' (Sher interview, 2007).

The newspaper headlines that resulted in early January 1983 could not have been worse for gay men in South Africa. On 4 January, the Cape Town newspaper *The Argus* reported on the new disease with the following headline: 'Homosexual' disease kills SAA staff.'[6] *The Sunday Times* coverage on 9 January was even more shrill: an article entitled, '"Gay" plague: More victims?' announced in a horrified tone that, 'Seven months before he became the first South African to die of the newly discovered disease – Ralph Kretzen, a self-confessed homosexual – still handled food on overseas flights.'[7] Gay men were very aware of and concerned about this negative coverage.

The South African Institute of Medical Research (SAIMR) was a key site of early AIDS research. Sher set up an AIDS department there with the director's blessing. The SAIMR had taken blood samples from over 200 gay men for another study and stored their serum. When they decided to test this serum for HIV with the newly developed tests in 1985, they found that 11.8 per cent of the samples were HIV-positive (Sher interview, 2007). Indeed, all the patients identified as being the first few cases of this new infectious disease in South Africa were white gay men. While heterosexuals were increasingly infected during the 1980s, as late as 1990 less than 1 per cent of the country's sexually-active population was estimated by the government to be infected (DoH 2005).

For much of the 1980s, AIDS was seen by South African epidemiologists as primarily affecting white gay men. By 1989, of the 98 cases voluntarily reported to the government's main AIDS policy-making body, the AIDS Advisory Group (AAG), 81 per cent were reported to have fallen into the 'homosexual/bisexual category' (Sher 1989). Similarly, in the mid-1980s it was estimated that 10–15 per cent of gay men in Johannesburg were infected with HIV (Sher 1989). The male/female ratio was 24:1 and only seven black patients had 'heterosexually acquired African AIDS' (Schoub et al. 1988: 153).

Some epidemiological studies from the early 1990s posited a 'two stage' theory of the South African AIDS epidemic (Schoub et al. 1988). Broadly speaking, this theory was that there was an epidemic among white 'homosexuals' which levelled off in the late 1980s and gave way to an 'heterosexual' epidemic which occurred mainly in the black population. For instance, in 1992 Alan Fleming, a professor in pathology, wrote that '…there have been two almost wholly separate epidemics, one in the male homosexual community who are predominantly white and the second in the heterosexual population with the majority black population being by far the worse affected so far' (Fleming 1992: 425). From early on there were indications that this model was flawed (Sher interview, 2007). Firstly, as Sher acknowledged, there was gay sex across the colour bar. Secondly, as early as 1986, blood transfusion data indicated that women were being infected (Sher interview, 2007). However, problematising the model in this way does not in any way dispute that the epidemic came in two waves involving two clades of the virus, the first being Clade B and the second being Clade C. What can be brought under critical scrutiny is whether cases of interracial gay sex or gay sex between black people may have been overlooked by epidemiologists due to stereotypes about gay sex being 'white'.

In particular, in the wake of social constructionist theories of scientific knowledge, it is worth problematising the sexual orientation and racial categories at work in this explanation of the epidemiology of AIDS. Firstly, as discussed above, social constructionists would argue that sexuality is not objectively fixed (Foucault 1976).

In a South African context, the dominant homophobic social construction of 'homosexuality' is that it is an 'un-African', 'white-import' (Epprecht 2004).

Epidemiology cannot be seen as objective and untainted by the social and cultural prejudices of the researchers conducting it, including the possibility that their research may have been influenced by the mistaken but widespread idea of homosexuality as an exclusively white phenomenon in South Africa.

As Simon Nkoli's infection with the virus shows, there clearly were cases of same-sex transmission of HIV to black males by the mid-1980s. In any event, more research is certainly required to test to what extent epidemiologists' biases about race and sexual orientation may have led to the phenomenon of same-sex male sexual transmission between races or among black people being overlooked in the period. Nevertheless, despite possible racial biases in epidemiologists' readings of 'gayness', their framing of AIDS as a 'gay' epidemic had important implications for how gay activists and society dealt with the issue in the period. As the epidemic was initially framed as a 'gay plague' in South Africa's media, in line with international trends, gay men bore the brunt of early AIDS-related discrimination in South Africa. In Natal in 1986, posters were put up by the blood transfusion service asking those who were gay or 'moffies' not to give blood.[8] Furthermore, the names of gay men living with AIDS were freely published in newspapers such as the *Cape Times* without their permission, while GASA 6010 had difficulty obtaining assistance from undertakers in removing the body of a gay man who had died from AIDS-related causes and in obtaining a Catholic burial for him (Pegge 1995).

From 1985, GASA published basic information about HIV transmission in its newsletter and arranged talks and seminars on AIDS.[9] According to the Triangle Project, this information was first developed by GASA 6010.[10] The easiest way for GASA 6010 to circulate information nationally would have been through GASA. So it can be surmised that much of the information on AIDS circulated by GASA nationally was developed by GASA 6010.

While GASA circulated information about AIDS through publications and meetings, it was not prepared to address the issue politically. Gevisser (1994) has argued that the organisation aimed to be 'apolitical' and was non-militant. This meant that even when it was denied representation on the AAG, which was the main AIDS policy-making body in the period, it did not protest. Far from it, while anti-apartheid organisations generally eschewed any 'collaboration' with the state, in 1985 GASA was content with recognition by the minister of health as the 'official mouthpiece of the gay community'.[11]

The AAG was founded by Ruben Sher and Jack Metz, the director of the SAIMR and a haematologist by training. They formed the AAG after successfully urging the government to establish an expert body to advise the government on AIDS. The AAG's members were from Johannesburg, Durban, Cape Town and Bloemfontein. They were mostly English-speaking professionals and came from disciplines such as epidemiology and microbiology (Sher interview, 2007).

According to Sher, the AAG came in for criticism from anti-apartheid health-worker organisations for being all white and for not including any gay people. Despite not having AAG representation, GASA was in regular contact with Sher right from the beginning. In these early years, Sher and his wife were invited to a GASA meeting in Hillbrow where they were given a cheque for R3 000 to fund AIDS research at SAIMR (Sher interview, 2007). In turn, he pleaded in the *South African Medical Journal* for tolerance to be exercised in relation to gay people and for them to be consulted more by doctors on the AIDS crisis (Sher 1989).

A significant barrier to gay organisations developing a more rigorous response to AIDS was that for much of the 1980s there appears to have been some disagreement about how serious the issue was among participants within the gay social scene and gay organisations. For instance, while GASA 6010 was very active around the issue, GASA's newsletter *Link/Skakel's* first headline on the issue was 'AIDS panic overstressed' (Gevisser 1994: 59).

Still, however limited their initial response was, at least gay organisations engaged with the issue; by comparison it was almost totally neglected by most other non-governmental organisations for most of the 1980s (even groups that would later become very active around the issue, such as progressive health-worker and women's organisations). For instance, speaking at the GASA Natal Coast branch's 1984/85 AGM, the branch chairperson argued that AIDS would mean a massive homophobic backlash which had to be addressed:

> Individually, some of us will be brought close to the reality of long term suffering and death, and collectively we will all be faced with caring for and dealing with people who are lonely and perhaps deserted by those closest to them. This is the kind of true gay spirit which I see developing out of the AIDS crisis. [12]

GASA 6010 in Cape Town is widely acknowledged as having been one of the most active non-governmental groups involved in AIDS work in the 1980s. It was founded in 1981 as a gay support and social group. In 1982, the year of its affiliation with GASA, it established its first 24-hour helpline staffed by volunteers and started an STD clinic for gay men which was also staffed by volunteers; most significantly, in that same year the first person living with AIDS used the clinic.[13] In 1984 (the year of Nkoli's jailing) an educational psychologist who was a member of GASA 6010 started going to gay clubs and bars in Cape Town two or three times a week to talk to men there about AIDS prevention. The volunteer was initially ridiculed and rejected and told not to spoil the club goers fun (Pegge 1995). According to Pegge, the nightclub project was only widely accepted around 1989 when it reached the point where most club goers accepted condoms and even asked for more.

In 1987, the Cape-based organisation was invited to hold South Africa's first AIDS candlelight memorial by Mobilize Against AIDS in San Francisco (Pegge 1995). Thirty men and three women gathered in GASA 6010's community centre, and Jewish and Christian prayers were said for the dead. The gay political tradition of the candlelight vigil was established following the assassination of Harvey Milk, the gay San Francisco city supervisor who was murdered in 1978 for pushing for reforms to end discrimination against gays and lesbians in that city. In the late 1980s and early 1990s, John Pegge of GASA 6010 associated the candlelight vigil with the militant American gay activism of the period.

Homophobia also created serious barriers to raising funds for social support and counselling for people living with HIV in the period. In 1988, GASA 6010 became the AIDS Support and Education Trust (ASET) to raise money for HIV prevention and care among sexual minorities. This was necessary as GASA 6010 was unable to legally fund raise without a fund-raising number, which it could not obtain due to it being an explicitly gay organisation. However, the name change/rebranding clearly did not help as ASET was also denied a fund-raising number. Homophobic laws thus had a disabling effect on gay AIDS activism by creating a sense of officially sanctioned taboo around any discussion or organising around gay sex, even when public health was at risk. In 1989, ASET managed to get around this by joining ranks with the Cape Mental Health Society to use its fund-raising number.[14]

There was certainly fracturing of the national gay movement in the mid-1980s, with differing views among gay men on the seriousness of AIDS and regionally varying responses. Nevertheless, in general terms, gay organisations did respond more comprehensively and earlier than other NGOs, even if it was in a regionally uneven way. As the final section of this chapter argues, this partially explains why later gay men were the first group of AIDS activists to be open about their HIV status and to push for a human rights-based approach to AIDS.

## Militant black gay lobbying in new political spaces

The largest political barrier to more effective lesbian and gay anti-apartheid organising around AIDS prior to 1990 was police harassment and the jailing of anti-apartheid gay activists, who would later go on to play a leading role in AIDS activism. Ivan Toms and Simon Nkoli were two such activists. The political transition to democracy which began in 1990 freed the political climate in ways that were conducive to more effective gay activism. In particular, it radically improved gay activists' ability to organise around AIDS. The first militant, relatively sustainable black-led gay organisations were formed.[15] Nothing symbolised the changing face of gay and lesbian politics as much as South Africa's first Gay Pride March held in

Johannesburg in 1990, which had more female and black participants than anyone had expected (Gevisser 1994).

Bev Ditsie met Nkoli, who influenced her to join his new organisation, GLOW:

> When the said dude [Simon] came back from jail he made an organisation with other gay people. He was influential especially because he was a political activist whose work encompassed other issues. I learnt from Simon and GLOW – they had books and knew how to chair meetings. I was doing things out of anger – no one was doing it in those days. I didn't understand discrimination. (Ditsie interview, 2006)

Ditsie dates the formation of the Township AIDS Project (TAP) as happening earlier than that of GLOW. Either way, both organisations seemed to have emerged around the same time and as interrelated processes. TAP was also very influential in the development of her political skills and confidence in talking about sexual and medical issues publicly: 'In terms of TAP, some of my first speaking engagements were as a TAP volunteer. It's where my self-esteem was groomed. We had to learn about HIV, the virus, its transmission and we knew how to articulate what was going on' (Ditsie interview, 2006).

Lesbians affiliated with GLOW, such as Ditsie, decided to get involved because some of their gay male friends were living with HIV and dying from AIDS-related causes, and they felt that they needed to take care of them. According to Ditsie, Nkoli had apparently always said that lesbian women would be the only people to take care of gay men with full-blown AIDS (Ditsie interview, 2006).

TAP had limited funding in the early days and also had to overcome legal barriers imposed by the sodomy laws. In the early 1990s, dildos – which were used in safer sex workshops – remained illegal. For related reasons, TAP did not enjoy government funding.

According to Luirink (2000), Simon Nkoli's analysis of government's failure to fund organisations such as TAP hinged on stigmatised and racialised perceptions of the disease: that it was first seen as a problem only affecting white gay men, then when it became seen as a black problem it was considered irrelevant, as it did not affect the National Party's constituency – the white population. Furthermore, sexual conservatism still exercised a stranglehold on government's efforts at AIDS awareness. For instance, its centrepiece strategy for AIDS education in school, which was commonly referred to as the 'yellow hand' campaign in AIDS activist circles, encouraged abstinence and barely mentioned condoms at all.

Despite its limited resources, TAP gave talks to different community-based organisations: 'We went to schools, NGOs, everywhere people said "come". We were educating nurses in clinics so we would go. We even spoke to little kids in crèches about sexual abuse' (Ditsie interview, 2006).

In a Western context, Dennis Altman (1993) has argued that lesbians faced 'dual oppression' within both the women's movement where they faced homophobia, and the gay rights movement where they faced sexism. While lesbians were expected to care for gay men with AIDS, in transition-era South Africa some lesbian activists felt dismayed by gay men not offering assistance in campaigning on gendered injustices which placed them at risk of HIV infection.

The limited research on lesbian transmission of HIV was noted by lesbian activists and scholars such as Vicci Tallis (1992). The lack of research acted as a key barrier to conducting AIDS education workshops among lesbians and was seen by Tallis as a consequence of the marginalisation of lesbians within gay AIDS activism and the 'AIDS world' more generally. The little research that was done, therefore, showed a lack of knowledge about dental dams used by lesbians to prevent HIV transmission or about how to use or obtain them (Tallis 1992).

As a consequence of limited research on the risks of transmission through lesbian sex, Ditsie struggled to adapt her AIDS education work to the needs of lesbians:

> I was trying to work out where do we, or I, fit in. Without research you speculate and you try to work out risk you take heed of blood, open sores and you work it out that way...So I would run safer sex workshops for girls and women emphasizing that sado-masochism could lead to infections. (Ditsie interview, 2006)

In addition to these gaps in research, the 'corrective' rape of lesbians to 'straighten them out' also placed lesbians at significant risk of contracting HIV. Ditsie found it hard to get gay men in GLOW/TAP to 'care' about the issue of 'corrective' rape (Ditsie & Newman 2002). Ditsie argues that this was for two reasons: firstly, gay men and lesbian women often had different gendered experiences of rape. She argued that whereas most lesbian women experienced deep trauma following a 'corrective' rape, some gay men saw it as 'just sex' and even 'fell in love' with their assailants afterwards (Ditsie interview, 2006). Lesbians' double oppression was also manifest in the sexism lesbians faced within gay rights activism. Discussing the early days of transition-era, multiracial, progressive gay activism, Ditsie has argued that, 'I don't think the men in GLOW saw lesbians as women...If they had seen us as women then they would have had to deal with their own sexism. Men are men, including most gay men' (Ditsie interview, 2006).

Despite the possible shortcomings of GLOW from a gender perspective, it represented a significant improvement on the apoliticism and non-militancy of GASA. In addition to which, it wasn't the only progressive movement which failed to be attuned to the needs of lesbians on prejudiced grounds. For instance, lesbians also experienced homophobia and a marginalisation of their issues in the women's movement.

Indeed, in most accounts of the history of GLOW, it is described as having been set up in conscious opposition to GASA's racism and apoliticism. This is certainly true, but there is an additional factor in GLOW's formation: gay men were increasingly coming together to organise around AIDS. In turn, the social networks which developed around AIDS also formed a basis for gay organising. Black gay rights activists saw AIDS and gay activism as mutually reinforcing, interlinked struggles, as would also be the case in a later period with the National Coalition for Gay and Lesbian Equality providing one of the bases for the formation of TAC (Treatment Action Campaign). For instance, both GLOW and TAP received the same donor funding and shared many of the same volunteers.[16]

According to Ditsie, GLOW's formation in 1989 (one year after Nkoli's release from jail) was a logical outflow of TAP. This was because TAP attracted gay men in numbers and when they came together around AIDS, they revealed the need for organising around socio-economic gay issues: 'GLOW emerged after TAP because when the numbers of gay men came through it made sense to have an organisation which was more socio-economically focused. . .These were the people that were threatened [by AIDS], they [AIDS activism and gay rights activism] came hand in hand' (Ditsie interview, 2006).

GLOW was much more politically powerful than any gay organisation that preceded it. It enjoyed greater legitimacy because of its mostly black membership and its close links with the liberation organisations. When GLOW started in 1989 it had a hundred members; by 1992 its ranks had swelled to about a thousand (Pandy 1992). The only obstacle to its further growth was the fact that many same-sex practising black people did not want to be open about their sexual orientation (Pandy 1992).

While a new, more militant form of lesbian and gay activism led by black people was taking hold in Johannesburg, Zackie and Midi Achmat were associated with the founding of the black-led Association for Bisexuals, Gays and Lesbians (ABIGALE) in Cape Town in 1992. As with GLOW, AIDS issues were central to ABIGALE's activities, and one of the aims set out in its constitution was to 'organise workshops and other educational initiatives for our community and particularly around the effects of AIDS' (Pandy 1992: 11).

Also like GLOW, and unlike GASA, ABIGALE was explicitly political and anti-racist. Whereas GASA's social functions had been racially segregated, ABIGALE organised a picket of 40 of its members outside the gay nightclub Strawbs, accusing the management of having a racist admissions policy and not admitting black patrons.[17] Similarly, while GASA was white dominated, ABIGALE claimed that of its 150 members, 99 per cent were black.[18]

This new form of gay activism was also evident in the case of Barry McGeary, a young man who lived in the small South African town of Brakpan. In 1991, he went to his doctor for an HIV test, as required by his insurance company. He was diagnosed as HIV-positive and his doctor then disclosed McGeary's status to two of his golfing friends. Within a week the whole town knew that McGeary was HIV-positive.

In this context, McGeary decided to sue his doctor for breach of confidentiality. He phoned advocate Edwin Cameron and asked him to be his lawyer, as by this stage Cameron had developed a public profile around AIDS. The case was later taken to the Supreme Court of Appeals in Bloemfontein. The Court found that the doctor had been wrong, that he had to pay damages to Barry McGeary, and it reaffirmed the principle of doctor–patient confidentiality in relation to AIDS (Dancaster & Dancaster 1995). The trial also showed what legal activism could achieve, an avenue that would only widen when a democratic Constitution was enacted. The trial made a deep impression on Edwin Cameron and made him decide that a charter had to be drafted on the rights of people living with HIV and AIDS. Around the same time, OLGA was drafting a charter on the rights of gay and lesbian people (Cameron interview, 2004).

## Gay rights and human rights activism in relation to HIV and AIDS

Edwin Cameron was pivotal to both the founding of the AIDS Consortium and drafting the Charter of Rights on AIDS and HIV (referred to as the AIDS Charter). His thinking in this regard was shaped by his experiences as a human rights lawyer, including that of defending Barry McGeary and opposing the closure of St Joseph's Hospice in Boksburg (Cameron interview, 2004).

Cameron convened a meeting of activists involved in AIDS policy-making at the University of the Witwatersrand. Mary Crewe, who was by then head of Johannesburg's AIDS Training, Testing and Counselling Centre, apparently suggested to Cameron that he initiate an AIDS consortium as a loose affiliation of AIDS organisations which could draft and endorse the AIDS Charter (Cameron interview, 2004). The final AIDS Charter was formally launched at the end of 1992. Gay AIDS activist Shaun Mellors revealed his HIV status at the NACOSA conference later that year, urging delegates to endorse the Charter.

Gay activists were devising the AIDS Charter while closely monitoring and lobbying parties to the negotiations that were drawing up South Africa's new Constitution. These negotiations were crucial in drafting the clause in the new Constitution's Bill of Rights which outlawed discrimination on the grounds of sexual orientation. The success of this gay rights activism was significant in terms of the history of AIDS activism in three ways:
- The non-discrimination clause led to the repeal of laws which had inhibited activist work to foster greater AIDS awareness.
- The clause paved the way for the rapid post-apartheid success of the legal reform agenda, and this freed up gay rights activists' time to focus on other issues such as HIV/AIDS.
- Thirdly, the success of legal activism based upon the clause provided lessons for legal activism which would be applied to later struggles for universal access to HIV treatment.

Gay activists and organisations such as OLGA and ABIGALE were closely engaged in efforts to have non-discrimination on the grounds of sexual orientation included in the country's new Constitution, which was being negotiated at Kempton Park. Gay and lesbian activists in ABIGALE felt that, 'It's now or never…we have the chance to make sure that lesbian, gay and bisexual rights are included in the new constitution…'[19]

Previous to the non-discrimination clause's inclusion in the country's new Constitution, AIDS activism was hampered by the sodomy laws. In addition, apartheid government censorship had blocked what publications gay activists could circulate. For instance, in 1993, the government's Committee on Publications banned two safer-sex videos made in South Africa called *For men who have sex with men* and *A lover's guide*.[20] This ban was confirmed when it was taken on appeal to the Publications Appeal Board, which ruled that the films featured 'long, drawn out scenes of sexual activity' which the Board saw as not in any way contributing to 'information about AIDS or safe sex', and argued that they aimed at '…provocation of lust and sexual stimulation'.[21]

Gay activists were totally outraged about the banning of the videos. ABIGALE covered the issue extensively in its newsletter, including a press clipping from the *Weekly Mail* (5–11 March 1993) of an article by gay activist and journalist Mark Gevisser. ABIGALE argued that it should challenge the ban: 'Sexuality is one of the last areas where self-appointed moral watchdogs feel they can prescribe to us what we may and may not read, view and do. Gays and lesbians are major victims of the censorship system.'[22] The South African branch of ACT-UP went even further in arguing that in the face of 500 infections a day, 'to deprive people of this kind of information is no different from infecting them; preserving the archaic, hypermoralistic attitudes of a handful of people is no excuse for genocide' (*Weekly Mail* 5–11 March 1993).

With the new Constitution and the legal reform it catalysed, after 1994 gay AIDS activists did not have to worry so much about issues of prudish censorship or sodomy legislation. Meanwhile, just as Gay Pride Marches marked greater public openness about being lesbian or gay, some gay activists started emerging from a 'second closet', disclosing that they were also living with HIV.

## Public openness about HIV status

White gay activists, such as Shaun Mellors, were open about their HIV status at big conferences debating the future shape of post-apartheid AIDS policy. Their revelations were personal and emotional, and had political impacts in that they meant that discussions about AIDS policy could no longer be argued in the abstract, without those most directly affected being present and vocal in expressing their interests in relation to it. They also added an emotional intensity to arguments for AIDS policy to be human rights-based, as set out in the AIDS Charter.

While the TAC is often seen as the first AIDS activist grouping which used openness about status in a radical mould to obtain specific political outcomes, there are a few important antecedents. The new, more militant black-led gay rights activists would start to draw upon anti-apartheid iconography and repertoires to combat homophobia and develop public awareness about AIDS. For instance, the 1993 funeral of activist Linda Ngcobo was perhaps the first 'political' AIDS funeral (Gevisser 1994). Gevisser characterises Ngcobo's funeral as having been political in that it was as much 'a memorial to a dead comrade as an impassioned plea for tolerance and a call-to-arms for rights' (1994: 16). Five years later, Zackie Achmat would call for the launch of the TAC at the funeral of AIDS activist Simon Nkoli. It was militant, black-led gay activism that laid the foundation for the later development of more militant AIDS activism led by people living with HIV.

## Conclusion

On the eve of the country's first democratic elections, gay AIDS activism had come a long way. Efforts to raise awareness and to provide social support to gay men living with and vulnerable to HIV infection had been sustained over many years. In addition, new strings had been added to the AIDS activists' bow. In particular, gay activists who focused on gay rights and those who focused on AIDS both used rights-based discourses to frame their campaigns. The country's first Gay Pride March showed that there was a new, more defiant, black-led gay and lesbian politics. Key gay anti-apartheid activists, such as Simon Nkoli and Ivan Toms, were also freed from jail. In this climate, gay AIDS activists were increasingly open about living with HIV. These were defiant actions given that the sodomy laws and Immorality Act (No. 5 of 1927) remained in full force, and that there was still enormous social stigma around AIDS and gay and lesbian sexuality in general.

This chapter has made the case for seeing these events against the historical and anthropological context of a diverse array of evolving same-sex sexual practices, identities and organisations in South Africa. Indeed, the 'apolitical', social-support nature of most 1980s gay AIDS activism only makes sense when viewed in the context of the general apoliticism and fragmentation of gay organisations at the time. To be precise, because there was no national gay organisation from the mid-1980s onwards, for much of the decade the strength of gay organisations' responses differed from region to region.

The chapter also problematised the production of early epidemiological knowledge around AIDS in South Africa by demonstrating that the two epidemiological theories encompassed the flawed assumption that homosexuality was a mostly white phenomenon. Conversely, a rich and growing literature demonstrates that same-sex sexual practices have a long history among black people in South Africa. In addition, some black gay men became infected with HIV in a very early period through interracial gay sex.

Charters for gay rights and the rights of people living with HIV had been drafted. These provided a powerful basis for advocacy at constitutional negotiations and at key AIDS policy-making forums, such as the NACOSA conference. In addition, they facilitated the formation of coalitions such as the AIDS Consortium and later the National Coalition for Gay and Lesbian Equality. Yet, struggles remained ahead for gay rights activists to have gay rights included in the country's final Constitution.

The advent of democracy allowed for a redirection of activists' energies and efforts. Anti-apartheid, gay rights activists who had previously been devoted almost exclusively to fighting apartheid were now partially freed up to fight AIDS. In the early 1990s, the epidemic also changed as an increasing number of cases were being found among black women and in the heterosexual 'general population', as tracked by annual antenatal clinic surveys (see for example Abdool Karim 1992).[23] And, rape and violence against women – which were issues of great concern to lesbian activists – would come to occupy a greater place in activist understandings of what drove new infections.

Gay rights activists actively and publicly owned AIDS as an issue and, from the late 1980s onwards, saw it as central to their increasingly vocal struggle for equal rights and dignity. Indeed, gay rights activism and AIDS activism grew so intertwined over the period that it is hard to understand the history of the one without reference to that of the other.

## Notes

1. There was much excitement when Dean Hamer announced in 1993 that he had found a genetic marker indicating the existence of a gene influencing male sexual orientation called Xq23. The gene has not been isolated or sequenced and another later study failed to confirm his finding. For more on this, see Agar (2004).

2. 'Moffie' is a derogatory word used to describe gay men. 'Dyke' is a derogatory term used in South Africa, and internationally, to describe lesbian women. '*Isitabane*' and '*ungqingili*' are isiZulu terms considered to be derogatory for gay people as they can also be used to describe hermaphrodites and reinforce the homophobic stereotype that all gay people are also intersexed or occupy some middle gender (Louw 2001). The term '*isitabane*' is also used in a derogatory way against lesbians (Keswa & Wieringa 2005).

3. Gay and Lesbian Memory in Action (GALA) archivist Anthony Manion referred to it as such when the author was a guest on GALA's Gay and Lesbian History Tour of Johannesburg in 2005.

4. As Gevisser notes, any three men disco dancing together at a nightclub could have been criminalised under this legislation.

5. Luirink (2000) asserts, for example, that anti-apartheid and gay rights activist Simon Nkoli was first informed of his status in 1985 when in jail, and that he had had his first white boyfriend in 1977.

6   This article was kept in a scrapbook made by Leon Eksteen who died in August 1986. He was the fifth Capetonian to die of AIDS. The scrapbook is now preserved in the Gay and Lesbian Memory in Action Archives under GASA/GASA 6010: Media Scrap Books Box.

7   This cutting is also included in a scrapbook of early press cuttings on AIDS kept by a member of GASA 6010 who was living with AIDS in the period. This scrapbook is now also kept in the GALA Archives under GASA/GASA 6010: Media Scrap Books Box.

8   Newspaper cuttings kept in a scrapbook made by Leon Eksteen now kept in the GALA Archive (GASA/ GASA 6010 Box, Media Scrap Books Vol 8.5): 'Row brews over "*moffie*" posters' (Unknown newspaper). 'Gays angry over blood transfusion poster' (*The Citizen*, 29 January 1986).

9   See the GALA Archives, Triangle Project Box: am2974/Triangle Project , C1.1.1–2; C1.2.1–2; C1.3; C1.4; C1.5.1.–2. Annual Reports, 'Triangle Project *Annual Review*', 1996, p. 13.

10  GALA Archives, Triangle Project, File C.1.5.1 Annual Reports, Triangle Project *Annual Review* 1996, p. 13.

11  GALA Archives, GASA, Gay Groups Minutes Etc Box, File A: National Gay Groups Minutes- Northern Cape, Eastern Cape, Natal Coast (Durban) and Port Elizabeth 1984-5, 'GASA Natal Coast: Chairman's Report 1984/5: Report of the Second AGM held on Friday 19th April 1985 at GASA Natal Coast Office 51 Williams Rd, Congella, Durban', p. 11.

12  See endnote 11.

13  GALA Archives, Triangle Project, File C.1.5.1 Annual Reports, Triangle Project *Annual Review* 1996.

14  See endnote 13.

15  There were antecedents such as the Saturday Group and the Rand Gay Organization but because of political repression, these were short-lived and limited in political impact and tactics compared to GLOW with its Gay Pride Marches and political funerals and ABIGALE (Association of bisexuals, gays and lesbians) with its pickets.

16  GALA Archives, Peter Tatchell Collection, AM2715; P Tachell Out and against apartheid *Him* 28: 12; Note also that Bjorn Ivensen and Beate Christiansen are noted as representatives of Norweigian funders (LLH Norway) and as cofounders of TAP and GLOW in: GALA Archive, Triangle Project Collection AM2974, Box B9.1.1-AIDS Consortium – Broader Community Liaison, Minutes of AIDS Consortium Meeting, 23 January 1993.

17  GALA Archive, ABIGALE materials, 'Strawbs: The struggle continues', p. 1. This article was part of an ABIGALE newsletter. Gevisser has noted that they picketed Strawbs in April 1993, so this article can be dated back to that period. (Gevisser 1994).

18  GALA Archives, ABIGALE materials, Mid-Year Chairperson's Report. This is obviously not an exact statistic, but it indicates that its chairperson's perception was that an overwhelming number of its members were black or coloured.

19  GALA Archives, ABIGALE materials, *Gay rights now!* p. 1.

20  Neither of these films was available at the time of writing. The only reference the author had was the news article cited in note 23.

21  GALA Archives, ABIGALE materials, *ABIGALE Newsletter* No. 3 (March 1993).

22  See endnote 21.

23  Abdool Karim notes a doubling of HIV infection rates within a six-month period among pregnant women attending antenatal clinics in rural KwaZulu-Natal.

## References

Abdool Karim Q (1992) *AIDS in SA: Epidemiology*. Report of the National AIDS Convention of South Africa, Johannesburg, 23–24 October

Agar N (2004) *Liberal eugenics: In defence of human enhancement*. Oxford, Malden and Victoria: Blackwell Publishing

Altman D (1993) *Homosexual oppression and liberation*. New York: New York University Press

Dancaster JT & Dancaster LA (1995) Confidentiality concerning HIV/AIDS status – the implications of the Appeal Court decision. *South African Medical Journal* 85(3): 141–144

Ditsie BP & Newman N (2002) *Simon and I* (documentary film). Johannesburg: Women Make Movies

DoH (Department of Health, South Africa) (2005) *Report: National HIV and syphilis sero-prevalence survey in South Africa*. Pretoria: DoH

Epprecht M (2004) *Hungochani: The history of a dissident sexuality in southern Africa*. Montreal: McGill-Queen's University Press

Fleming AF (1992) South Africa and AIDS: Seven years wasted. *Current AIDS Literature* 5(11): 425

Foucault M (1976) *The history of sexuality: An introduction* (translated by R Hurley). Harmondsworth: Penguin

Gevisser M (1994) A different fight for freedom: A history of South African lesbian and gay organization from the 1950s–1990s. In M Gevisser & E Cameron (Eds) *Defiant desire: Gay and lesbian lives in South Africa*. Johannesburg: Ravan Press

Gevisser M & Cameron E (1994) Defiant desire: An introduction. In M Gevisser & E Cameron (Eds) *Defiant desire: Gay and lesbian lives in South Africa*. Johannesburg: Ravan Press

Keswa B & Wieringa S (2005) Chapter Six. In R Morgan & S Wieringa (Eds) *Tommy boys, lesbian men and ancestral wives: Female same-sex practices in Africa*. Johannesburg: Jacana Media

Louw R (2001) Mkhumbane and new traditions of un(African) same-sex weddings. In R Morrell (Ed.) *Changing men in southern Africa*. Pietermaritzburg: University of Natal Press

Luirink B (2000) *Moffies: Gay and lesbian life in southern Africa*. Cape Town: David Philip

Malan M (1986) AIDS in the USA and RSA – An update. *South African Medical Journal* 70: 119

Nkabinde N & Morgan R (2005) 'This has happened since ancient times…it's something you are born with': Ancestral wives amongst same-sex sangomas in South Africa. In R Morgan & S Wieringa (Eds) *Tommy boys, lesbian men and ancestral wives: Female same-sex practices in Africa*. Johannesburg: Jacana Media

Pandy T (1992) Gay and proud. *SPEAK* December: 11

Pegge JV (1995) Living with loss in the best way we know how: AIDS and gay men in Cape Town. In M Gevisser & E Cameron (Eds) *Defiant desire: Gay and lesbian lives in South Africa*. Johannesburg: Ravan Press

Reid G (2006) How to become a 'real gay': Identity and terminology in Ermelo, Mpumalanga. *Agenda. Empowering Women for Gender Equity* 67(13): 137–145

Safai B, Arnett K, Gallo RC, Groopman JE, Popvic M, Sarngadharan MC, Schüpbach J & Sliski A (1984) Seroepidemiological studies of Human T-Lymphotropic Retrovirus Type III in Acquired Immune Deficiency Syndrome. *The Lancet* 30(1)(8392): 1438–1440

Schoub BD, Johnson S, Lyons SF, Martin DJ, McGillivray G & Smith AN (1988) Epidemiological considerations of the present status and future growth of the acquired immunodeficiency syndrome epidemic in South Africa. *South African Medical Journal* 74(4): 153–157

Sher R (1989) HIV infection in South Africa 1982–1989: A review. *South African Medical Journal* 76: 4–8

Stein E (1990) Introduction. In E Stein (Ed.) *Forms of desire: Sexual orientation and the social constructionist controversy*. New York & London: Routledge

Tallis V (1992) Lesbians and AIDS. *Agenda* 15: 69–80

Vilmer E, Barre-Sinoussi F, Cherman JC, Dauguet C, Fischer A, Gazengel C, Griscelli C, Manigne P, Montagnier L, Rouzioux C & Veziret Brun F (1984) Isolation of new lymphotropic retrovirus from two siblings with haemophilia B, one with AIDS. *The Lancet* 323(8380): 753–757

## Archival sources

Gay and Lesbian Memory in Action (GALA) archive, Historical Papers Department, William Cullen Library, University of the Witwatersrand, East Campus, Johannesburg

## Interviews

Beverley Palesa Ditsie, activist, film maker and friend of the late Simon Nkoli, Gay and Lesbian Organisation of the Witwatersrand, Johannesburg, 14 September 2006

Edwin Cameron, former human rights and AIDS activist and Supreme Court of Appeals judge, Johannesburg, 4 October 2004

Ruben Sher, Immunologist, Johannesburg, 30 January 2007

## CHAPTER EIGHT

# Sexing women: Young black lesbians' reflections on sex and responses to safe(r) sex

Zethu Matebeni

Women in same-sex relationships exist in societies that are laden with heterosexuality, sexism and, in some situations, homophobia. Such societies inhibit women's right and opportunity to develop and shape their own identities and freely practise their sexual preferences. Adrienne Rich (1993) argues that many women find themselves in what she terms 'compulsory heterosexuality', which exists in most societies and imposes heterosexuality on women. She argues that 'heterosexuality is the presumed "sexual preference" of most women either implicitly or explicitly' (Rich 1993: 229). Some women reject this 'compulsory heterosexuality' and choose to engage in same-sex relationships or alternative sexual relationships.

There are various ways in which 'lesbian' is defined and these definitions point to the fact that women's same-sex practices do not necessarily fit neatly in a 'lesbian' category. For example, Doan (1994) argues that while there are women who engage in same-sex behaviour who do not identify themselves as lesbian, there are also women who do not engage in sex with women and consider themselves 'lesbian'. Some of the women in the latter grouping are found in feminist political circles and others have had relationships with women in the past.

The question of lesbian identity or who the lesbian is and what 'lesbian' means, has not been sufficiently explored in South Africa. While some see identities such as 'lesbian' as problematic in African contexts (Kendall 1998), many women in same-sex erotic relationships do adopt and identify themselves as lesbians, or variations of 'lesbian' such as 'tommy boys', 'Galla man', 'dyke', '*manvrou*', 'butch and femme' (Blyth 1989; Dirsuweit 1999; GALA archives; Gevisser & Cameron 1994; Morgan & Wieringa 2005). With the adoption of the South African Constitution, many South Africans have the privilege of claiming a range of identities and openly choosing experiences with which they are comfortable, knowing that they will be protected by the law. This chapter looks at sexual identities among a group of women who self-identify as lesbian or homosexual, and how their sexual identities affect their sexuality and their decisions around sex.

Whether women in same-sex relationships choose to identify as lesbian or not, Swarr and Nagar (2003) demonstrate that such women, especially if they are poor, face numerous struggles. They argue that identity categories such as race, gender, class, sex and sexuality are essentially interrelated and simultaneously experienced.

This is evident in how 'women experience, analyse and articulate their daily struggles around sexuality in relation to other material and symbolic struggles central to their lives' (Swarr & Nagar 2003: 493). The authors go on to argue that resource access and material survival versus sexuality, identity, intimacy and community, should not be seen in isolation from each other. They argue that women in same-sex relationships are constantly reminded of the social structures, social power, patriarchal societies and the economic limitations they live in (Swarr & Nagar 2003).

There are legitimate reasons why some women find it difficult to identify with or adopt a lesbian identity when in a same-sex relationship. These difficulties include, as Kitzinger and Wilkinson (1995) argue, internal and external constraints such as invisibility and silence surrounding lesbianism; incompatibility between self-perceptions and stereotypes of lesbians; awareness of the social consequences of adopting a lesbian identity (including potential rejection and violence); fear and horror invested in the word 'lesbian'; and believing that continued sexual attraction to men is incompatible with being a 'real lesbian'.

Among many black South Africans, homosexuality is regarded as un-African and a Western import. This belief is perpetuated by the lack of visibility of black people, as opposed to white people, who are openly in same-sex relationships; the fact that while same-sex relationships are taking place, they are not termed 'gay' or 'lesbian'; and the outright rejection of same-sex relationships among many people in black communities. Those in same-sex relationships in these communities feel the impact of this belief, as many end up experiencing violent attacks (Gevisser 1994).

## Sexuality in post-apartheid South Africa

During the apartheid era the South African government was 'deeply invested in questions of racial reproductive heterosexual sexuality' (Hoad et al. 2005: 16), to the extent that policies such as the Immorality Act of 1950, the Prohibition of Mixed Marriages Act of 1949, the Immorality Act of 1957, and the amended Immorality Act of 1969 prohibited sexual mixing between different race groups, as well as homosexual acts (Hoad et al. 2005). During the 1980s the gay and lesbian movement, along with some political leaders and sympathetic journalists, continually put pressure on the state to ensure that gay and lesbian rights were included in the 1994 Interim Constitution delivered by the Constitutional Assembly and ratified by Parliament in 1996 (De Waal & Manion 2006). The South African Constitution now includes a clause prohibiting discrimination on the grounds of sexual orientation.

As argued by Posel (2004), since the demise of apartheid and the ratification of the Constitution and its Bill of Rights in 1996, sex and sexuality have become topics for public debate and argument. Freedom of sexual practices, identity and expression has become a protected right accessible to all. There has also been an explosion of sexual imagery, display and debate, evident in the booming sex industry, explicit television programmes, and various media promoting and selling sex. Discourse on social and political concerns, including the alarming levels of sexual violence in both the public and private spheres as well as debates on HIV/AIDS, have gained much public attention and have made sex and sexuality important public issues.

Posel (2004) also argues that the issue of HIV/AIDS has been largely a post-apartheid problem and HIV/AIDS campaigns and public health education programmes have been promoting, although some not very successfully, awareness on how the virus is transmitted. The pandemic has emphasised the need to talk about sex and sexuality, and has encouraged national conversations about these two topics, as well as about risk and protection. However, the sex talked about is mostly heterosexual or focuses mainly on male experiences.

With the emergence of the HIV and AIDS epidemic as the major public health concern and crisis on the subcontinent, much debate on sexuality in South Africa has taken place in the context of the epidemic and levels of sexual violence (Shefer & Potgieter 2006). Yet many people in same-sex erotic relationships have escaped neither the epidemic nor the endemic sexual violence affecting South Africans. While much has been written about gay men's sexuality and its interplay in HIV and AIDS debates, there continues to be a silence about female same-sex relationships and how HIV and AIDS affect women in these relationships. The belief that women in same-sex relationships are at no or low risk of contracting HIV and other sexually transmitted infections (STIs) continues to dominate. This belief also takes for granted or ignores many women who are in both same-sex relationships and heterosexual relationships and the risks of infection in these relationships.

The effects of sexual violence are widely felt within the lesbian community in Johannesburg, as large numbers of lesbian women fall victim to hate crimes and violent sexual attacks, some of which lead to HIV infection or even death (Muholi 2004). The black lesbian community in Johannesburg has experienced numerous deaths of active and young lesbian women who have died from AIDS-related complications. Debates on HIV and AIDS and on surviving hate crimes and rape continue to be difficult and very emotive discussions in lesbian and women-centred circles, as we continue searching for spaces and resources that are directed at us and our daily experiences. These spaces do not exist despite the Constitution's protection of sexual rights and recognition of homosexual relationships. South Africa remains highly homophobic, patriarchal and heterosexist, and this translates into heterosexuality being seen as the ideal and being privileged above other forms of sexuality (Wells & Polders 2006a). This privilege directs much attention and resources to heterosexual norms, while ignoring and rejecting the existence of other sexualities that face the same challenges as the heterosexual ideal.

Fear and 'forced' silence among many black lesbians has led many to remain voiceless about their sexuality and experiences. Efforts to encourage black lesbian women to claim their space and talk about their sexualities are minimal and, when efforts are made, these women require, among other things, constant encouragement to talk about these issues, strict measures to protect anonymity and confidentiality, and the creation of safe spaces where black lesbian women can gather and engage in such dialogue without fear, victimisation or forced visibility.

## Understanding women's same-sex sexuality and lesbianism

There is still no consensus on what and who is lesbian in the international literature. For some, lesbianism is seen as the emotional and psychological identification of women with other women, which has existed for centuries among women. For example, Faderman (1981) defines 'lesbian' as a relationship in which two women's strongest emotions and affections are directed toward each other. In this relationship, she adds, sexual content may be a part of the relationship to a greater or lesser degree, or it may be entirely absent. The two women prefer to spend most of their time together and share most aspects of their lives with each other.

In another instance, being lesbian is put on a 'continuum' which includes 'a range – through each woman's life and throughout history – of woman-identified experience, not simply the fact that a woman has had a consciously desired genital experience with another woman' (Rich 1993: 239). In this sense, 'lesbian' can be expanded to embrace many more forms of 'primary intensity between and among women, including the sharing of a richer and inner life, the bonding against male tyranny, the giving and receiving of practical and political support' (Rich 1993: 239). Proponents of this definition argue that such an inclusive definition suggests various interconnections existing in ways women bond together. Those who criticise it argue that such all-inclusive definitions blur the distinction between lesbian relationships and non-lesbian female relationships, or between lesbian identity and female-centred identity. Zimmerman (1981) argues that this understanding of lesbianism eliminates 'lesbian' as a meaningful category.

Faderman and Rich are not very concerned about the sexual relationships that lesbian women engage in. Kitzinger (1987) and Farquhar (2000), on the other hand, put sex and sexuality at the core of their definitions or understanding of 'lesbian'. Kitzinger understands lesbian identity as 'intended to characterize the set of meanings ascribed by a woman to whatever social, emotional, sexual, political or personal configuration she intends when she describes herself as lesbian' (Kitzinger 1987: 43). Farquhar (2000) takes an extra step by focusing particularly on the sexual practices between lesbian women. She notes that, among lesbians in the United Kingdom in the 1970s and 1980s, lesbian authenticity was ascribed to interpretations of sexual practices such as 'butch–femme' roles; the use of dildos or penetrative sex; lesbian sex with men; 'safer' sex; and other forms of sex. Importance was placed on particular forms of sexual practice, rather than on the practices themselves. The forms of sexual practice were then related to constructions of subjectivities and identities.

Sexual experiences and the sexuality of lesbian women often become almost completely invalidated, because lesbian sexual experiences frequently hide under the emotional, affective and political relations between women (as seen in Rich and Faderman above). One other reason for this is that lesbian sex and sexuality are generally understood in relation to a heterosexual paradigm of oppositional duality, which prescribes gender roles and gendered social codes. Some contributors to lesbian scholarship, including Rich and Faderman as well as Potgieter (1997) in the South African context, have contributed to the desexualisation of lesbians. In the only extensive study of black lesbians in South Africa, *Black, South African, Lesbian: Discourses of Invisible Lives* by Potgieter (1997), the author fails to define lesbian in the South African context or to fully explore issues of sexuality. Instead, she refers to feminism's definition of lesbian as 'women who love women', which desexualises lesbian identity. Potgieter rather engages in the sexual identity versus homosexual behaviour debate. This resonates within the historical context of lesbian and gay people in South Africa, where identity-claims as a collective took prominence for political reasons (for more on this, see Gevisser & Cameron 1994). Potgieter (1997) does not question or explore 'who is lesbian', but rather puts lesbianism under feminism and takes for granted the meaning of the category in the South African context.

Calhoun (1995) argues that when lesbianism is understood under feminism only, sexual desire hides under 'love', and the sexual aesthetics of 'butch and femme' roles are denied. Furthermore, the 'woman-identified woman' (or 'lesbian' as defined by some feminists) has no distinct sexuality, to the extent that one might say 'she has no sexuality at all' (Calhoun 1995: 11). Calhoun sees a problem when lesbianism is desexualised and argues that 'when feminist woman loving replaces lesbian genital sexuality, lesbian identity disappears into feminist identity and sexual difference between heterosexual women and lesbians cannot be effectively represented' (1995: 10).

Many scholars argue against the desexualisation of lesbian identity (see Newman 2002). Ferguson (1981) argues that the ability to take one's own sexual needs seriously is a necessary component of an egalitarian love relationship. So, a definition that fails to highlight sexual agency undermines lesbians' challenges to the dominant heterosexual ideology. The possibility of a sexual relationship between women is an important challenge to patriarchy because it acts as an alternative to the heterosexuality so strongly endorsed by patriarchy. It also shows that not all women are dependent on men for sexual or romantic love and physical satisfaction. This chapter highlights the importance of bringing sex, and the performance and negotiation of lesbian sex, back into the category 'lesbian'.

## Methodology

Studies show that lesbian women tend to be relatively inaccessible to researchers and are thus difficult to 'sample' (Zimmerman 1981). Lesbians traditionally have been less visible than homosexual men – in the past few of them were (publicly) politically involved, they tend to be quiet about their sexual identity or socially isolated, and they utilise space in different ways to gay men (Leap 2005). To access numbers of lesbian women at the same time, lesbian organisations or (private and public) functions catering for lesbian women are spaces that researchers can enter to get a 'sample' of lesbian women. It was in such spaces that this research was undertaken.

A venue in central Johannesburg attracts a number of lesbian women or women who are known to have been, or are, in relationships with women. Approximately 100 women of different races and age groups frequent this space, but for this research, black women were recruited. Each respondent was individually introduced to the research and given a self-administered questionnaire, which guaranteed anonymity and confidentiality. Each respondent collected a questionnaire and walked to a private area where they filled in the questionnaire on their own. Respondents were encouraged to answer the questions in their own language or a language they felt comfortable with. In many cases, respondents collected the questionnaires, took them home and, upon completion, sent them back to the researcher.

Two copies of an informed consent form and information sheet accompanied each questionnaire, one to be given back to the researcher and another to be kept by the respondent. To ensure anonymity, these were not attached to the questionnaires. The study defined its target population as women who currently are, or have been, in sexual relationships with other women. A total of 23 out of 30 distributed questionnaires were returned. Four of the 30 respondents completed an informed consent form but never sent back the questionnaire and there was no follow-up on these. All the respondents were from the Johannesburg area.

As an insider, it is easier for me to access a diversity of lesbian women, many of whom are friends or acquaintances. Because lesbian circles tend to be small, many of us know each other or socialise in the same spaces, which also makes it easier to approach people or even to learn about each other's sexual relationships and various aspects of our intimate lives. Although it is difficult for researchers to broach sex-related topics with lesbian women, as an insider this is much more possible.

## Findings

### Who is lesbian? Self-identification and gender-related roles

Although Johannesburg has a fairly large 'lesbian community', many of the visible black lesbian women are below the age of 40 years. Lesbian women older than 40 tend to meet in different places to those frequented by their younger counterparts.
- The age of the respondents ranged from 19–34 years with an equal distribution of respondents in the following age groups: 18–21 years, 22–25 years and 26–29 years. Four respondents were 30–33 years old and one respondent was 34 years old.
- With regards to occupation, roughly a third were employed and a third were studying. Of those studying, four had part time jobs and three were full-time students. The remaining four respondents were unemployed.

- More than half of the respondents were currently in relationships or had a sexual partner. Only six respondents reported that they were single but in many cases these women had casual partners. Those who were in relationships were usually referred to as 'partnered'.[1] However, being partnered did not necessarily mean that the respondent had only one partner.

To elicit expressions of self-identity, respondents were asked, 'What word do you use most to describe your sexual orientation?' Various options were included. Almost all respondents (n=19) identified themselves as lesbian. Unlike in other African countries, where women apparently do not use the category 'lesbian' to express their sexual feelings towards other women (Gay 1985; Kendall 1998; Morgan & Wieringa 2005), women in Johannesburg seem to use this category.

Of the 19 respondents who identified themselves as lesbian, only two stated that they preferred to call themselves 'a woman-loving woman' (WLW) (although they also ticked lesbian), a commonly used term among certain (feminist) circles of women in same-sex relationships in Johannesburg. Two other respondents preferred to describe themselves as homosexual, with the same number preferring not to describe themselves or choosing the category 'other'. Table 8.1 details the demographics of respondents.

Respondents were also asked if they adopted any (gender-related) roles or used other ways to describe themselves. Six out of 20 respondents who answered this question described themselves as 'butch', and nine respondents described themselves as 'femme'.

In Johannesburg, many women claim a lesbian identity once they have been sexually involved with another woman. Also, women tend to be perceived as lesbian if they are seen with or known to have been sexually involved with a woman who is already known within the 'lesbian community'. Among younger women who identify as lesbian, butch and femme roles tend to be emphasised. These roles relate to gender roles of masculinity and femininity and present a very strong sexual style in a relationship (Wieringa 2005). It is common for these women to openly refer to themselves as femme or butch and it also tends to be easy to distinguish between butch and femme based on dress code, walk, mannerisms and who they are attracted to. A butch usually prefers a femme, and two butches or two femmes together are not seen as 'ideal'.

Similar to what Nestle (1981) describes, Johannesburg's butch–femme relationships are complex, erotic statements, not phony replicas of a heterosexual model. Butch–femme dynamics are 'filled with a deeply lesbian language of stance, dress, gesture, loving, courage and autonomy...courage to feel comfortable with arousing another woman...A butch sexuality and femme sexuality...a developed lesbian specific sexuality that has a historical setting and a cultural function' (Nestle 1981: 100). Butch–femme relationships in Johannesburg have also been researched by Busi Kheswa (cited in Morgan & Wieringa 2005).

**Table 8.1:** Respondent demographics

| Variable | n |
|---|---|
| **Age** | |
| 18–21 | 6 |
| 22–25 | 6 |
| 26–29 | 6 |
| 30–33 | 4 |
| 34–37 | 1 |
| **Self-identify as…** | |
| Lesbian | 19 |
| Homosexual | 2 |
| Woman-loving-woman | 2 |
| **Role play** | |
| Butch | 6 |
| femme | 9 |
| No role/other | 6 |
| **Occupational status** | |
| Employed | 8 |
| Unemployed | 4 |
| Student | 3 |
| Employed student | 4 |
| Other | 1 |
| **Relationship status** | |
| Single | 6 |
| Partnered | 13 |
| Other | 4 |

Note: N = 23

## Sex and the self: Emotions on sex with women

There are various 'ideals' and ideas about how lesbian women think about and give meaning to sex. The narrative on sex is presented as positive – something that is enjoyed, pleasurable and intimate. Phrases and concepts such as 'sexy', 'passion', 'pleasure', 'bonding and closeness', 'fulfilment', 'intimate', 'expression of love', and 'sharing between two people' were used by most respondents to give meaning to what they thought and felt about sex. Only one respondent felt that sex could include more than two consenting individuals. Another respondent felt that sex was private 'between me and my partner'. The same respondent also felt that she should not talk to others about the sex she has. A few respondents felt that sex was related to who they are. As one respondent put it, 'it [sex] affirms my sexual orientation', and another stated that sex means 'being myself' (referring to the way she has sex).

Respondents were asked to recall the first time they had sex with a woman and what this was like. Most respondents reported that their first sexual encounter with a woman happened when they were between the ages of 14 and 17 years. Only two respondents had initiated sex with a woman before the age of 13 years. In describing their first sexual experience with a woman, a few respondents recalled that it was 'shocking'; others reported that it was 'scary', as they did not know what to do.

> T'was scary, I was not sure if I was going to satisfy her, but it turned out beautifully. (26-year-old lesbian)
>
> Shocking and foreign but it identified who I am and motivated me to be myself. (21-year-old femme)
>
> Shocking to me that she made me feel that way. (26-year-old butch lesbian)

Most of the respondents remembered 'nice', 'great', 'wonderful' experiences. Some respondents felt that because they did not know what to do, they had been nervous or scared.

> Great. Something I never experienced before. It was fireworks. (30-year-old femme)
>
> Wonderful and relaxing but a bit scary if you don't know what to do. (20-year-old femme)
>
> I was scared, it was painful and I cried. (23-year-old femme)

**Table 8.2** Respondent sexual information and activity

| Variable | n |
| --- | --- |
| **Age at first sex with a woman**[a] | |
| 13 or less | 2 |
| 14–17 | 8 |
| 18–21 | 4 |
| 22–25 | 3 |
| **No. of sexual partners in lifetime**[b] | |
| 1–5 | 8 |
| 6–10 | 4 |
| 11–15 | 5 |
| More than 20 | 4 |
| Lost count/not sure | 2 |
| **No. of current sexual partner(s)**[b] | |
| 1 | 13 |
| 2 | 3 |
| 3 | 4 |
| 4 or more | 3 |

Notes: a. n = 17; b. N = 23

**Table 8.3** Current sexual partner(s) per relationship status and role play

|  | No. of current sexual partners | | | | Role performance/play | | |
| --- | --- | --- | --- | --- | --- | --- | --- |
|  | 1 | 2 | 3 | 4+ | Butch | Femme | other |
| Single | 3 | 3 | – | – | 1 | 3 | 2 |
| Partnered | 9 | – | 1 | 3 | 4 | 6 | 3 |
| Other | 1 | – | 3 | – | 1 | – | 1 |

To gain an understanding of sexual history and sexual partners, respondents were asked about the number of sexual partners they had. Respondents were not asked if they had ever been, or were currently in, a sexual relationship with a man. Table 8.2 provides more information about respondents' sexual experiences.

Among the respondents, a majority had had between one and five sexual partners in their lifetime. Six respondents had had more than 20 partners, two of whom could not remember or had lost count of the number of sexual partners they had had. Contrary to popular belief about lesbians in Johannesburg, most respondents (more than half) reported having one current sexual partner, rather than multiple partners, that is, they were monogamous. Three respondents reported that they had four or more sexual partners at the time.

When looking at differences with regards to role-playing lesbians, more femme lesbians (6) compared to butch women (4) reported being in relationships. Of those who reported that they were single, the ratio of butch to femme was 1:3. Table 8.3 provides details of current sexual partners of respondents and roles.

The number of sexual partners was higher among those who reported to be partnered than among those who were single. Of the 13 respondents who were partnered, four had three or more concurrent partners. As mentioned earlier, those who were single also had casual sexual partners.

Respondents were asked to talk about the first time they had sex with their latest sexual partner. There were various ways in which sex was initiated with the latest partner. In some situations, respondents reported that sex was planned. This happened mainly in situations where the individuals had been dating for a while and then decided to have sex. In other situations it was not planned, it just happened after a night out, or the time was right or the space was conducive. When asked if there was any negotiation about sex and when these negotiations took place, most respondents (n=11) reported that sex was negotiated before and after it took place. Eight respondents reported that no negotiations or discussions took place about sex, and four reported that they talked about sex only after it had happened. Of those who had talked about sex, respondents reported that the main discussions included: pleasing each other; what each person likes and how sex could be improved; safety and protection against STI and HIV transmission; discussions around penetration; and how to have sex with a woman. These are important discussions as some women do not like penetration.

Sex seems to be an important indicator of same-sex relationships among women in Johannesburg. This is evident from the findings, as none of the respondents reported not being sexually active or never having had sex with a woman. This is in contrast to previous studies looking at female same-sex relationships. In particular, Gay's (1985) and Kendall's (1998) studies of 'mummy–baby' relationships and *'motsaolle'* (special friends) in Lesotho, show that although there were physical and sometimes sexual acts between women, these were not seen as sexual or even 'lesbian' in nature. This is because sex was perceived as only happening between a man and a woman and as requiring a penis (*koai*) and penetration – no *koai*, no sex. Among the respondents in my study, sex between women included emotions as well as the physical act. A few respondents were quite specific that sex between women meant 'sexual intercourse' and others focused more on orgasm and the satisfaction that each partner experiences during sex. This finding is important in that it disqualifies the notion of desexualised lesbian women. It is clear here that lesbian women do have sex and do identify the physical and emotional act between them as sex. It is also no coincidence that the women in this study described themselves as lesbian and were having sex with women.

In a previous section it was discussed that there are women who engage in sex with women, but who do not identify as 'lesbian' (see Doan 1994). This was not found to be the case in my research. My findings also contrast with those of Kendall, who quotes Frye's ironic statement, 'lesbians don't have sex at all. There is no male partner whose orgasm and ejaculation can be the criterion for counting times' (Kendall 1998: 230). My findings reassert that there can be sex between black South African lesbian women in Johannesburg without the presence of a male or a penis. Furthermore, orgasm and sexual satisfaction between black South African women does take place.

## Sex and HIV: The dynamic of aesthetics

Traditionally, lesbian women were thought to be free from the risk of STIs and HIV and AIDS. Findings from a study conducted among gay men and lesbian women in South Africa show that this is not the case. Self-reported HIV rates among lesbian women in this study show that 8 per cent of those who had been tested for HIV were HIV-positive (Wells & Polders 2006b).

In light of current discussions about safe sex, HIV transmission and AIDS, respondents gave diverse responses when asked, 'What does it mean for you to have safe sex with a woman?' One respondent said it meant 'no bisexuals'. Some lesbian women prefer to stay away from openly bisexual women as they worry about transmission of STIs and may 'fear becoming known' to the male partner. Some respondents talked about 'using protective means' and expressing their love in ways that are safe. Others referred to knowing and understanding the risks if safe sex is not practised. Nine respondents reported that they had never practised safe sex with a woman. Most of those who reported ever practising safe sex mentioned dental dams and condoms as the most commonly used barrier methods. A few of the respondents who reported practising safe sex with a woman cited the following methods:

> No preventative measure, just hands and tongues. (21-year-old femme)

> Foreplay and thigh sex. (20-year-old WLW)

> Mostly used fingers, but everything two women do, we do. (20-year-old femme)

> ...avoid exchange of fluids. (30-year-old femme)

Those not practising safe sex reported that they do not because they:

> Don't know places where to get safety measures from. (23-year-old butch)

> Trust [each other]. (27-year-old butch)

> Ignore that we can be infected. (26-year-old butch)

> Know I'm safe and my partner is not sleeping around; only with one partner. (30-year-old femme).

Others felt that there are:

> No resources for safe sex for lesbians. (31-year-old WLW)

> Lesbian protection is hard to find unless you improvise. (23-year-old femme)

> [I am] taken by a moment – I don't think at that time. (29-year-old 'other')

In conversations about safe sex between women, many lesbians mention that the existing safe-sex techniques available for lesbian women are 'not sexy; they are too clinical; they spoil the moment; are very ugly/unattractive, and impossible to use'. One respondent agreed with these sentiments and wrote, 'Dental dams – they're a disaster, they just don't work!'

AIDS has triggered discourses of danger regarding sex and how danger relates to people's sexuality. With high rates of HIV infection in Gauteng and South Africa as a whole, one has to think twice before engaging in unprotected sex and is constantly reminded of HIV. Writing in the *Mail & Guardian Online* and citing Professor Alan Whiteside of the University of KwaZulu-Natal, a journalist reported that 'HIV prevalence in Gauteng is well over 30 per cent', and it is even higher in some other provinces; and 'HIV prevalence among women and among people between 20 and 24 years continues to increase, with 29 per cent of South African women being infected'.[2]

All respondents were asked if they ever think about HIV and AIDS, and what their thoughts are. Almost all (19) reported that they think and worry about the epidemic. Some of the thoughts and concerns that respondents had include the issue of multiple partners and unfaithfulness:

> If one…is HIV-positive then there's unfaithfulness. (27-year-old butch)
>
> My partner slept around a lot. It worried me till I got tested. (19-year-old femme)
>
> I had many partners and…thinking about contracting the virus. (20-year-old butch)

Others mentioned that they were aware of people who have HIV or have died of AIDS-related illnesses and wanted to protect themselves and their partners.

> In my family six members died of HIV. (31-year-old WLW)
>
> Since I'm HIV-positive I worry about infecting my partner. (28-year-old femme)

There were those who felt that while they did think and worry about the epidemic, they still did not know their status and do little to protect themselves. They reported:

> I did (think) about it, but it did not bother us that much. (26-year-old lesbian)
>
> I don't know my status. (20-year-old lesbian)
>
> Most of the time I don't use protection. (24-year-old lesbian)
>
> I know I can contract sexual infections but have not done anything to protect myself. (21-year-old femme)

The rest reported that they do not really worry because 'it's for heteros' and 'I'm in constant check of status and practise safe sex'.

These findings are not in total contrast to those where 57 per cent of lesbian women reported that they have never been in a situation where they could have contracted HIV, and 53 per cent said that they don't think they are at risk of being HIV-positive (Wells et al. 2006). However, high rates of HIV are still present within the 'lesbian community'. These could be attributed to rape, sexual violence, bisexual partners, and unsafe transactional sex with men.

### Sex, pleasure and performance

With all the concerns that respondents have about getting infected or infecting each other, one may wonder how this concern expresses itself in sexual activity and behaviour. The study investigated whether there were times when respondents felt that sex was not as 'rosy and beautiful' as they portrayed it at the beginning. When asked what bad sex was and if they had ever experienced it, more than half (14) of the respondents said they had experienced bad sex. Many described bad sex as 'not mutual pleasure'; 'painful and rushed'; 'when the other partner is forced to engage in it'; 'when my partner inserts her fingers in my vagina'; 'sleeping with a robot'; 'having it with someone who does not know what's going on'; 'one-sided sex'; 'selfish partner: when she's done she doesn't want to be touched or comes before me'.

Those who had experienced bad sex said that they felt 'used', 'irritated', 'unsatisfied', 'horrible and dirty', 'bad', and some 'questioned what was going on'. A few gave accounts of the consequences or how bad sex happened with their partner. Some mention 'cheating' as a result. Others said it was related to performance and enjoyment, which meant that there was no orgasm or pleasure: 'I was powerless and stopped before the other person was satisfied' (20-year-old lesbian). 'I felt like I'm giving everything and receiving nothing' (28-year-old femme).

Respondents continued to talk about their concerns about sexual performance. Of those who said that they have worried about their performance (10), reasons such as 'thinking too much', 'being drunk', 'being sober', 'concerns about pleasing a new sexual partner', 'not in the mood', 'silence during sex', 'stress and tiredness' were given as obstacles to optimum sexual performance.

When asked to comment on their sexual performance, most respondents felt that they were 'very good' and, without being prompted, some even rated themselves out of a score of 10. The lowest rating was 7.5, with most respondents ranging between 8 and 10. However, while many boasted about their excellent performance, a few reported that they are concerned when their partner is not satisfied or when they are not doing their best sexually.

One concern was related to not practising safe sex:

> When I see, feel or sense she was not satisfied or she tells me there's something I didn't do well. (30-year-old femme)

> Most of the time I worry 'cos we're having sex without protection and I'm not giving it all. (28-year-old femme)

The previous sections reiterate the importance of sex in lesbian relationships. When sex takes place, issues relating to HIV and AIDS, as well as performance, have to be constantly negotiated. Lesbian sex can be risky, particularly when protective measures such as dental dams, gloves or condoms are not used. What emanates from the above discussions is that it is difficult to negotiate safety within a lesbian sexual relationship, as protective measures are not only unavailable, but also unpleasant and not 'sexy'. So, many women are compromised and some delay finding out their HIV status or ignore an infection when something has 'gone wrong'. There continues to be a gap in public health education and campaigns focusing on sexual relationships. Most public health campaigns target heterosexual couples, and marginalise same-sex relationships. There is a need for such campaigns to address women who have sex with women, as clearly many lack sufficient information and resources and thus engage in sexual practices that can put them at risk.

## Conclusions

There is a huge gap in lesbian research in South Africa about what it means to be a lesbian. Studies that have looked at lesbians have assumed homogeneity among this very diverse group. Women in same-sex erotic relationships define and identify themselves in various ways. While some choose to identify as lesbian, others take on more gender-related roles as their forms of identification. These forms of identification have various meanings and practices with regards to sex, sexuality and sexual performance.

While the gap in lesbian research widens, an even larger gap continues to grow in relation to studies on lesbian sexuality and safe sex. The limited research in this area has only looked at HIV testing practices and HIV prevalence in the gay and lesbian community. Such research shows high rates of HIV infection in the lesbian community, but does not explore why this is the case. Because lesbian women are not thought to be at risk, they are not targeted in the numerous HIV prevention campaigns in the country. This has an impact on testing practices, access to information about HIV transmission among lesbian women, and the practising of safer sex.

Respondents in this study show that there is a general concern about HIV and safety with regards to sex with a woman. Because many people do not know their status, and because there is a lack of (sexy and pleasant) protective methods for lesbian women, HIV continues to be a concern and affects pleasure and performance.

## Notes

1. 'Partnered' is a term used in the lesbian circles in Johannesburg to distinguish between those who are available and open to casual sexual partners and those generally not available (that is, already in a sexual relationship).
2. Y Rampersadh, 'HIV/AIDS rate in Gauteng at 30%'. *Mail & Guardian Online*, 6 October 2005. Accessed October 2007 at http://www.mg.co.za/article/2005-10-06-hivaids-rate-in-gauteng-at-30.

## References

Blyth S (1989) An exploration of accounts of lesbian identities. MA thesis, University of Cape Town

Calhoun C (1995) The gender closet: Lesbian disappearance under the sign 'women'. *Feminist Studies* 21(1): 7–34

De Waal S & Manion A (Eds) (2006) *Pride, protest and celebration*. Johannesburg: Jacana Media

Dirsuweit T (1999) Carceral spaces in South Africa: A case study of institutional power, sexuality and transgression in a women's prison. *Geoforum* 30(1): 71–83

Doan L (1994) What's in and out there? Disciplining the lesbian. *American Literary History* (Curriculum and Criticism) 6(3): 572–582

Faderman L (1981) *Surpassing the love of men: Romantic friendship and love between women from the renaissance to the present*. New York: William Morrow & Co

Farquhar C (2000) Lesbian in a post-lesbian world? Policing identity, sex and image. *Sexualities* 3(2): 219–236

Ferguson A (1981) Patriarchy, sexual identity and the sexual revolution. *Signs* 7(1): 158–172

Gay J (1985) 'Mummies and babies' and friends and lovers in Lesotho. *Journal of Homosexuality* 11(3–4): 97–116

Gevisser M (1994) A different fight for freedom: A history of South African gay and lesbian organizations from the 1950s to 1990s. In M Gevisser & E Cameron (Eds) *Defiant desire: Gay and lesbian lives in South Africa*. Johannesburg: Ravan Press

Gevisser M & Cameron E (Eds) (1994) *Defiant desire: Gay and lesbian lives in South Africa*. Johannesburg: Ravan Press

Hoad N, Martin K & Reid G (Eds) (2005) *Sex and politics in South Africa: Lesbian and gay rights under the new Constitution*. Cape Town: Double Storey Books

Kendall J (1998) When a woman loves a woman in Lesotho. In S Murray & W Roscoe (Eds) *Boy–wives and female husbands: Studies of African homosexualities*. New York: St Martin's Press

Kitzinger C (1987) *The social construction of lesbianism*. London: SAGE Publications

Kitzinger C & Wilkinson S (1995) Transitions from heterosexuality to lesbianism: The discursive production of lesbian identities. Special issue: Sexual orientation and human development. *Developmental Psychology* 31(1): 95–104

Leap W (2005) Finding the centre: Claiming gay space in Cape Town. In M van Zyl & M Steyn (Eds) *Performing queer: Shaping sexualities, 1994–2004* (Vol. 1). Cape Town: Kwela Books

Morgan R & Wieringa S (2005) *Tommy boys, lesbian men and ancestral wives*. Johannesburg: Jacana Media

Muholi Z (2004) Thinking through lesbian rape. *Agenda* 61: 116–125

Nestle J (1981) Butch-femme relationships: Sexual courage in the 1950s. *Heresies* 12 (reprinted in J Nestle [1987] *A restricted country*. New York: Firebrand)

Newman S (2002) Silent witness? Ailleen Palmer and the problem of evidence in lesbian history. *Women's History Review* 11(3): 505–530

Posel D (2004) Getting the nation talking about sex: Reflection on the discursive constitution of sexuality in South Africa since 1994. *Agenda* 62: 53–63

Potgieter C (1997) Black, South African, lesbian: Discourses of invisible lives. PhD dissertation, University of the Western Cape

Rich A (1993) Compulsory heterosexuality and lesbian existence. In H Abelove, MA Barale & DM Halperin (Eds) *The lesbian and gay studies reader*. New York: Routledge

Shefer T & Potgieter C (2006) Sexualities. In T Shefer, F Boonzaier & P Kiguwa (Eds) *The gender of psychology*. Cape Town: University of Cape Town Press

Swarr AL & Nagar R (2003) Dismantling assumptions: Interrogating 'lesbian' struggles for identity and survival in India and South Africa. *Signs: Journal of Women in Culture and Society* 29(2): 491–516

Wells H, Judge M & Kruger T (2006) *Experiences and dimensions of power: Discussions with lesbian women.* Pretoria: OUT LGBT Well-being

Wells H & Polders L (2006a) Anti-gay hate crimes in South Africa: Prevalence, reporting practices, and experiences of the police. *Agenda* 67(2–3): 20–28

Wells H & Polders L (2006b) *HIV and sexually transmitted infections (STIs) among gay and lesbian people in Gauteng: Prevalence and testing practices.* Pretoria: OUT LGBT Well-being

Wieringa SE (2005) *Globalization, love, intimacy and silence in a working class Butch/Fem community in Jakarta.* Amsterdam School for Social Science Research, Working Paper No. WP0508, University of Amsterdam

Zimmerman B (1981) What has never been: An overview of lesbian feminist literary criticism. *Feminist Studies* 7(3): 451–475

## Archival sources

Gay and Lesbian Memory in Action (GALA) archive. Life Histories. Historical Papers Department, William Cullen Library, University of the Witwatersrand, East Campus, Johannesburg

CHAPTER NINE

# Creating memory: Documenting and disseminating life stories of LGBTI people living with HIV

Ruth Morgan, Busi Kheswa and John Meletse

The GALA (Gay and Lesbian Memory in Action) Archives, currently housed at the University of the Witwatersrand in Johannesburg, is in many ways an activist archive striving to construct and record memory related to same-sex experience and practices in South Africa.[1] Since the archive was established in 1997 we have been collecting material related to HIV in the lesbian, gay, bisexual and transgender and intersex (LGBTI) sector. We have extensive coverage from the early 1980s onwards, including press clippings, individual collections – such as the Simon Nkoli collection and the Barry McGeary collection – and organisational records from the Township Aids Project in Soweto and the Triangle Project in Cape Town.

In 2002 we realised that there was a huge gap in the records regarding personal narratives that could convey the complexity of living with HIV for LGBTI individuals. GALA's HIV oral history project was thus initially established in conjunction with Mpumi Njinge (a talented young gay film maker) to bring these voices into the archive. Our aim was to engage meaningfully with people and to promote dialogue at different levels, focusing not only on the telling of personal stories but also on repackaging the information for our LGBTI communities, by creating products such as a community theatre performance and educational comics based on the narratives, in order to break the silence and stigma surrounding living with HIV.

## Documenting life stories

Less than a year before he died, Mpumi – who refused to disclose his own HIV status in the LGBTI community – discussed the urgency he felt in collecting the stories of other people he knew living with HIV. One of these people was Tshidi, a well-known drag queen in Soweto who owned a shebeen. Mpumi was shocked to see how ill Tshidi was and was determined to get his life story because Tshidi had been his mentor and role model when they were 'coming out' as young teenagers in Kwa Thema. A couple of months later Tshidi died and, needless to say, Mpumi never got his story. Mpumi then managed to do some interviews documenting his own life but unfortunately he got ill and died before we recorded his full story. At that point we realised we had to do something in order to break the silence and stigma in the LGBTI sector and start a dialogue around HIV. We had to find a way to engage our community.

In 2003 GALA staff members Busi Kheswa and the Reverend Paul Mokgethi, from the Hope and Unity Metropolitan Community Church, started collecting life stories as part of our HIV outreach and oral history project. Paul has collected life stories from gay men and Busi has focused on lesbians. Ruth Morgan interviewed GALA colleague John Meletse who is Deaf, gay and HIV-positive. The interview process proved difficult in many ways – people would repeatedly cancel scheduled interviews. Even people who had openly disclosed their status seemed very resistant to being interviewed. When interviews did take place, some women felt traumatised as their interviews re-evoked the experience of being raped and the interviewers also often felt traumatised by the issues raised in the interviews and the fact that the people they interviewed were their friends.

Despite these difficulties, GALA had collected a total of 23 life story interviews by December 2006, including 15 from gay men and 8 from lesbians living with HIV. This is a significant accomplishment given the continued stigma and silence around HIV. A few of these stories are outlined below.

Two young lesbians – Buhle Msibi and Busi Sigasa – both of whom were involved with the Forum for the Empowerment of Women, contracted HIV after being raped. Buhle died in 2006 and Busi died in early 2007. Buhle was date-raped by a man she knew well who couldn't accept she was a lesbian. Her life story highlights the problems she had accessing her social grant as a result of the social worker's homophobia – the latter was a devout Christian. Busi's life story focuses on her reluctance to go to an HIV clinic due to the stigma attached to being identified as an HIV patient. As a result, she delayed receiving antiretroviral treatment for a period of at least six months, at a time when she needed medication that may have saved her life.

The life story of a gay man – Paul Mokgethi – focuses on the issue of disclosure to his family of being HIV-positive, and the quadruple stigma of being a priest who is gay, HIV-positive, and involved in a relationship with a white man. He described how his family had to come to terms with all these aspects of his life.

John Meletse is employed by GALA. His testimony is of a man who, as mentioned, is Deaf, gay and HIV-positive. The first time he went for an HIV test, he tested negative and was determined to practise safe sex and use preventative measures. He was later date-raped by his hearing boyfriend who mixed alcohol into his drink without his knowledge. They then had unprotected sex without John's knowledge and John only discovered what had happened the following morning. He does not remember anything about the actual experience.

His second HIV test was conducted by a hearing heterosexual doctor at a clinic in Soweto who gave him no pre- or post-test counselling. The nursing sisters were

## LIFE STORIES OF LGBTI PEOPLE LIVING WITH HIV

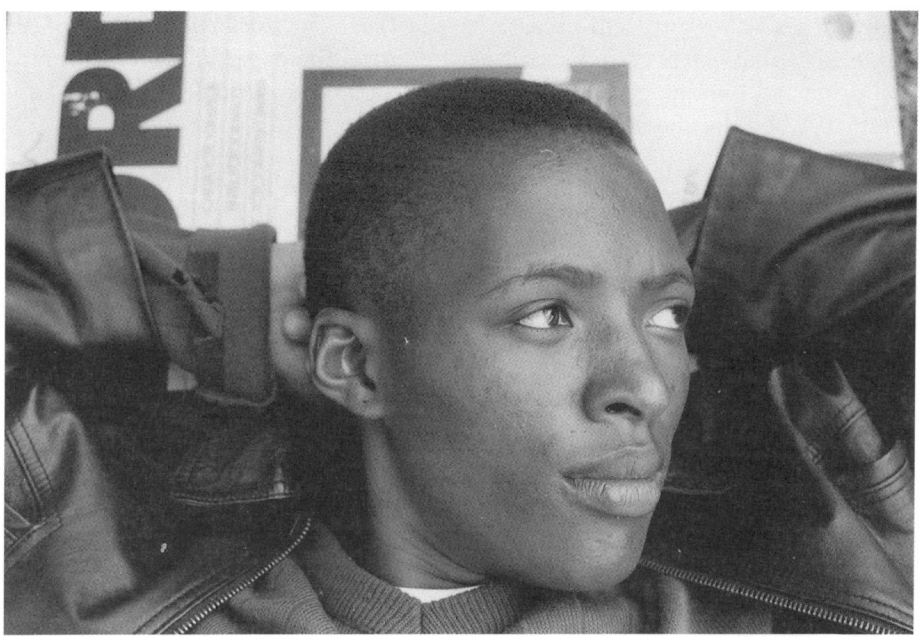

The life stories of these two young lesbians, Buhle Msibi (above) and Busi Sigasa (below) were recorded by GALA. Both women were involved with the Forum for the Empowerment of Women and both contracted HIV after being raped. Buhle died in 2006 and Busi died in early 2007.

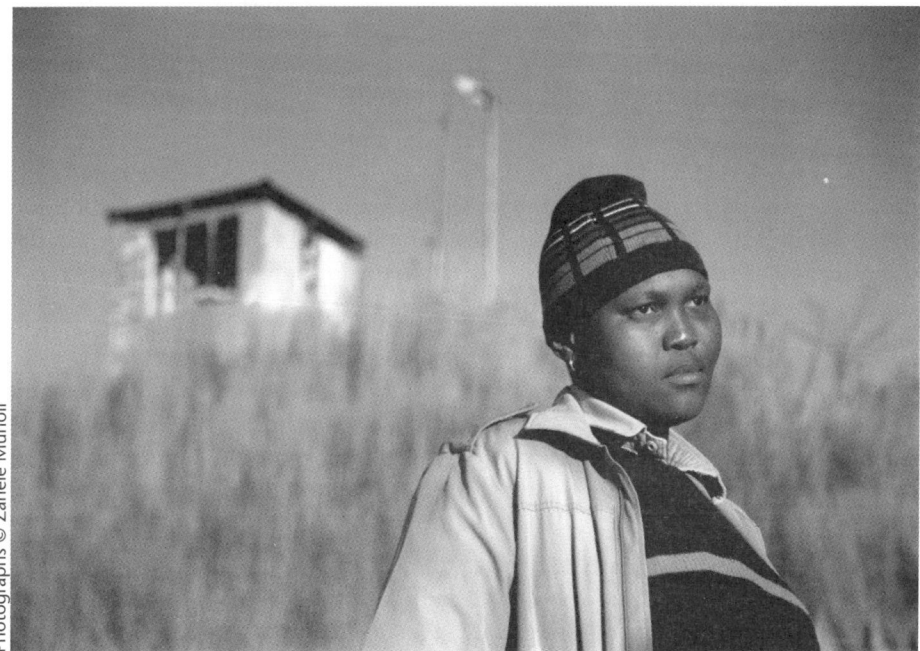

Photographs © Zanele Muholi

also patronising towards him because he was Deaf. The doctor wrote 'YOU ARE HIV+' in capital letters on a piece of paper, shoved the paper in front of his face and dismissed him. No sign language interpreters were available. He was totally traumatised by the diagnosis.

Fortunately, his grandmother was very supportive during this time, as were his GALA colleagues. As a gay, Deaf person living with HIV, John wanted to be a role model for Deaf LGBTI and heterosexual youth, and all Deaf HIV-positive people. He currently conducts training workshops on sexual diversity and HIV for Deaf adults and Deaf youth and discloses his HIV and gay status to his audiences. John emphasises that there is still a lot of stigma in the Deaf community and in Deaf schools around HIV and about being LGBTI.[2]

## Disseminating HIV-related outreach materials

Once we had collected a number of life stories, in 2005 the focus of our project shifted to repackaging the material into a number of outreach products for the LGBTI community in order to continue and deepen the dialogue.

### Coming Out Again (2005/06)

In 2005, GALA, in collaboration with various directors, artists and media organisations, developed a community theatre production called *Coming Out Again*. The aim of the production was to share the stories of HIV-positive people in the LGBTI community. This theatre production was performed in 2005 and 2006. It reflected the stories of real South African people and their wider struggle for human rights by highlighting aspects of the life stories of HIV-positive and LGBTI people. It depicted their experiences with HIV, such as coping with loved ones who are positive, remaining HIV-negative, and life after learning one is HIV-positive. Each performance lasted approximately 45 minutes and was followed by a facilitated post-performance discussion, led by Jason Wessenaar of the Centre for the Study of AIDS. Each performance had South African Sign Language (SASL) interpretation, both for Deaf actor John Meletse and for the audience. An additional five performances of *Coming Out Again* were presented during a national tour of Durban, Pietermaritzburg and Cape Town.

### Talking About Us (2006/07)

In 2006/07 GALA started to film a documentary called *Talking About Us*, based on *Coming Out Again*. The production team included film maker Donne Rundle and GALA trainee film maker and staff member Busi Kheswa. The documentary shows six ordinary young people telling their stories. The autobiographical element is essential, but the film is also infused with daily life, depicting people who are in the process of deepening their self-awareness while at the same time facing complex conflicts peculiar to their generation. The film shows a part of the microcosm of the new society in South Africa.

Due to lack of funding, this documentary has never been completed.

## *Eyes Wide Open* and *Are Your Rights Respected?* (2006)

The LGBTI community has been left out of most development communication programmes in the country, and so a comic book called *Eyes Wide Open* was designed as a fun, informative way to reflect the stories and experiences of the gay and lesbian community. The comic is based on the issues raised in the theatrical production, as well as additional issues and feedback raised during various consultative workshops.

A storyline was developed which was first tested with LGBTI organisations and members of the community. Once the storyline had been refined, it was then expressed in graphic images and text, and two pages of information were included. The comic was then tested again via two focus group sessions, and changes were made to the storyline and language to reflect the feedback from this process.

In August 2006, an educational comic *Are Your Rights Respected?* was launched. The comic aimed at raising awareness among Deaf youth and deals with the issue of sexual rights, including LGBTI and HIV issues. The project was funded by the Foundation for Human Rights, HIVOS and Atlantic Philanthropies. The comic incorporates SASL, and is specifically aimed at Deaf people. Given the failure of Deaf education in South Africa and the fact that the average literacy level of Deaf adults here is at Grade 4, the comic book format was seen as being the most accessible medium of communication. The comic has minimal English text.

John Meletse was instrumental in creating this comic, which included a narrative around a schoolboy 'coming out' to his friend and his teacher. This mainstreaming of gay issues into broader sexual rights issues was very successful. The comic is being used by the World Bank as evidence of good practice, and as part of its work on the intersection between disability and HIV/AIDS.

## A pilot project in life orientation for Deaf learners

In 2007, GALA commissioned an HIV training consultant to pilot *Are Your Rights Respected?* at Sizwile School for the Deaf in Soweto.

The pilot project consisted of:
- Two HIV and AIDS information sessions for all teaching staff at Sizwile.
- Six HIV and AIDS training sessions with five Deaf facilitators, including two Deaf teaching assistants, two Deaf teachers from Sizwile School, and GALA staff member John Meletse.

- The development of supplementary learning material for Deaf learners (three worksheets were developed focusing on HIV and AIDS, harming and helping, and sexual orientation and friendship).
- Twelve lessons with learners from Grades 7 to 12 co-facilitated by John Meletse, teaching assistants and teachers, and monitored by the consultant.

A lot of discomfort was experienced by the learners when they discussed issues of homosexuality. A large proportion of male and female learners expressed negative views towards homosexuals. Although there were learners who were willing to accept a friend who was gay, the majority (of those who expressed opinions) felt that they would not be able to accept a gay friend, that they did not understand why people would 'choose' to be gay, and many questions were posed about gay sex. As a result, the project was continued in 2007 by John Meletse, who conducted weekly sensitisation sessions focusing on issues of sexuality, HIV and tolerance at Sizwile School for learners in Grades 8 to 12.

## Digital story projects (2006/07)

GALA staff member Busi Kheswa's digital story *I Have Listened, I Have Heard* was produced as part of a WomensNet digital story project, *Digital Stories for Transformation*,[3] focusing on violence against women, including lesbians. Her story focuses on her experiences interviewing lesbians who are now HIV-positive as a result of hate crimes involving rape. In early 2007 the Open Society Institute for Southern Africa ran a digital story project with an HIV focus for southern Africa. GALA colleagues John Meletse and Paul Mokgethi participated in this project and produced digital stories based on aspects of their lives as HIV-positive gay men.

## Conclusion

GALA's HIV oral history and outreach project aims to construct memory around the complexity of the issues surrounding being both HIV-positive and LGBTI. Our outreach work ensures that this information is repackaged into innovative products which reach both the LGBTI and the Deaf community.

## Notes

1. For more information on GALA's approach to documenting memory using oral history projects, see Manion and Morgan (2006); Morgan (2003).
2. For an in-depth discussion of John's experiences of 'coming out' as a gay man and being diagnosed as HIV-positive, see Meletse and Morgan (2006).
3. Digital stories are stories produced, stored and disseminated using various digital media such as mobile phones, email and the internet.

## References

Luczak R (Ed.) (2007) *Eyes of desire 2: A Deaf GLBT reader*. Minneapolis: Handtype Press

Manion A & Morgan R (2006) The Gay and Lesbian Archives: Documenting same-sex sexuality in an African context. *Agenda:* 67(2–3): 29–35

Meletse J & Morgan R (2006) I have two! Personal reflections of a Deaf HIV positive gay man in South Africa. In C Schmaling & L Monaghan (Eds) *HIV/AIDS and Deaf communities* (A special issue of *Deaf Worlds*) (Reprinted in shortened form in Luczak 2007)

Morgan R (2003) 'So it is African although they were hiding it': Same-sex sangomas and the indigenous oral archive. *Archives and Indigenous Peoples* (A special edition of *Comma – The International Journal on Archives*)

Morgan R (2008) *Deaf me normal: Deaf South Africans tell their stories*. Pretoria: University of South Africa Press

# PERSPECTIVES FROM SUB-SAHARAN AND SOUTHERN AFRICA

There is a politics called public health politics, which gets you published in prestigious journals and in those journals you would use phrases like MSM: 'MSM venues', 'township MSM', 'younger MSM', 'MSM who have both male and female partners' and 'MSM who bridge with women'. That is the language of those journals and good luck to you in your future careers when you publish in them. But is that the language that does justice to the realities here in South Africa? I have no doubt it is the language that does justice to some realities in the USA although actually among real American men I talked to, it doesn't do much justice to their realities. It does justice to academic careers. And I really wonder what South Africa, southern Africa and Africa in general deserves. Does it deserve the frames, the tropes, the illusions of the North, of America, of Europe, perhaps of the south of Australia? Or does it actually deserve respect and the kinds of language and conceptual struggles that might allow us all to be surprised? *Peter Aggleton, conference delegate*

People who participate in research should get their information back. Once we signed agreements with researchers stating that the study findings would make their way back to us. One of the researchers sent an electronic version via the internet – a 150-page document to people who have hotmail addresses…to people who access the internet from internet cafes where they pay per half hour and anything between R1 and R2.50 a page. So now people have received the information, but there is nothing they can do with it. In fact they can't even open the document properly, forget about read it. The other thing is that the information is written…by an academic. The language is such that people can do very little with it.

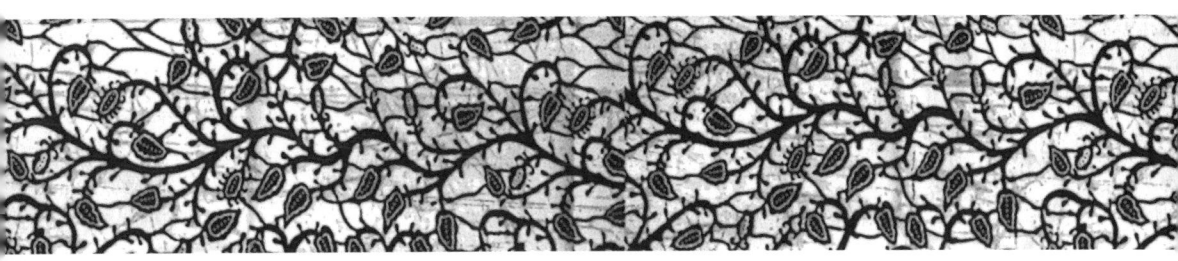

And so what we do now is agree on how the information is going to make its way back. That researchers promise to come back to us…that they do a little presentation. And if there are too many people, then they train people…to go out and do that presentation to others. But get the information out so that it has meaning and so that people can really benefit from *Ian Swartz, conference delegate*

## CHAPTER TEN

# What we know about same-sex practising people and HIV in Africa

Cary Alan Johnson

By the mid-1980s, AIDS in Africa was being referred to as a 'heterosexual epidemic', in contrast to the association of the disease in other parts of the world with gay men (and later with other marginalised groups, such as Haitians, intravenous drug users, and haemophiliacs). Early African male AIDS patients claimed that they had never engaged in sex with other men, and the world was eager to believe them. The facile acceptance of these claims was, I argue, the product of a racist belief in the hypersexuality (and, furthermore, the hyper-*heteronormative* sexuality) of African men.

The construction of a universally heterosexual African HIV/AIDS epidemic has led to a 'sloppy and ideological science', according to historian Marc Epprecht (2004). Scientists and policy-makers have been slow to acknowledge the possibility that same-sex male transmission is playing an important role in HIV transmission in Africa and have put little effort into understanding the links between hetero- and homosexual HIV transmission.

In March 2005, Cáceres et al. (2005) reviewed 561 studies on HIV and men who have sex with men in non-Western settings. Of these, 224 focused on Latin America and 235 on Asia, with only eight addressing same-sex transmission in Africa. The paucity of research on HIV and same-sex practices in Africa is the result of a multiplicity of factors that include:
- The hesitancy of those who engage in same-sex practices to expose themselves to potentially judgemental researchers;
- Resistance by African research review panels to approve research on homosexuality;
- A general unwillingness among otherwise rigorous scientists to address same-sex transmission due to their discomfort with homosexuality;
- Homophobic stigma faced by HIV researchers themselves when addressing issues of homosexuality;
- Denial of the frequency of same-sex behaviour in Africa;
- The misconception that same-sex practising women face no significant HIV-related health threats.

Opportunities for collecting data on homosexual behaviour and attitudes toward homosexuality are consistently neglected. While behavioural surveillance surveys are conducted throughout Africa by governments and their partners – mainly non-governmental organisations, UN agencies, and academic institutions – in order to collect data for public health and economic development programmes, these studies have avoided including questions related to same-sex conduct. The 2001 study Sexual Behaviour of Young People in Botswana (SIAPAC 2001), conducted by UNICEF, UNAIDS, Population Services International, the government of Botswana, and the African Youth Alliance of Botswana, provides a large and useful database for public health enquiries, but asked not a single question on the issue of homosexuality. The behavioural survey conducted by the National AIDS Control Programme of Tanzania and UNAIDS, designed to 'track trends in HIV/AIDS-related knowledge, attitudes, and behaviors in subpopulations at particular risk of HIV infection', failed to ask about behaviour, identity, or attitudes related to same-sex desire (Tungaraza n.d.). These examples represent lost opportunities to broaden our knowledge of sexual behaviour and attitudes among young people in Africa.

Similarly, the Guttmacher Institute (2006) asked more than 20 000 young people from four African countries questions related to sexuality, family life and health, but failed to ask a single question that might have provided data about same-sex behaviour. While Guttmacher researchers asked important questions about (heterosexual) anal sex, they and their local partners felt that their respondents were too young to be questioned about sexual orientation. If questions related to same-sex identity and behaviour are never asked, there will never be any relevant data collected, and claims that homosexuality doesn't exist in Africa will continue unchallenged.

Scholars who undertake research on non-heteronormative sexuality may face derision and 'gay-baiting', defined as the practice of using ideas or prejudices about someone's sexuality to intimidate or silence them (Rothschild 2005). Researchers at the universities of Nairobi in Kenya and Cheikh Anta Diop in Senegal experienced significant stigma while conducting research on men who have sex with men (MSM). One of the leading researchers on the topic, Dr Amadou Moreau of the Population Council in Senegal, reported that 'because homosexuality is so stigmatized, as a researcher I am stigmatized as well, by family, friends, and community'.

## Some of the key studies

### Behavioural research

The Horizons Program was the first international NGO to recognise that the HIV-related vulnerabilities of MSM in Africa deserved serious attention. Horizons is a USAID-funded programme, implemented by a consortium of organisations including the Population Council, International Center for Research on Women, International HIV/AIDS Alliance, Program for Appropriate Technology in Health, Tulane University, Family Health International, and Johns Hopkins University. Horizons has produced two ground-breaking studies on MSM in Africa, based on research conducted in Dakar, Senegal, in 2002, and in Nairobi, Kenya, in 2005. These studies have provided important information about stigma, violence, identity, secrecy, and sexual practices among MSM, particularly younger men in urban settings.

Horizons collaborated with a number of local partners, including government agencies, academic institutions and organisations of MSM, creating a broad base of interest and support for this work at the country level. The Senegal research was conducted in collaboration with Cheikh Anta Diop University and the Senegalese National AIDS Control Programme. The Kenya research was undertaken in partnership with the University of Nairobi Institute of African Studies.

In March 2004, a study was conducted by the Ghana National AIDS Control Programme, using questionnaires completed by 156 MSM in the greater Accra area as an assessment tool with which to guide future programming (Attipoe 2004). In Uganda, Semugoma (2005) conducted ethnographic research to identify the health needs of same-sex practising men and women. In 2003, the University of California at San Francisco's (UCSF) Center for AIDS Prevention Studies (CAPS), in collaboration with Makerere University in Kampala, conducted research with more than 300 MSM in Uganda, but the results have yet to be made public. A participatory community assessment was conducted in Algeria, Morocco and Tunisia between September 2005 and June 2006 in which 193 MSM engaged in an analysis of their HIV-related needs and situations and proposed a number of solutions (International HIV/AIDS Alliance 2005). This research was conducted by three African AIDS service organisations, including the Association de Lutte Contre le SIDA (Morocco) in collaboration with the International HIV/AIDS Alliance. OUT LGBT Well-being (OUT) in Gauteng, South Africa, has answered critical questions about the attitudes and sexual health of same-sex practising men and women in South Africa in their reports *Research Findings on the Sexual Practices of Young Gay Men in South Africa* (OUT 2005), and *Gay and Lesbian People's Experience of the Health Care Sector in Gauteng* (OUT n.d.). The UCSF CAPS (Lane et al. 2006) and OUT (Wells & Polders 2005) in South Africa have both conducted important research on the uptake of voluntary counselling and testing by lesbian, gay, bisexual and transgendered (LGBT) people.

Understanding how LGBT people perceive their access to healthcare is an important aspect of designing effective sexual health interventions. The health-seeking behaviour of African LGBTs is described in OUT's (n.d.) *Gay and Lesbian People's Experience of the Health Care Sector in Gauteng* and by Ehlers et al. (2001) in *The Well-being of Gays, Lesbians and Bisexuals in Botswana*. In the latter, data from 47 questionnaires completed by gay, lesbian and bisexual respondents in Botswana were analysed in order to examine issues related to treatment at healthcare facilities, alcohol and drug use, and perceived HIV risk.

Researchers have begun to examine the sexual aspects of various homosocial situations and settings, such as among mineworkers, prisoners, soldiers, boys living on the streets, and in the context of certain initiation rituals. Additional research is needed in order to understand this previously hidden male–male sexual behaviour, and the levels of HIV-related risk. Many of the men involved may unwittingly become what Semugoma (2005) refers to as 'amplifying populations' with regard to the spread of HIV in the larger community.

Sadly, the marginalisation that many same-sex practising people experience in their daily lives is reflected in research related to the impact of HIV on their lives (and again in the implementation of HIV/AIDS programmes based on that research). While African MSM were involved in the research that has been conducted in Ghana, Nigeria, Kenya and Senegal, they mainly functioned as research assistants, brought in to provide 'access to MSM communities'. They played little role in conceptualising the research, developing the research instruments or, ultimately, in analysing the results.

This has led to bias and misinterpretation of data. To cite but one example, the author of this chapter was told by the non-LGBT director of a West African research team that most of the MSM whom he had interviewed during a pre-project assessment had engaged in their first homosexual experience with a foreigner. When the author examined the data together with the researcher, it became clear that less than one-third of the respondents reported an initial homosexual encounter with an expatriate. The researcher's bias had caused him to read his own perception, that homosexuality was externally imposed, onto the data, despite evidence to the contrary.[1]

There are few openly gay or lesbian African social scientists or biomedical specialists involved in AIDS research, and most African LGBT organisations lack the capacity to conduct robust scientific research without technical assistance. LGBT communities express great appreciation for the efforts of non-LGBT researchers, without whom even this small amount of data would not exist. Nevertheless, researchers must find creative, meaningful ways of involving same-sex practising men and women in the design, analysis, dissemination and implementation of scientific research.

## Seroprevalence research

Abdoulaye Wade, chief of the STI/AIDS Level Two Division at the Senegalese Ministry of Health, conducted the first seroprevalence study of same-sex practising men in Africa in 2005 (Wade et al. 2005). The research protocol consisted of the implementation of a questionnaire, physical examination, and detection of HIV through serum samples of MSM in five Senegalese cities. Of 442 respondents, Wade et al. found HIV infection serology in the blood samples of 96 (21.5 per cent). By comparison, the overall seroprevalence rate for adult males in Senegal is 0.2 per cent while the seroprevalence rate for female sex workers is 27.1 per cent (UNAIDS 2006).

Similarly, unofficial results from seroprevalence studies of MSM conducted by the HIV Vaccine Initiative in Kenya suggest a seroprevalence rate of 40 per cent or higher, while the general seroprevalence rate for Kenya is 6.1 per cent among adults aged 15 to 49.[2] A behavioural and seroprevalence survey among MSM in Ghana has revealed similar early results.[3] Tim Lane of CAPS interprets this data to suggest that seroprevalence among MSM could also be much higher than that of the general population in the higher seroprevalence countries of southern Africa, for which no same-sex specific HIV surveillance has been conducted. According to Lane, 'We should not be surprised if we see 40 or 50 per cent of MSM infected in countries like South Africa and Zimbabwe.'[4]

All of the available HIV seroprevalence data for women who have sex with women in Africa is self-reported, and therefore is likely to be under-represented. In a survey of 123 women who identified as lesbian in Tshwane (formerly Pretoria), South Africa, 9 per cent of black and 5 per cent of white women reported that they were HIV-positive. In a 2002 study conducted by the Human Sciences Research Council in South Africa, 13 per cent of lesbian women (15–49 years of age) self-reported a positive HIV test result (cited in Wells & Polders 2005: 2). While this rate is lower than seroprevalence rates for heterosexual South African women, it still represents a substantial number of people for whom there currently exist no targeted HIV prevention, treatment or care services.

One caution is necessary when interpreting the research that has been conducted on same-sex practising men and women in Africa: the use of 'snowball' (non-random) sampling relies on respondents to recruit peers for participation in the research, who in turn recruit their peers, and so on. This technique may lead to an overly homogenised sample and a potential skewing of the data in ways that random sampling can avoid. Instances of unprotected sex, violence and sex work, for example, are likely to be higher among a cohort of MSM who are young, urban and economically marginalised, than in the larger population of MSM.

As of 2007, seroprevalence research was being conducted among MSM by LGBT groups in five southern African countries, with technical assistance from Johns Hopkins University and funding from the Open Society Institute. This research should provide governments, donors and NGOs with irrefutable proof of the need to increase prevention, treatment and care projects specifically targeting gay and bisexual African men.

## What the available research indicates about HIV and same-sex practices in Africa

Though limited in scope, depth and duration, the research that has been conducted has revealed some consistent findings that provide critical information for understanding homosexualities in Africa and for launching effective HIV interventions. Some of the more salient results are discussed below.

Most African MSM have also engaged in sexual relations with women. Among MSM interviewed in Dakar and Nairobi, 88 per cent and 69 per cent respectively had had sexual relations with a woman at least once in their lives. Of those respondents in Nairobi who had had sex with a woman, 20 per cent had engaged in heterosexual vaginal sex in the last month.

MSM harbour some significant misperceptions that may increase vulnerability to HIV infections. These include the false beliefs that HIV and sexually transmitted infections (STIs) cannot be transmitted through anal sex or through sex between men; or that only the receptive partner in anal intercourse is at risk of contracting STIs; and that washing the genitals and anus with disinfectants after unprotected sex is an effective way of preventing STI and HIV transmission (International HIV/AIDS Alliance 2005).

Economic exchange plays a role in sex among the men surveyed. Two-thirds of the men interviewed in Senegal and 52 per cent of those in Kenya had 'received money' in exchange for sex with other men during the last 12 months. Twenty-nine per cent of the respondents in Kenya also reported paying for sex. No comparisons were made, however, with economic exchange among heterosexuals.

Condom use is inconsistent among MSM. Fewer than 60 per cent of same-sex practising men surveyed in Kenya reported using condoms 'always' during anal sex. In Senegal, only 23 per cent of the sample reported condom use during insertive anal sex and 14 per cent during receptive anal sex. Even fewer MSM consistently used condoms in their heterosexual encounters.

Contrary to the belief that same-sex behaviour is taught to Africans by Westerners, most respondents engaged in their first homosexual experience with another African male, mainly fellow students, neighbours or extended family members (Semugoma 2005). Fewer than 3 per cent of respondents in Kenya and less than one-third in Mali had had their first homosexual experience with a foreigner or tourist. The first homosexual experience occurred on average at age 15 years in Senegal, and 17 years in Kenya.

In research conducted in South Africa by OUT, sexual abuse of both lesbians and gay men was common. The perpetrators of this violence include police officers, neighbours, schoolmates and family members.

## HIV vulnerabilities of women who have sex with women

The myth that sexual activity between women poses no risk for HIV transmission exists among healthcare professionals as well as among many women who have sex with women (WSW), themselves. HIV has been isolated in vaginal secretions, cervical biopsies, menstrual blood and breast milk (Hughes & Evans 2003). Sexual practices, such as digital-vaginal or digital-anal contact, as well as sex with shared penetrative toys, may well serve as a means for transmission of HIV-infected cervicovaginal secretions (Marrazzo 2004).

The details surrounding the first case of female-to-female transmission were released only in February 2003 in the journal *Clinical Infectious Diseases*.[5] In this case, a 20-year-old woman with no additional risk factors other than her sexual relationship with a female partner tested positive for HIV; the infecting strain matched that of her partner. The route of transmission was determined to most likely have come from the use of sex toys (Kwakwa & Ghobrial 2003).

The lengthy delay in the verification of the first case of female-to-female transmission, and the lack of subsequent research on this transmission vector, highlights the need for additional research on the HIV risks tied to sex between women and increased sensitivity in the conduct of such research. Same-sex practising women participating in HIV research may not self-identify as lesbian or bisexual, and many studies fail to even ask female participants about their involvement in same-sex practices. In most studies, if a woman has engaged in other behaviours considered to be higher risk behaviours, the fact that she also engages in same-sex behaviour will be subsumed and ignored, therefore contributing to the invisibility of same-sex female transmission. The US Centers for Disease Control and Prevention (CDC 2006) reported that of the 246 461 cases of women found to be HIV seropositive up to December 2004, information on whether the women had had sex with women was missing in more than 60 per cent of the case reports.

In addition to the biosexual risk of HIV transmission between women, various social factors also increase exposure to HIV and challenge women's efforts to protect themselves from infection. Many WSW are pressured or forced into arranged marriages to fulfil perceived responsibility to family and/or to 'cure' homosexual behaviour. While same-sex oriented men are also forced into heterosexual marriages, women have far less ability to negotiate sex, and particularly to refuse unprotected sex. Same-sex practising and gender non-conforming women are also subjected to 'corrective' rape and other forms of sexual abuse, which in their violence and brutality pose a disproportionate risk for HIV transmission. Some same-sex attracted women may also choose relationships with men at various points in their lives as a result of economic necessity or sexual and/or romantic desire. Other risk factors for same-sex practising women include the effects of alcohol and drug abuse, including intravenous drug use, which is a very real concern for many women who lead lives characterised by marginalisation and discrimination.

According to Alicia Heath-Toby of the Lesbian AIDS Project at Gay Men's Health Crisis in New York, the information, technology, and research capabilities for studies on female-to-female transmission exist today, but obstacles such as government homophobia still stand in the way. No African women's organisations are addressing the issue of female–female transmission of HIV and, with the exception of efforts by a few LGBT groups, no prevention programming for lesbians is under way. As a result, WSW may be the most 'at risk' group of all, not due to biological susceptibility, but to sheer neglect.

## The impact on HIV/AIDS programming of minimal research on same-sex practising people

HIV prevention programmes for MSM are under way in most Asian countries, many with US government funding. Efforts to prevent HIV transmission among MSM are under way in Bangladesh, Cambodia, Vietnam, Thailand, Hong Kong, India, Indonesia and China, through the combined efforts of local LGBT groups and international NGOs, such as the Naz Foundation, Family Health International, and the International HIV/AIDS Alliance.

In September 2006, the Naz Foundation hosted a conference for organisations throughout the region engaged in work with same-sex practising men. According to Kevin Frost, Vice President for Clinical Research and Prevention Programs at the American Foundation for AIDS Research (AmFar), having good epidemiology about the impact of HIV on MSM in Asia was essential to overcoming resistance and to obtaining increased funding for programs to address same-sex transmission. AmFar manages a clearing house for HIV prevention work among MSM for organisations working in the Greater Mekong Region of Southeast Asia. Similarly, programmes for MSM in Latin America have been functioning with both national and international assistance since the early 1990s.

The failure to undertake research on HIV and same-sex practising people in Africa – particularly the lack of seroprevalence data – has undercut efforts to advocate for targeted programming. AIDS policy, planning and resource allocation is driven by statistics. While a human rights framework upholds the right of every individual to equal access to healthcare and health-related information, governments are often forced into action only when it can be proven that a statistically significant number of people in a social group are affected and in need of targeted attention. Given the continued criminalisation of consensual same-sex acts, and the absence of compassion within various African national discourses for gay men and lesbians, clear seroprevalence data are needed to effectively advocate for an increase in HIV-related services.

## Working with what we've got

There are still important gaps in our knowledge of HIV and same-sex practices in Africa. We need more seroprevalence data on both men and women, as well as answers to many unanswered questions. Are female condoms and microbiocides important tools in HIV prevention among same-sex practising men? What role is sexual violence playing in HIV transmission among same-sex practising men and women? Are there cultural differences in the sexual behaviour of same-sex practising men and women throughout the African continent that impact on HIV vulnerability? Are same-sex practising men and women playing a significant role in HIV-orphan care that could be scaled up for the benefit of affected communities?

The few HIV interventions for same-sex practising people currently under way in countries like Ghana, Senegal and Kenya would provide a rich and useful set of information if they were properly reviewed and evaluated. Best practices can also be drawn from HIV interventions targeting gay men and lesbians of African descent in other parts of the world. Work with South Asian and Latin American same-sex practising communities may also provide relevant strategies. While additional research on Africa is essential, this research gap cannot be used to justify a failure on the part of African governments and international donors to provide services to respond to the HIV-related needs of same-sex practising people.

## Acknowledgement

This chapter first appeared as Chapter 2 in *Off the map: How HIV/AIDS programming is failing same sex practicing people in Africa*, by Cary Alan Johnson, published by the IGLHRC, New York in 2007. It is reproduced here with minor amendments with kind permission from the IGLHRC.

## Notes

1. Gay men who have been subjects of HIV research also complain that insufficient effort is made to make the results of the research available to the community.
2. International Gay and Lesbian Human Rights Commission (IGLHRC) interview with staff of International HIV Vaccine Initiative, Mombasa, Kenya, 15 June 2006.
3. IGLHRC interview with Anonymous, 11 November 2006.
4. IGLHRC interview with Tim Lane, PhD, University of California San Francisco Center for AIDS Prevention Studies, 25 May 2006.
5. Other cases of female-to-female transmission had been reported in the past – as early as 1984 – but attributions of these cases were based on the absence of a history of alternative risks for HIV infection, and seem not to have been fully accepted as evidence by the medical community. For a history of case studies, see K Morrow 'Say It! Women get AIDS! HIV among lesbians', *Selfhelp Magazine* 28 May1998. www.selfhelpmagazine.com/articles/glb/womenhiv.html.

## References

Attipoe D (2004) *Fighting HIV in Ghana requires addressing homosexuality.* Accra: Ghana AIDS Commission

Cáceres CF, Konda K & Pecheny M (2005) Review of the epidemiology of male same-sex behavior in low and middle-income countries. In *Review of HIV prevalence and the epidemiology of preventive and bridging behavior among MSM in low and middle-income countries.* Geneva: UNAIDS

CDC (Centers for Disease Control and Prevention, USA) (2006) *HIV/AIDS among women who have sex with women.* Accessed June 2006, http://www.cdc.gov/hiv/topics/women/resources/factsheets/wsw.htm

Ehlers VJ, Zuyderduin A & Oosthuizen MJ (2001) The well-being of gays, lesbians and bisexuals in Botswana. *Journal of Advanced Nursing* 35(6): 848–856

Epprecht M (2004) *Hungochani: The history of dissident sexuality in southern Africa.* Montreal: McGill-Queens University Press

Guttmacher Institute (2006) *Protecting the next generation: Understanding HIV risk among youth.* Accessed October 2006, http://www.guttmacher.org/pubs/PNG-data.html

Hughes C & Evans A (2003) Health needs of women who have sex with women. *British Medical Journal* 327: 939

International HIV/AIDS Alliance (2005) Meeting the sexual health needs of men who have sex with men in North Africa and Lebanon (MSM/MALE project): International HIV/AIDS Alliance

Kwakwa HA & Ghobrial MW (2003) Female-to-female transmission of Human Immunodeficiency Virus. *Clinical Infectious Diseases* 36(3): e40–41

Lane T, McIntyre J & Morin S (2006) HIV testing and stigma among black South African MSM. Center for AIDS Prevention Studies' poster presentation to the International AIDS Conference, Toronto, Canada

Marrazzo JM (2004) Barriers to infectious disease care among lesbians. *Emerging Infectious Diseases* 10(11): 1974–1978

OUT (OUT LGBT Well-being) (2005) *Research findings on the sexual practices of young gay men in South Africa.* Johannesburg: OUT

OUT (n.d.) *Gay and lesbian people's experience of the health care sector in Gauteng.* Johannesburg: OUT

Rothschild C with Lang S & Fried (Eds) (2000/2005) Written out: How sexuality is used to attack women's organizing. New York: IGLHRC & CWGL

Semugoma P (2005) Same-sex sexual behavior, HIV, and health care in Uganda. Unpublished study

SIAPAC (Social Impact Assessment and Policy Analysis Corporation) (2001) *2001 BTW: The sexual behaviour of young people in Botswana. UNICEF evaluation report.* Accessed 2001, http://www.unicef.org/evaldatabase/index_15342.html

Tungaraza FSK (n.d.) Youth behavioral surveillance survey in Tanzania. Power Point presentation on the BSS research conducted by the National AIDS Control Programme of Tanzania and UNAIDS

UNAIDS (2006) *Report on the global AIDS epidemic.* Geneva: UNAIDS

Wade AS, Kane CT, Diallo PAN, Diop AK, Gueye K, Mboup S, Ndoye I & Lagarde E (2005) HIV infection and sexually transmitted infections among men who have sex with men in Senegal. *AIDS* 19(18): 2133–2140

Wells H & Polders L (n.d.) *Gay and lesbian people's experience of the health care sector in Gauteng.* (A research initiative of the Joint Working Group, conducted by OUT LGBT Well-Being and Unisa's Centre for Applied Psychology) Pretoria: OUT & JWG

Wells H & Polders L (2005) *HIV & sexually transmitted infections among gay & lesbian people in Gauteng: Prevalence and testing practices.* Pretoria: OUT LGBT Well-Being

CHAPTER ELEVEN

# Same-sex sexuality and HIV/AIDS: A perspective from Malawi

Daveson Nyadani

The 15th International AIDS Conference held in Bangkok, Thailand, in July 2004 called for:

> ...the creation of a supportive social, policy, and legal environment to enable MSM [men who have sex with men], as well as those with differing sexual and/or gender orientation, to more effectively respond to the HIV/AIDS epidemics in their own respective settings as equal partners in the struggle against the spread of AIDS...[1]

This plea is particularly relevant for Malawi. In this chapter I will sketch the situation around same-sex sexuality in Malawi in general, and in relation to HIV/AIDS. I will end with an overview of steps that should urgently be taken to accomplish for Malawi what the participants of the 15th International AIDS Conference called for.

## Historical background

After having been under British control in the first half of the twentieth century, Malawi became a republic and was declared a one-party state in 1966. The country was ruled by the dictator Dr Hastings Kamuzu Banda. During Banda's rule, human rights violations were rampant. Imprisonment without trial was the order of the day. In 1993, a referendum led to the establishment of a multiparty democracy with free national elections. This referendum came about after increasing domestic unrest and pressure from Malawian churches and the international community. The political transition was accompanied by accelerated economic liberalisation and structural reform.

From its colonial period, Malawi inherited the Westminster legal and constitutional framework. 'Typical of all Westminster Constitutions, they provide basic minimum structures and leave functional issues to discretion and tradition. In Africa, however, discretion has often held sway and has led to unusual and unhappy stories of plunder, genocides and ill-fated prescribed economic antidotes' (MISA 1999: 179).

## Legal situation and same-sex sexuality

In Malawi, the sexual activities of men and women with same-sex desires are criminalised according to sections 153 and 156 of the Malawian Penal Code.

Section 153 prohibits 'unnatural offences', which include sodomy, while section 156 concerning 'public decency' is used to punish homosexual acts. Foreigners who engage in same-sex sexual practices with locals can be prosecuted under article 156 and expelled as 'undesirable aliens'.

Surprisingly, these prohibitions are completely at odds with the Constitution of the Republic of Malawi. Section 20(1) of the chapter on Human Rights states that:

> Discrimination of persons in any form is prohibited and all persons are, under any law, guaranteed equal and effective protection against discrimination on grounds of race, colour, sex, language, religion, political or other opinion, nationality, ethnic or social origin, disability, property, birth or other status.

For some reason, however, sexual orientation is not considered to be included in 'other status'.

The Malawi Human Rights Resource Center has argued against this anomaly and proposed changing the Penal Code to be consistent with protecting the rights guaranteed in the Constitution. The Malawian government has, however, never taken any official position regarding issues of homosexuality. The minister of health, Marjorie Ngaunje, and the minister of information, Patricia Kaliati, have given contradictory views and Parliament has shelved proposals to amend the Penal Code on six occasions.

## Denial, culture of silence, stigmatisation and homophobia

The Malawian Penal Code reflects the existing social and cultural stigmas regarding same sex intimacy. 'We don't have homosexuals in Malawi' is a popular statement used by most people in influential positions to deny the existence of people who are gay. Malawian culture presupposes that men will marry women and women will marry men. Often this forces men and women who desire same-sex intimacy into false marriages, resulting in self-denial and denial to friends, family and spouses.

Malawian society seldom recognises the existence of sexual activity or emotional relationships between individuals of the same sex. When recognised, same-sex activities and relationships are seen as an influence (often described as a 'disease') of Western society. The denial of these activities and relationships increases the stigma surrounding these men and women, and subverts the needs and rights of these individuals, forcing many into hidden and overlooked lives.

Religion and the media are at the forefront of preaching anti-gay messages to the public. Homophobic and hate-provoking sentiments have been voiced from Christian churches, Islamic quarters, and media houses. These institutions brand homosexuality as unnatural, against the order of nature, immoral, against Malawian culture and un-African. Civil society has been strangely silent on the rights of minority groups, one of which is the gay community.

There are some indications that the situation is changing, though. In 2006, the Anglican Diocese of Lake Malawi declined to ordain a pro-gay priest and since then the Anglican Church of Lake Malawi has been divided over the issue of homosexuality. The two factions, one for the pro-gay priest and the other one against, now have mass at different times on Sundays, suggesting some support for the people with same-sex desires.

## Little is known about same-sex sexuality

Given a climate of denial and stigmatisation, it is understandable that little is known about persons with same-sex desires. In November 2006, the Centre for the Development of People (CEDEP) did the first survey of knowledge, attitudes and practices of persons with same-sex desires in five of the 29 districts of Malawi. The main objective of the study was to document that there actually are gay people in Malawi and also to gain an understanding of issues relating to same-sex relationships in the Malawian context. In total, 100 gay, lesbian and bisexual people were interviewed for the study.

Preliminary data from this survey confirmed the difficult situation in which persons with same-sex desires live. Of all respondents, 66 per cent reported that they do not reveal their sexual orientation to third parties. The most frequently given reasons for not disclosing were fear of stigma and negative reactions from society (60 per cent) and fear of how people would react (58 per cent). These reasons were followed by fear of parents' and relatives' responses (55 per cent) and fear of religious authorities (29 per cent). Fear of losing friends was mentioned in 25 per cent of responses (CEDEP 2006).

Although CEDEP did this baseline survey on same-sex sexuality in Malawi, the number of respondents (100) was too small to qualify as a representative sample of a population of 12 million people. However, the study does dispel the myth that there are no gay people in Malawi. There is a need for further research on which to base the frequency of same-sex conduct and to estimate the number of people who claim homosexual identities. General health surveys should also include issues of same-sex relationships and the challenges that gay people encounter.

## HIV/AIDS

According to UNAIDS and the World Health Organisation (UNAIDS & WHO 2007), Malawi's AIDS epidemic appears to have stabilised, and is declining in some areas. There is some evidence of behavioural change that could account for the reduction in new HIV infections. HIV prevalence, based on a population survey, is estimated at 12.7 per cent. There is, however, no information about HIV prevalence among persons who engage in same-sex practices; it is also unclear what the role is of homosexual or bisexual transmission in Malawi's epidemic. Of the 100 people interviewed by CEDEP, 59 per cent reported that they had been for voluntary counselling and testing (VCT). This, however, leaves 41 per cent who had never gone for VCT. The data collection instrument did not provide for further questions on the respondents' serostatus (CEDEP 2006).

In Malawi, same-sex sexuality is also absent from HIV prevention campaigns. CEDEP reviewed messages disseminated via radio, TV and newspapers as well as HIV/AIDS education materials that are distributed by the National AIDS Commission, the Ministry of Health and the Ministry of Education. None of these give any messages targeted at people in same-sex relationships (CEDEP 2006).

## Changing climate

There are indications that the climate in Malawi is changing. In December 2006, while opening a conference for ministers of health of the Southern African Development Community (SADC), Malawi's minister of health, Marjorie Ngaunje, said:

> To make advances in prevention, we must begin to tackle honestly the difficult questions that the epidemic raises…addressing positively the needs of sex workers and of men who have sex with men. We must address the real drivers of the epidemic and target groups that are most vulnerable…Let's be open and start talking about prostitutes and homosexuals because its only South Africa among the SADC states that recognizes homosexuals.[2]

Furthermore, in 2003 the National AIDS Commission (NAC) modified Malawi's *National HIV/AIDS Policy* to include MSM and WSW (women who have sex with women). Section 5.10 of this government policy states:

> People who engage in same-sex sexual relations are socially and culturally vulnerable to prevailing attitudes. If they are not accorded access to HIV/AIDS prevention education, treatment, care and support, they may endanger others as a result of their ignorance…Furthermore, the government, through the NAC, undertakes to put in place mechanisms to ensure that HIV and STI prevention, treatment, care and support can be accessed by all without discrimination, including people engaged in same-sex sexual relations. (Government of Malawi 2003)

## What is needed to move forward?

In order for the NAC to be able to effectively implement its policies, several things are needed, namely research, empowerment and social change.

First of all there is a need for research to:
- establish the prevalence of HIV/AIDS and other sexually transmitted infections (STIs) among same-sex practising people;
- understand the personal, social and structural determinants of their sexual risk behaviours;
- explore the variety of ways in which same-sex sexuality is expressed.

This information is critical for the development of effective interventions.

In relation to HIV/AIDS there is an urgent need to educate and create awareness among men and women with same-sex desires about behaviours that promote the spread of HIV and other STIs. More broadly, there is a need to initiate discussions among men and women with same-sex desires on social issues, sexual rights, life experiences and 'coming out' issues, in order to empower them to make informed decisions for their lives. Such empowerment will enhance their confidence and interpersonal skills, and consequently enable them to negotiate confidently for safer sex with their sexual partners.

Change is needed that goes beyond people with same-sex desires. There is a need to educate the general public, the health sector and civil society about the existence of gay people and their rights. The culture of silence regarding the existence of same-sex sexuality and the absence of health-relevant information targeting them give this population a false picture that they are safe from the HIV/AIDS pandemic and other STIs. The absence of community dialogue on same-sex sexuality robs the minority population of life skills and of involvement in the programmes that affect them. Stigmatisation and homophobia make life difficult for persons with same-sex desires to come out and fight for their rights. The human rights issues that are tackled by civil organisations are selective in nature, as they do not include issues affecting minority groups. The print media publish very homophobic and hate-provoking articles regarding same-sex sexuality, so much so that it is difficult for most persons with same-sex desires to be visible as they risk being stigmatised, beaten up or losing friends. Because of these problems and many others, there is a need to develop and disseminate information on human rights and the law affecting minority groups in order to educate, inform and advocate for the rights of minorities via the media. This will eventually change public attitudes, influence policies and put an end to discriminatory laws.

## Notes

1. Leadership statement: Males who have sex with males. 15th International AIDS Conference, Bangkok, Thailand, 11–16 July 2004. Accessed December 2008, http://www.unaids.org/bangkok2004/docs/leadership/LS_MSM.pdf
2. Cited in *Pukaar* 56 (Jan. 2007): 11. *Sex workers and gays roped in to fight AIDS*. Accessed December 2008, http://www.nfi.net/NFI%20Publications/Pukaar/2007/JanPukaar07new.pdf

## References

CEDEP (Centre for the Development of People) (2006) *Knowledge, attitudes and practice study (KAP) of people in same-sex relationships in Malawi.* Blantyre: CEDEP

Government of Malawi (2003) *National HIV/AIDS policy: A call for renewed action.* Accessed May 2007, http://www.who.int/hiv/Malawi-HIVAIDS-Policy.pdf

MISA (Media Institute of Southern Africa) (1999) *So this is democracy: The state of the media in southern Africa.* Windhoek: MISA

UNAIDS & WHO (World Health Organisation) (2007) *AIDS epidemic update.* Geneva: UNAIDS & WHO

CHAPTER TWELVE

# A bird's-eye view of HIV and gay and lesbian issues in Zimbabwe

Samuel Matsikure

Zimbabwe is classified as a low-income country in southern Africa, with a per capita income of US$363 (UNDP 2006). The country has an estimated population of 12.9 million, with 35.4 per cent in urban areas and the majority living in rural areas (UNDP 2006).

Gays and Lesbians of Zimbabwe (GALZ) operates as a voluntary association. Its membership is clustered into what are called 'affinity groups' where members within the same geographical setting come together and form small groups that have a minimum of 10 members. Affinity groups exist in urban and rural areas, such as Mutare, Chipinge, Bulawayo, Banket, Bindura, Beatrice, Chiredzi, Chitungwiza, Kariba, Mt Darwin, Masvingo, Victoria Falls and Gweru. Other members are scattered in Bindura, Chinhoyi, Wedza, Mtoko, Checheche, Kwekwe, Kadoma, Penhalonga, Rusape, Marondera and other rural areas.

The affinity groups organise educational activities on HIV and AIDS and other events and GALZ provides resources and training for these groups to function and operate. The activities are strictly for those who are affiliated to the organisation. This is done for security reasons and to abide by the laws that govern 'social clubs', which GALZ is registered as. GALZ also distributes condoms and other HIV prevention materials to lesbian, gay, bisexual, transgender and intersex (LGBTI) individuals.

This chapter highlights HIV and AIDS among the LGBTI community in Zimbabwe, and concludes with key recommendations based on the work of GALZ.

## HIV and AIDS among the gay community

The now infamous 1995 speech by Zimbabwean President Robert Mugabe, in which he argued that 'gays and lesbians were unnatural, subhuman' and 'behave worse than dogs and pigs', is probably the best-known example of hate speech by any African head of state (Johnson 2007). The stigma against and dehumanisation of gays and lesbians continues and state-led homophobia in Zimbabwe is holding back the potentially positive impact of interventions related to curtailing the spread of the HIV/AIDS pandemic. In general, healthcare service providers, including those in the counselling field, are not willing to address the issues faced by men who have sex with men (MSM) and women who have sex with women (WSW).

A number of specific challenges are faced, which are summarised in Table 12.1.

**Table 12.1** Challenges faced by gays and lesbians in Zimbabwe

| | |
|---|---|
| Political | • Criminalisation of MSM. |
| | • State-led and endorsed homophobia and dehumanisation of same-sex practising people. |
| Health-seeking behaviour | • Members do not go for voluntary counselling and testing for fear of the results. |
| | • Reluctance to access healthcare due to fear of being ridiculed. |
| | • Positive individuals worry about where to seek treatment. |
| | • In Zimbabwean culture, counselling as a form of therapy is still new to many. They view counselling as a process for people who wish to join GALZ and hence it is not fully utilised. |
| Health systems issues | • Confidentiality is of grave concern, as counsellors have been known to disclose the status of gay individuals. |
| | • Sex kits are very expensive, especially KY jelly and other lubricants, dental dams, etc. none of which are locally manufactured. |
| Social and behavioural | • Denial and stigma: members are dying without disclosing their HIV status for fear of rejection and ridicule from other members of the gay community and from their families. |
| | • Partners hide their sexual problems and pretend all is well to friends and relatives. |
| | • Many who are HIV-positive are not willing to disclose their status for fear of not finding sexual partners and fear of rejection. |
| | • Complacency about risk: there have been a few cases of wilful transmission and risk-seeking behaviour among members due to denial of HIV status and lack of awareness about HIV transmission. |
| | • Reaching out to those who are not GALZ members but are part of the gay community is hampered by the lack of support from other stakeholders. |
| | • Forced marriages to protect the family and the family name has led many gay men and lesbian women to lead double lives. |
| | • Double disclosure (sexuality and HIV status) is very daunting, and often avoided. |

## Discrimination and stigma from multiple sources

Non-governmental organisations (NGOs) working on HIV and AIDS often do not offer information to or about MSM or WSW, nor do they do any research linked to these groups or sexual practices. While on the one hand they recognise MSM and WSW when networking, on the other hand they downplay LGBTI issues, largely due to the homophobia perpetrated by the government. Some of these NGOs fear losing their registration or donor funds if they include LGBTI issues on their agendas.

Similarly, human rights groups dismiss LGBTI issues on the grounds that Zimbabwe has no consensus on the issue of homosexuality and the president is against it. So the issue cannot be discussed, even though there may by sympathy towards the community.

Yet HIV and AIDS affects us all as, in Africa, communities intersect.

Homophobia among staff in social services affects the delivery of services to people who identify as gay or bisexual. Many affected people do not seek assistance or psychosocial support from the health services, for fear of being ridiculed.

Discrimination and stigma also come from family and communities, from schools, churches and social clubs that struggle with social acceptance and add to the alienation of and discrimination against LGBTI in Zimbabwe.

## Recommendations and conclusions

My recommendations focus on four areas, as explained briefly below.

### Improve information, education and communication

There has been increasing media focus, including radio talk shows and discussions, on homosexuality, which has at least brought the issue into the public domain. This creates an opportunity to educate Zimbabwean society on human rights issues. There is a need for more funding for locally produced educational materials on the LGBTI community, which can be included in general HIV and AIDS programmes. These materials should also be distributed to health institutions, HIV and AIDS NGOs, LGBTI and other communities.

### Focus on HIV prevention

A key emphasis must be on HIV prevention. Access to condoms, latex-compatible lubricants and dental dams is key in this regard.

### Increase access to resources

There must be access to resources and dedicated funds for prevention, care and treatment.

There is a resource gap between health education programmes and practical follow-up due to the lack of person-power and resources. There is a need for more volunteers to go into communities and distribute information and safer-sex kits.

## Explore and satisfy the need for research and training

There is need for more research on the impact of HIV and AIDS on MSM and WSW. The counselling and testing centres should collect statistics on same-sex activities so as to implement appropriate interventions. There is a need for training in ways of designing HIV and AIDS programmes within environments that are hostile to LGBTI, and clear guidance on how to implement and manage HIV and AIDS intervention programmes in these contexts.

### References

Johnson CA (2007) *Off the map: How HIV/AIDS programming is failing same sex practising people in Africa.* New York: International Gay and Lesbian Human Rights Commission

UNDP (United Nations Development Programme) (2006) *Human Development Report, 2006.* New York: UNDP

CHAPTER THIRTEEN

# Epidemiological disjunctures: A review of same-sex sexuality and HIV research in sub-Saharan Africa

Kirk Fiereck

This chapter reviews five recent studies of same-sex practising (SSP) individuals in sub-Saharan (but excluding southern) Africa that have also investigated issues related to HIV and sexually transmitted infections (STIs). The following discussion serves as an observational analysis and will interpret findings reported across the studies. The chapter will also discuss these cross-cutting themes in relation to other relevant literature in order to suggest additional directions for community response, intervention and future research. In stating that I will compare findings across sites, a brief mention of the utility and the limits of this exercise is helpful before beginning. Each study reports on a group of individuals that exist within particular historical and social contexts that should be taken account of in future research and when designing interventions. As such, this chapter does not attempt a thorough discussion of the local implications of these overarching themes. However, by looking at these studies in aggregate, it is helpful to tease out commonalities among them as they pertain to SSP individuals in sub-Saharan Africa generally. Drawing attention to these themes, while general in scope, will help inform future interventions and research regarding SSP individuals in sub-Saharan African contexts, while also highlighting sexual health issues SSP people may be facing in areas of sub-Saharan Africa that have not yet been researched or documented.

## Overview

I will limit the focus of this review primarily to five recent survey studies conducted in East and West Africa. I chose these particular studies based on their focus on both same-sex sexuality and HIV and sexually transmitted disease (STD) risk. In addition, their geographic placement outside of southern Africa lends a complementary focus to other chapters presented in this volume. Countries where the studies were conducted include:
- two in Senegal – one of which was based in Dakar (Niang et al. 2002, 2003) while the other was conducted in five cities throughout Senegal (Wade et al. 2005);
- one in Accra, Ghana (Attipoe 2004);
- one in Nairobi, Kenya (Onyango-Ouma et al. 2005); and
- one in Nigeria (mainly an urban study) (Allman et al. 2007).

All the studies, with the exception of the Nigerian one, were surveys based on convenience samples or a snowball (respondent-driven) sampling strategy. While the Nigerian study presented qualitative data, the report is based on formative research that informed a survey study that was implemented in 2007. The study samples varied in size and represented wide age ranges (see Table 13.1). All reports highlight both behavioural (such as condom and lubricant use) and structural (such as stigma, discrimination and violence) determinants of STI risk.

In this chapter, I will focus on reviewing data from these studies that was available regarding: (1) sexual behaviour; (2) STI protective behaviours; (3) commercial and exchange sex; (4) stigma, discrimination and violence; and (5) HIV and STIs. While I will focus my discussion on these five main themes within the five studies, I will also draw on relevant historical and anthropological literature where this helps to contextualise the data, as well as suggest and inform directions for future research.

All studies in this review regarding SSP individuals and STI risk have focused on SSP men. This points to a dearth of information available regarding SSP women in these contexts and what particular issues and risks these women face with regard to HIV and STI infection. While there has been widespread consensus by health experts that sexual transmission of HIV between women is rare or unlikely, others have argued that there are risks for HIV and STI transmission among SSP women (Dworkin 2005; Friedman et al. 2003; Johnson 2007; Lemp et al. 1995; Marrazzo 2004).

While a recent report of female-to-female transmission of HIV involving the use of sex toys has been substantiated (Kwakwa & Ghobrial 2003), reports in Western contexts indicate that SSP women have other risks for HIV transmission, which include having sexual intercourse with men who have sex with men (MSM) and drug use, among others (Dworkin 2005; Friedman et al. 2003; Lemp et al. 1995). In narrative accounts among SSP women in Namibia (Lorway 2005) and South Africa (Morgan & Reid 2003; Nkabinde & Morgan 2005), SSP women report experiencing rape as well as engaging in sex with SSP men.

With regard to reporting HIV and STD transmission among SSP women, researchers have called attention to a potential epidemiological blind spot (Dworkin 2005). They point out that STI risk behaviour among SSP women is not routinely recorded, and when it is, SSP women can be disregarded as an epidemiological category for STI transmission. If women report risk behaviours that have traditionally been considered to be higher risk (for example, sex with men or injecting drugs), they will be categorised as an intravenous drug user or heterosexual instead of an SSP woman in epidemiological surveys (Dworkin 2005; Marrazzo 2004). Given the socio-cultural specificity and complexity of STI risk among SSP women, there has been an epidemiological bias against researching STI risk among these groups, highlighting the disjunctures that exist between

**Table 13.1** Summary of studies

| Study | Sample size (N) | Age range (mean) | Recruitment strategy |
|---|---|---|---|
| Senegal (Niang et al. 2002, 2003) | 250 | 18–53 (25) | Convenience sample (snowball) |
| Senegal (Wade et al. 2005) | 463 | 18–52 (24 median) | Convenience sample (snowball) |
| Ghana (Attipoe 2004) | 150 | 15–40 (not available) | Convenience sample (snowball) |
| Kenya (Onyango-Ouma et al. 2005) | 500 | 18–55 (26 median) | Convenience sample (snowball) |
| Nigeria (Allman et al. 2007) | 58[a] | 16–48 (27) | Convenience sample (snowball & self-selection) |

Note a. Small sample size due to this study being qualitative/formative research conducted prior to a larger survey study of the same population.

sexual practice and sexual identity in many contexts. Therefore, a commitment by researchers and activists to address the under-researched health issues and HIV and STD prevention needs of SSP women, particularly in African contexts, is needed. This is especially important since provisional reports of HIV infection among SSP women in South Africa have suggested significant rates of seroprevalence (Wells 2006; Wells & Polders 2004).

# Results

## Sexual behaviour

Sexual behaviour of SSP males was reported across the studies. Reviewing reported sexual behaviour is important since the existence of same-sex behaviour among men in sub-Saharan Africa has been difficult to ascertain due to the historical reluctance to investigate the existence of SSP behaviour in these contexts (McKenna 1996, 1999; Parker et al. 1998). In addition, a number of other studies have chronicled social and political processes that have contributed to contestations surrounding non-heteronormative sexuality in the region (Allman et al. 2007; Attipoe 2004; Cameron 2002; Cock 2005; Donham 1998; Epprecht 1998, 2005; Hoad 1999, 2000; Lorway 2006). These studies have brought to light important issues regarding post-colonial discourses, racism, gender regimes, cultural imperialism, and the globalisation of sexual identity constructions as they relate to sexuality and SSP people. While the literature on SSP sexuality in sub-Saharan Africa is substantial and growing, this chapter will focus on reviewing the results of the aforementioned behavioural surveys.

All studies (aside from the qualitatively focused Nigerian study) recruited significant numbers of respondents who had self-identified as SSP men (Table 13.1). Of note, the study conducted in Nairobi, Kenya, was able to recruit 500 men to take part in its survey within two months, indicating that same-sex behaviour among men in Kenya is significant (Onyango-Ouma et al. 2005). All studies used convenience sampling as their recruitment strategy. Generally, studies reported that this approach to obtaining a survey sample was necessary given the significant levels of stigma and discrimination that SSP men experience in these contexts. Thus, in these environments, the ability to recruit a representative sample is more difficult than it would be where same-sex behaviour is legalised or there is less social stigma. While this limits the ability to make wide-ranging conclusions about same-sex sexuality in these contexts, the samples do afford important information regarding SSP people in these regions of sub-Saharan Africa.

Across studies, SSP men frequently reported engaging in a range of sexual behaviours, including anal intercourse and oral sex (Table 13.2). With regard to anal sex, in the more recent Senegal study, large proportions of men had engaged in insertive (43.0 per cent) and receptive (34.3 per cent) anal sex with another man within the past month (Wade et al. 2005). In the Kenya study, almost all men (89 per cent) reported anal sex with another man within the past month (Onyango-Ouma et al. 2005). In the same study, when asked whether they had 'ever had' anal sex with another man, 100 per cent reported this behaviour. Similar to the Kenyan study, virtually all men (98 per cent) in the Ghanaian study had reported 'engaging in anal sex' (Attipoe 2004). In the more recent Senegal study, only disaggregated figures (for example, insertive and receptive) were reported for anal intercourse. This explains why figures in this study may seem lower than in others.

**Table 13.2** Summary of sexual behaviour of SSP men

| Study | Anal intercourse | Vaginal intercourse | Oral sex |
|---|---|---|---|
| Senegal (Niang et al. 2002, 2003) | ~20.0% with women[a] | 88.0% 'ever had' | n/a |
| Senegal (Wade et al. 2005) Within past month | 43.0% – insertive  34.3% – receptive | 32.8%  (94.1% –'ever had') | 25.5% – insertive  24.0% – receptive |
| Ghana (Attipoe 2004) | 98.0% 'engage in anal sex'[b] | n/a[c] | 73.0% 'engage in felatio' |
| Kenya (Onyango-Ouma et al. 2005) Within past month | 89.0%  (100%–'ever had')[b] | 14.0%  (69.0%–'ever had') | 63.0% 'sexual practices include oral sex' |

Notes a. No aggregate data reported for anal intercourse with men in this study (data only reported regarding condom use and anal sex).
b. Figure does not differentiate between insertive or receptive anal intercourse.
c. In the Ghana survey, 46% of men surveyed described themselves as 'bisexual' (Attipoe 2004: 29).

Concerning sex with women, most studies reported directly on whether study respondents engaged in vaginal intercourse (Table 13.2). In both Senegal studies, the overwhelming majority of men reported ever having had vaginal sex (Niang et al. 2002; Wade et al. 2005), while in the Kenya study 69 per cent of men reported ever having had vaginal sex (Onyango-Ouma et al. 2005). While the Ghana study did not report on the proportion of men who had engaged in vaginal sex directly, the author did report that 46 per cent of men described themselves as being 'bisexual' (Attipoe 2004). When asked whether respondents had engaged in vaginal sex during the past month, 32.8 per cent and 14 per cent of men responded that they had in the recent Senegal and the Kenya studies respectively (Onyango-Ouma et al. 2005; Wade et al. 2005). These figures indicate that SSP men also have sex with women, and that these sexual behaviours are neither isolated nor rare. The first Senegal study and the Kenya study both reported on men engaging in anal sex with women. In Senegal, nearly a fifth [of the survey sample] had had anal sex with a woman (Niang et al. 2002). In Kenya, 7 per cent and 3 per cent of men who reported sex with women, reported anal intercourse with a woman in the past month and week, respectively (Onyango-Ouma et al. 2005).

Three of the studies also reported on men engaging in oral sex with other men. In Ghana, 73 per cent of men surveyed reported that they 'engage in felatio' (Attipoe 2004), while in Kenya, 63 per cent of men indicated that their 'sexual practices included oral sex' within the past month (Onyango-Ouma et al. 2005). In the 2005 Senegal study, roughly a quarter of the sample reported that they had engaged in insertive oral sex, with an equal proportion of the sample reporting engaging in receptive oral sex.

In addition to anal, vaginal and oral sex, 25 per cent of men in the Kenyan study also reported ever having had group sex. Here, group sex was defined as 'any sexual encounter with two or more men at the same time' (Onyango-Ouma et al. 2005: 26). However, once a time frame was included in the question regarding group sex (for example, within the past month/week), the proportion of men reporting this behaviour lessened (10 per cent in the last month and 3 per cent in the past week).

## STI protective behaviours

Information regarding STI protective behaviours was also reported, including data on condom and lubricant use. Before discussing these findings, it is important to highlight the findings regarding condom knowledge that were reported in two of the studies. In Kenya 77 per cent and in Senegal 80 per cent of men reported that they knew condom use helped to prevent HIV and STIs (Niang et al. 2002; Onyango-Ouma et al. 2005). Despite this knowledge, use of condoms was inconsistent across studies.

**Table 13.3.** Summary of STI protective behaviour (condom use)

| Study | Condom use (with men) | Condom use (with women) |
|---|---|---|
| Senegal (Niang et al. 2002, 2003) % at last sex reporting condom use of those reporting the behaviour | 23.0% – insertive anal<br>14.0% – receptive anal | 37.0% – vaginal |
| Senegal (Wade et al. 2005) % within past month reporting inconsistent condom use of those reporting the behaviour | 55.3% – insertive anal<br>57.9% – receptive anal<br>94.1% – insertive oral<br>84.7% – receptive oral | 53.9% – vaginal |
| Ghana (Attipoe 2004) % reporting condom use of those reporting the behaviour | 11.6% – always<br>88.4% – inconsistent<br>(n=147) | 30.4% – always<br>60.8% – inconsistent<br>8.8% – not stated<br>(n=69) |
| Kenya (Onyango-Ouma et al. 2005) % at last sex reporting condom use of those reporting the behaviour | 75.0% – insertive anal<br>75.0% – receptive anal<br>(58.0% reported 'always use'; 11.0% reported 'never use') | n/a |

Table 13.3 summarises the rates of condom use reported by men across studies. With regard to anal sex, condom use across studies was low or inconsistent with the exception of the results reported from Kenya. Inconsistent condom use (ICU) was defined across studies as 'most of the time', 'sometimes' or 'never', as opposed to 'always'. In the first Senegal study, rates of condom use at last sex were very low, with only 23.0 per cent and 14.0 per cent of men engaging in insertive anal sex and receptive anal sex, respectively, reporting that they had used a condom (Niang et al. 2002). In the 2005 Senegal study, more than half of men engaging in insertive and receptive anal sex within the past month reported ICU (Wade et al. 2005). In the Ghana study (Attipoe 2004), 88.4 per cent of men reported ICU during anal sex (insertive or receptive – no time frame specified). Conversely, in Kenya, a large proportion of the sample (75 per cent) reported using a condom at last anal sex (insertive or receptive) with another man (Onyango-Ouma et al. 2005).

Condom use during vaginal sex was also reported in all studies except for the Kenya and Nigeria studies. In general, proportions of men reporting condom use during vaginal sex were higher than corresponding proportions for anal sex among the samples and rates of ICU were lower (see Table 13.3). Whether the differences between these proportions were significant was not reported. The more recent Senegal study was the only study to report on condom use during oral sex. Rates of ICU reported were extremely high, with 94.1 per cent and 84.7 per cent of men reporting ICU for insertive and receptive oral sex respectively, within the past month (Wade et al. 2005).

In addition to condom use, lubricant use was also reported in most studies. The 2002 Senegal study reported that informants mentioned that there was generally 'poor access to water-based lubricants' (Niang et al. 2002: 2). Supporting this observation, in the 2005 Senegal study, 91.4 per cent of men reported inconsistent use of lubricants during the past year. In this study, inconsistent use corresponded to 'often', 'sometimes' or 'never', as opposed to 'always'. In Kenya, lubricant use was high, with 92 per cent of men reporting that they used lubricants (Onyango-Ouma et al. 2005). However, 84 per cent of men also reported that they used petroleum-based lubricants.

## Commercial sex/exchange sex

One commonality found across most of the studies (for example, in Ghana, Kenya and Senegal) is that high proportions of SSP men in these surveys engaged in sex-for-money exchanges. In the first Senegal study, the authors stated that 'two-thirds' (approximately 67 per cent) of men reported they 'received money' and 9 per cent reported they 'paid money' at their most recent sex encounter (Niang et al. 2002). Lower proportions of men receiving money for sex were reported in the 2005 Senegal study, where 22.5 per cent of men reported this behaviour during the previous month (Wade et al. 2005). One explanation of the difference between these two Senegal studies might be an increased sample size and the inclusion of four additional cities in the more recent sample, in addition to Dakar. Outside of Dakar, the prevalence of sex-for-money exchanges may vary or respondents may be less likely to report them, which may explain this difference. The figures for the Kenya study were based on recall during the previous year, with 52 per cent of men reporting that they 'received something', and 29 per cent reporting that they 'paid something' for sex (Onyango-Ouma et al. 2005: 28). In Ghana, 53.3 per cent of men reported that they engaged in sex with other men for 'economic reasons' (Attipoe 2004: 15).

In the Kenya study, the authors did not specify exchange of money in their survey but included a discussion regarding the various commodities that were exchanged by men, including alcohol and housing payments (e.g. rent) (Onyango-Ouma et al. 2005). The authors reported that there was a higher median amount of money exchanged at last sex reported by men receiving payment for sex than by those paying for sex. They propose that this disparity could indicate an under-representation of foreign or professional SSP men in the sample who might be more likely to be the 'higher-paying partners of men in the sample' (Onyango-Ouma et al. 2005: 28). Attipoe (2004: 15) also briefly discussed global aspects of exchange sex in Ghana, reporting that men who are involved in same-sex sexual relationships for 'purely economic reasons' give priority to customers from wealthier countries. A narrative account from an unemployed Liberian bisexual man indicated that a number of refugees engage in exchange sex for economic survival (Attipoe 2004).

In two studies there was a deliniation reported between self-identified sex workers and other respondents who did not self-identify as sex workers but did engage in sex-for-money exchanges. Fourteen per cent of the Kenyan sample self-identified as 'sex workers', although there were higher proportions of men in the study reporting that they had received or paid something for sex during the previous year (Onyango-Ouma et al. 2005). Similarly, only 1.3 per cent (2 respondents) of the sample in the Ghana study reported that they considered themselves to be 'commercial sex workers', while 53.3 per cent of that sample reported that their sexual relationships with other men included some sort of economic exchange (Attipoe 2004). This study also included narrative accounts of a range of men who engage in exchange sex with other men but that may not necessarily identify as sex workers. One self-identified gay student reported that he had sex with men for pleasure, but also to 'get money for school' (Attipoe 2004: 16). Some men in this study reported that they received gifts from other men of things they needed and other non-necessity items, such as trips abroad, in exchange for having sex.

The existence of exchange-sex relationships that are differentiated from commercial sex work have been chronicled elsewhere throughout sub-Saharan Africa and have primarily focused on women engaging in exchange sex with men (Hunter 2002; Meekers & Calves 1997; Standing 1992; White 1988; Wojcicki 2002). Hunter (2002) and Wojcicki (2002) both point out that in primarily black South African communities, sex work as a profession is highly stigmatised, whereas more informal forms of sex-for-money exchange are not. In fact, Wojcicki (2002) points out that much literature that focuses on describing sex-for-money exchange in sub-Saharan Africa indicates that women have been able to move in and out of various forms of exchange sex without being stigmatised, and that many of the reasons for entering into exchange sex are the same for when individuals enter into commercial sex work. In this context, sex work tends to be differentiated from more informal exchange sex by many aspects, depending on the region or locality in question.

In the South African context, sex workers self-identify as such, wear more sexually suggestive clothing, do not tell their families about their work, tend to sell sex as a primary means of income generation, and have set prices for various services. Alternatively, women involved in exchange sex do not identify with the sex worker label, they contribute resources gained through exchange sex to their families, do not have set prices for sex and, often their families know that they are engaging in these activities and accept the situation (Hunter 2002; Wojcicki 2002). According to Standing (1992), specifically in sub-Saharan Africa it is important to understand that what is described as prostitution, or sex work as I have referred to it here, is 'embedded in a wider nexus of socioeconomic exchanges, which are not static through time' and highlights 'the importance of not transferring meanings derived from a western context to an African one without proper scrutiny' (1992: 478).

There are similar pitfalls when uncritically transposing a framework regarding sex-for-money exchanges constructed to explain the sexual realities of heterosexual women, onto SSP men, given differing gender norms and gendered opportunity structures. However, it is instructive to use this framework as a way to interpret these preliminary data and suggest future avenues for enquiry.

## Stigma, discrimination and violence

All studies identified issues of stigma, discrimination and violence as major problems for SSP men in sub-Saharan Africa. These were the most discussed problems reported by men in the Kenya study, with 63 per cent of men reporting that these were issues of concern (Onyango-Ouma et al. 2005). A full third of the respondents in this study also reported that they had experienced some form of stigmatisation or discrimination during the previous year. This included public forms of aggression/humiliation and alienation/humiliation by family, friends or neighbours.

In the 2005 Senegal study, the authors reported that these issues affected the way in which they conducted the study and were particularly salient when trying to work among populations of SSP men in Senegal (Wade et al. 2005). The first study conducted in Senegal also highlighted the stigma that SSP men faced when interacting with health workers (Niang et al. 2002). Men would go to clinics to seek treatment for penile symptoms but not anal symptoms, due to the stigma attached to anal sexual health issues by health workers.

In Ghana, almost a quarter of men surveyed reported 'stigmatisation' in their lives and 16 per cent reported that they experienced 'rejection' (Attipoe 2004: 19). The majority of men (58 per cent) in this study also reported that they could not be open about their sexual involvement with other men. Workplace discrimination among SSP men was also reported in Kenya and in narrative accounts among men surveyed in Nigeria (Allman et al. 2007; Onyango-Ouma et al. 2005). A major theme covered in the Nigerian study focused on the stigmatisation that many SSP men encounter in their interactions with families, religious groups and an extremely religious Nigerian society (Allman et al. 2007). The authors reported that these social processes of stigmatisation in the Nigerian context led many SSP men to lead double lives that involved living a publicly heterosexual life, while privately engaging in same-sex practices.

Violence was also reported across the studies and included verbal, physical and sexual violence. In the first Senegal study, reported sources of verbal and physical abuse included families, communities and the police (Niang et al. 2002). Interestingly, the largest proportions of SSP men reported that their family was the source of these types of violence, with 49 per cent and 28 per cent of men respectively reporting familial verbal and physical abuse. In Kenya, 22 per cent of men reported that they had experienced some type of violence during the previous year (including verbal, physical, sexual and 'other') (Onyango-Ouma et al. 2005). With regard to sexual violence, both Senegal samples and the Kenya sample reported these experiences. In the first Senegal study, 37 per cent of men reported being forced to have sex during the previous year, and 43 per cent of men reported being forced to have sex ever (Niang et al. 2002). The second Senegal study found that 30 per cent of men surveyed reported ever having been forced to have sex with another man, and 10 per cent of men had reported that their first sex with another man was forced (Wade et al. 2005). In Kenya, only 5 per cent of men reported sexual violence (Onyango-Ouma et al. 2005). Of note, roughly half of the men in the Kenya sample who experienced sexual violence were self-identified sex workers. Friends, partners, clients or other sex workers were often the reported sources of this violence.

## HIV and STIs

Only one study reported on the seroprevalence of HIV among SSP men. In the more recent Senegal study, the authors reported that 21.5 per cent of the survey sample had tested positive for HIV (95 per cent CI: 17.8–25.6) (Wade et al. 2005). This figure included those found to be positive with HIV-1 and HIV-2, and those who were found to have dual infection (both HIV-1 and HIV-2). The factors that were most strongly associated with risk for HIV infection in this study were being infected with Herpes Simplex Virus-2 (HSV-2), being older than 28 years, having had 10 or more sexual partners, working as a waiter or bartender, and living in Dakar.

This study also looked at the prevalence of STIs. Just over 22 per cent of the sample was infected with HSV-2, while 4.1 per cent and 5.4 per cent of men in this study were infected with chlamydia and gonorrhoea respectively (Wade et al. 2005). Of the participants who answered questions regarding reported symptoms of STIs during the previous year, 34.9 per cent reported they had had at least one symptom.

Other studies did not report directly on the prevalence of STIs, but did present results on reported STI symptoms. In Kenya, 47 per cent of the sample reported ever having experienced one of the eight common STI symptoms listed in the structured interviews, and 24.8 per cent of the sample reported having had one of these symptoms within the last year (Onyango-Ouma et al. 2005). The study also ascertained risk factors for STI symptoms. After adjusting for other factors, having oral sex and being a victim of stigma or discrimination during the past year were significantly associated with reporting at least one STI symptom (Onyango-Ouma et al. 2005).

In the first Senegal study, questions regarding STI symptoms were asked and 42 per cent of men reported that they suffered discharge and burning in the penis (Niang et al. 2003). The same proportion reported bleeding and discharge from the anus (Niang et al. 2003). Data on STI symptoms were also reported in Ghana, with 33 per cent of those surveyed reporting penile discharge and just over 18 per cent reporting anal discharge (Attipoe 2004).

## Discussion

### Sexual behaviour

Generally speaking, the ability of these studies to recruit these samples calls into question the assumption that SSP individuals and populations do not exist or that the prevalence of same-sex behaviour is insignificant in African contexts. With regard to sexual behaviour, the data across studies demonstrate that the majority of men frequently engage in a range of sexual behaviours with other men as well as with women. In total, these findings indicate that SSP men in these contexts are not exclusively engaging in same-sex behaviour. This clearly demonstrates that sexualities of SSP men may not necessarily be explained using Western-defined sexual categories, such as homosexual, gay or bisexual. If men in these contexts self-identify using these terms, their meaning cannot implicitly be assumed to coincide with their Western definitions or constructions.

These empirical results tend to follow Foucault's (1978) theoretical argument for the socially constructed nature of sexuality; that these are historically- and culturally-specific sexualities that are not necessarily encompassed by pre-existing terms. However, Foucault's framework precludes an understanding of how sexualities are also intertwined and understood within local gender norms and constructions. In the Thai context, Jackson (2000) argues against understanding non-Western eroticisms in terms of sexuality alone (for example, gay, bisexual or any other label that intends to describe a person's sexuality) without acknowledging how gender is also conceived as an aspect of sexuality and vice versa. Given the developmental and historical particularities of African contexts and the diversity of sexual practices exhibited by SSP men in the region, Western-defined terms should be used cautiously and critically examined. Their localised meanings should be determined and should include an understanding of their relation to localised gender constructions. Indeed, some studies' qualitative and initial ethnographic findings indicate that local sexualities are understood and are imbricated with local gender constructions (Niang et al. 2002, 2003; Onyango-Ouma et al. 2005). For example, in a number of studies of SSP men in African contexts, local identities for insertive and receptive participants in anal sex have existed that connote one's sexual identity, but that have also connoted aspects of an individual's locally understood gender (Amory 1998; Donham 1998; Niang et al. 2003; Onyango-Ouma et al. 2005). These studies also indicate that individuals' sexualities, erotic potentialities, and identity constructions are in flux and are being refigured depending on various social and historical transitions, including globalisation, migration and the emergence of mass-mediated cultures.

### STI protective behaviours

The major finding across these studies regarding STI protective behaviours was that rates of ICU were high, despite high proportions of men who knew that condom use prevented HIV and STIs. Use of lubricants was also troubling and of considerable importance when considering the design and implementation of HIV and STI prevention programmes. Of note in the Kenya study is that while there were high percentages of condom use, there were also high proportions of men who reported use of oil-based lubricants that can cause condoms to degrade during sex and compromise their integrity. As such, these data call into question the effectiveness of the high rates of condom use among the Kenyan sample with regard to HIV and STI prevention.

Future research that focuses on STI protective behaviours among SSP men in these contexts should attempt to focus on what sorts of determinants are the root causes of the disjuncture between these high proportions of knowledge of condom use protecting against STIs and the comparatively low use of condoms during sex. Additionally, given the data presented on high rates of exchange sex, stigma, discrimination, violence and sexual violence among SSP men in these contexts, knowledge of the extent to which these types of issues structure STI risk behaviours would be very useful for HIV and STI prevention programming and community-based advocacy.

### Commercial sex/exchange sex

Hunter (2002) makes the case, citing a recent review by Lurie (2000), that in South Africa today much of the HIV epidemic may not be due to sex work, but rather to the more informal modes of exchange sex that are structured by prevailing gendered and racialised economic and social inequalities. In this regard, sex workers or those who are involved in exchange sex can become labelled incorrectly as an HIV risk group. Anthropologists have warned against the uncritical application of epidemiologic methods, stating that this can result in 'oversimplified constructions that deny variation and mask the underlying social influences on individual behaviour' (Brown et al. 1996: 211). Ultimately, this sort of uncritical epidemiology can exacerbate existing social inequalities by reinforcing prevailing power dynamics. This occurs by labelling a certain community a 'risk group' while neglecting the social processes that structure this risk, such as racism, gender (or sexuality)-based and economic inequalities, or political marginalisation. Ultimately, this can result in well-intentioned but maladaptive HIV prevention interventions that can do more harm than good.

This also raises questions for future research when looking at exchange sex behaviours among SSP individuals in sub-Saharan Africa. In particular, what sorts of social, political and historical contexts structure commercial and exchange sex in these contexts and what implications will this have for HIV and STI prevention programming, sexuality and gender research and community activism? Specifically, Lurie's (2000) epidemiological review, when placed within Hunter's (2002) analysis of the differentiation of exchange and commercial sex in South Africa, problematises a research agenda and HIV prevention approach that only targets sex workers as a 'risk group'. This approach neglects acknowledging culturally specific aspects of exchange sex in African contexts and risks overlooking the social, economic and sexual health needs of men and women who are involved in, and impacted by, exchange sex. Additionally, given that these more informal forms of exchange sex are occurring across these studies in large proportions, the role that exchange sex plays in the day-to-day erotic realities of SSP men in these contexts needs to be more fully investigated in order to understand the ways in which these relationships mediate risk for and transmission of HIV and STIs among SSP men.

## Stigma, discrimination and violence

Issues of stigmatisation and violence faced by SSP people are evident across studies. While some of the analyses investigated ways in which stigma and violence mediate risk of HIV and STI transmission in these contexts, the social processes and mechanisms that sustain and reproduce them, and their effects on health in these contexts, require greater research. The way in which stigma operates as a social process in these contexts will impact on the implementation of STI prevention on initiatives among SSP people.

Parker and Aggleton (2003) point out that addressing stigmatisation as something that individuals do to other individuals is a uniquely western understanding of this concept, and does not necessarily translate to localities in the global south. In these contexts, 'bonds and allegiances to family, village, neighbourhood and community make it obvious that stigma and discrimination…are social and cultural phenomena linked to the actions of whole groups of people' (Parker & Aggleton 2003: 17). This echoes the finding in the 2002 Senegal study that the highest proportions of verbal and physical abuse experienced by SSP men are from individuals' families. Similarly, in Nigeria, social rejection of SSP men 'began and was experienced in the family, it was then common for this rejection to be subsequently experienced from other social institutions, such as organized religion, or from the broader Nigerian society' (Allman et al. 2007: 160). However, by looking closely at the social relationships that underpin these experiences of stigma and the power dynamics at play, interventions that address the necessary dual-life constructions of SSP men, or that address the power relationships that exist between SSP individuals and these social institutions, can be addressed. Additionally, Parker and Aggleton (2003) describe stigma as having 'a history which influences when it appears and the form it takes' (Parker & Aggleton 2003: 17).

Instructive analyses that look at the history of stigma processes in southern Africa include Epprecht (1998, 2005), Hoad (1999) and Phillips (2004). Each of these analyses looks at the social, political and historical forces that are at play regarding lesbian and gay human rights, stigma, violence, homophobia and gendered economic and social disparities in these contexts. Similar studies that deconstruct and tease out the forces at play behind the reports of stigma reviewed here would be invaluable to designing interventions and responses that can effectively address these issues.

## HIV and STIs

In spite of the wide reporting of STI symptoms, it was a common finding that SSP men were reluctant to openly address issues of HIV and STIs with medical staff. Reported rates of STIs and STI symptoms were said to be much higher among groups of SSP men than among the general population (Niang et al. 2002; Onyango-Ouma et al. 2005; Wade et al. 2005). In a study of SSP male and female youth in a South African township community, respondents reported feeling uncomfortable or unable to discuss sexual health issues openly with local clinic staff, demonstrating a lack of health services available to sexual minority populations (Graziano 2004). The need to develop sexual health initiatives that are non-discriminatory and non-stigmatising for SSP individuals will be an important issue when designing future HIV and STI prevention and care programmes throughout sub-Saharan Africa. Unfortunately, HIV seroprevalence data were only reported in one of the Senegal studies. However, the stark disparity between the prevalence reported in this study (21.5 per cent) and that of the general Senegalese population (1–2 per cent) is alarming (Wade et al. 2005). Whether this sort of disparity is present in other contexts is unclear and the need for epidemiological serosurveys of SSP individuals with regard to HIV and STIs throughout the region is imperative.

## Limitations

One of the main limitations of this review is related to the inability to make cross-study comparisons based on variations in evaluative criteria. For example, due to the small number of studies and their limited scope, many of the themes discussed here were not uniformly reported across studies. There were also differences in recall time frames and terminology used for many questions regarding STI risk and protective behaviours across studies, which limits comparability of the results. Additionally, the samples in these studies were convenience samples, indicating that the findings are not necessarily representative of the wider populations of SSP people from which the study participants were selected.

## Conclusion

Aside from these limitations, this review provides an instructive critique and highlights areas that require further clarification and study. Of particular note, the ongoing study of same-sex sexualities in sub-Saharan Africa will need to take account of the various complex social, political and historical forces that continue to shape and construct erotic possibilities in these contexts. Without question, accurate (or inaccurate) understandings of these sexualities will have manifold implications for the structure and shape of future health and sexuality research, as well as for designing and implementing interventions to address health and developmental issues of SSP people. In addition, some studies point out that local sexual identities are also influenced by global flows of Western same-sex identities that have impacted on sub-Saharan African contexts (Amory 1998; Attipoe 2004; Donham 1998; Onyango-Ouma et al. 2005). These sorts of hybridised identity constructions, or creolised identities as typified by Anderson (2006), can have significant historical and social implications and should be given consideration when discussing issues of sexual identity construction of SSP people in sub-Saharan Africa. In particular, a theoretical framework that includes both sexuality and gender in understanding the social construction of sexuality of SSP individuals in these contexts may prove important (Jackson 2000; Butler as quoted in Osborne & Segal 1994).

It is important to understand sexual and gender constructions in relation to the other themes discussed in this chapter. Certain gender or sexual identities may correspond to specific constellations of HIV and STI risk and to social conditions that may structure HIV risk behaviours, such as engaging in exchange or commercial sex, which may mediate one's ability to successfully negotiate safer-sex practices in various situations. While much current research on SSP people in sub-Saharan Africa has unproblematically used terms like MSM and women who have sex with women (WSW) to describe generalised STI risk categories, Young and Meyer (2005) have raised cautions against the erasing of the 'sexual minority person' within these broad categories. They, and others (Dworkin 2005; Muñoz-Laboy 2004) argue that these categories can result in epidemiological blind spots and hamper HIV prevention efforts by under-allocating resources to groups within these broad categories that may be at increased risk of HIV and STI infection. Given the possibility that many SSP individuals in sub-Saharan Africa do not take on sexual identities, epidemiological categories such as MSM and WSW may erase particularly at-risk sexual subgroups in these contexts. As such, these categories should be used cautiously and critically.

Overall, this review indicates that there is a diversity of sexual and erotic expression among SSP individuals in sub-Saharan Africa and that future research and HIV and STI interventions must be aware of and responsive to this diversity. Additionally, issues related to the local delineations between exchange sex and commercial sex may prove important to the epidemiology of HIV and STIs among the SSP men represented in these surveys. Likewise, the processes that structure stigma, violence and discrimination among SSP individuals are important to HIV and STI prevention efforts and will require in-depth research and structurally-based interventions to address their deeply socially embedded nature. While these studies are ground-breaking in that they have highlighted the existence of same-sex sexuality in sub-Saharan Africa, they also leave a number of important questions unanswered. This review has attempted to outline a number of these in order to suggest future directions for research, public health intervention and advocacy.

## Acknowledgements

I would like to thank the South African Human Sciences Research Council (HSRC) and the HIV Center for Clinical and Behavioral Studies, and particularly Vasu Reddy and Theo Sandfort, for organising the conference From Social Silence to Social Science, as well as for giving me the opportunity to present this chapter during the proceedings. I would also like to thank Theo Sandfort for his intuitive guidance in the formative stages of this presentation and the Columbia University Mailman School of Public Health Student Travel Fund for sponsoring my travel expenses to attend the conference. In addition, thanks to all of the organisations that provided financial support for the conference.

## References

Allman D, Adebajo S, Meyers T, Odumuye O & Ogunsola S (2007) Challenges for the sexual health and social acceptance of men who have sex with men in Nigeria. *Culture, Health & Sexuality* 9(2): 153–168

Amory D (1998) *Mashoga, mabasha,* and *magai:* 'Homosexuality' on the East African Coast. In SO Murray & W Roscoe (Eds) *Boy-wives and female husbands: Studies in African homosexualities.* New York: Palgrave

Anderson B (2006) *Imagined communities* (Revised edition). London & New York: Verso

Attipoe D (2004) *Revealing the Pandora's box or playing the ostrich? A situational appraisal of men having sex with men in the Accra metropolitan area and its environs.* Ghana: West African Project to Combat HIV/AIDS and STI

Brown PJ, Inhorn MC & Smith DJ (1996) Disease, ecology, and human behavior. In TM Johnson & CF Sargent (Eds) *Medical anthropology: A handbook of theory and method.* New York: Greenwood Press

Cameron E (2002) Constitutional protection of sexual orientation and African conceptions of humanity. *South African Law Journal* 188(4): 642–650

Cock J (2005) Engendering gay and lesbian rights: The equality clause in the South African Constitution. In N Hoad, G Martin & G Reid (Eds) *Sex & politics in South Africa: The equality clause/gay and lesbian movement/the anti-apartheid struggle.* Cape Town: Double Storey Books

Donham DL (1998) Freeing South Africa: The 'modernization' of male-male sexuality in Soweto. *Cultural Anthropology* 13(1): 3–21

Dworkin SL (2005) Who is epidemiologically fathomable in the HIV/AIDS epidemic? Gender, sexuality, and intersectionality in public health. *Culture, Health & Sexuality* 7(6): 615–623

Epprecht M (1998) The 'unsaying' of indigenous homosexualities in Zimbabwe: Mapping a blindspot in an African masculinity. *Journal of Southern African Studies* 24(4): 631–651

Epprecht M (2005) Black skin, 'cowboy' masculinity: A genealogy of homophobia in the African nationalist movement in Zimbabwe to 1983. *Culture, Health & Sexuality* 7(3): 253–266

Foucault M (1978) *The history of sexuality, Volume 1: An introduction.* New York: Random House

Friedman S, Bailey S, Case P, Des Jarlais D, Diaz T, Garfein R, Hollibaugh A, Hudson S, Maslow C, Morse E, Ompad D, Perlis T & Young R (2003) HIV prevalence, risk behaviors, and high-risk sexual and injection networks among young women injectors who have sex with women. *American Journal of Public Health* 93(6): 902–906

Graziano KJ (2004) Oppression and resiliency in post-apartheid South Africa: Unheard voices of black gay men and lesbians. *Cultural Diversity and Ethnic Minority Psychology* 10(3): 302–316

Hoad N (1999) Between the white man's burden and the white man's disease: Tracking lesbian and gay human rights in southern Africa. *GLQ: A Journal of Lesbian and Gay Studies* 5(4): 559–584

Hoad N (2000) Arrested development or the queerness of savages: Resisting evolutionary narratives of difference. *Postcolonial Studies* 3(2): 133–158

Hunter M (2002) The materiality of everyday sex: Thinking beyond 'prostitution'. *African Studies* 61(1): 99–120

Jackson P (2000) An explosion of Thai identities: Global queering and re-imagining queer theory. *Culture, Health and Sexuality* 2(4): 405–25

Johnson CA (2007) *Off the map: How HIV/AIDS programming is failing same-sex practising people in Africa*. New York: International Gay and Lesbian Human Rights Commission

Kwakwa HA & Ghobrial MW (2003) Female-to-female transmission of Human Immunodeficiency Virus. *Clinical Infectious Diseases* 36(3): e40–e41

Lemp G, Anderson L, Jones M, Katz M, Kellogg T, Nieri G & Withum D (1995) HIV seroprevalence and risk behaviors among lesbians and bisexual women in San Francisco and Berkeley, California. *American Journal of Public Health* 85(11): 1549–1552

Lorway R (2005) 'Vulnerable' desires: Contesting Namibian (homo)sexuality in the era of HIV/AIDS. *Anthropology*. Toronto: University of Toronto

Lorway R (2006) Dispelling 'heterosexual African AIDS' in Namibia: Same-sex sexuality in the township of Katutura. *Culture, Health & Sexuality* 8(5): 435–449

Lurie M (2000) Migration and AIDS in southern Africa: A review. *South African Journal of Science* 96(6): 343–347

Marrazzo JM (2004) Barriers to infectious disease care among lesbians. *Emerging Infectious Diseases* 10(11): 1974–1978

McKenna N (1996) *On the margins: Men who have sex with men and HIV in the developing world*. London: The Panos Institute

McKenna N (1999) *The silent epidemic: HIV/AIDS and men who have sex with men in the developing world*. London: The Panos Institute

Meekers D & Calves AE (1997) 'Main' girlfriends, girlfriends, marriage, and money: The social context of HIV risk behaviour in sub-Saharan Africa. *Health Transition Review* 7(Supplement): 361–375

Morgan R & Reid G (2003) 'I've got two men and one woman': Ancestors, sexuality and identity among same-sex identified women traditional healers in South Africa. *Culture, Health & Sexuality* 5(5): 375–391

Muñoz-Laboy M (2004) Beyond 'MSM': Sexual desire among bisexually-active Latino men in New York City. *Sexualities* 7(1): 55–80

Niang CI, Castle C, Diagne M, Gomis D, Moreau AM, Niang Y, Tapsoba P, Seck K, Wade AS & Weiss E (2003) 'It's raining stones': Stigma, violence and HIV vulnerability among men who have sex with men in Dakar, Senegal. *Culture, Health & Sexuality* 5(6): 499–512

Niang CI, Diagne M, Diouf M, Gomis D, Moreau A, Niang Y et al. (2002) Meeting the sexual health needs of men who have sex with men in Senegal. *Horizons Final Report.* Washington, DC: Population Council

Nkabinde N & Morgan R (2005) 'This has happened since ancient times...it's something you are born with': Ancestral wives amongst same-sex sangomas in South Africa. In R Morgan & S Wieringa (Eds) *Tommy boys, lesbian men and ancestral wives: Female same-sex practices in Africa.* Johannesburg: Jacana Media

Onyango-Ouma W, Birungi H & Geibel S (2005) *Understanding the HIV/STI risks and prevention needs of men who have sex with men in Nairobi, Kenya.* Nairobi: The Population Council

Osborne P & Segal L (1994) Gender as performance: An interview with Judith Butler. *Radical Philosophy* 67: 32–39

Oswin N (2006) Decentering queer globalization: Diffusion and the 'global gay'. *Environment and Planning D: Society and Space* 24(5): 777–790

Parker R & Aggleton P (2003) HIV and AIDS-related stigma and discrimination: A conceptual framework and implications for action. *Social Science and Medicine* 57: 13–24

Parker R, Aggleton, P & Kahn S (1998) Conspicuous by their absence? Men who have sex with men (MSM) in developing countries: Implications for HIV prevention. *Critical Public Health* 8(3): 329–346

Phillips O (2004) (Dis)Continuities of custom in Zimbabwe and South Africa: The implications for gendered and sexual rights. *Health and Human Rights* 7: 83–113

Standing H (1992) AIDS: Conceptual and methodological issues in researching sexual behaviour in sub-Saharan Africa. *Social Science and Medicine* 34(5): 475–483

Wade AS, Diallo PAN, Diop AK, Gueye K, Kane CT, Mboup S, et al. (2005) HIV infection and sexually transmitted infections among men who have sex with men in Senegal. *AIDS* 19(18): 2133–2140

Wells H (2006) *Levels of empowerment among lesbian, gay, bisexual and transgender [LGBT] people in KwaZulu-Natal, South Africa.* Pretoria: OUT LGBT Well-being

Wells H & Polders L (2004) *Levels of empowerment among lesbian, gay, bisexual and transgender [LGBT] people in Gauteng, South Africa.* Pretoria: OUT LGBT Well-being

White L (1988) Domestic labour in a colonial city: Prostitution in Nairobi 1900–1952. In SB Stichter & JL Parpart (Eds) *Patriarchy and class: African women in the home and the workplace*. Boulder: Westview Press

Wojcicki J (2002) Commercial sex work or *Ukuphanda*? Sex-for-money exchange in Soweto and Hammanskraal area, South Africa. *Culture, Medicine, and Psychiatry* 26: 339–370

Young R & Meyer I (2005) The trouble with 'MSM' and 'WSW': Erasure of the sexual-minority person in public health discourse. *American Journal of Public Health* 95(7): 1144–1149

# NEEDS, PROGRAMMING, POLICY & DIRECTION FOR FUTURE RESEARCH

It's very important for lesbians to talk about sexual pleasures before safer sex, because if people keep the whole sex thing a secret, it's difficult to have a way forward... Like I mean, I find gay guys...at least they're much more flexible and they have spaces, they can cruise. You can't cruise as a lesbian – you know, it's the whole sin thing. If we create spaces where we could express freely, people could open up. And if it's there then we'll hear about a lot more than just two cases of lesbian this or that, or of lesbians who are positive, because there are a lot of lesbians who are positive. What really disturbs me is when people talk on our behalf... And also, until the service providers are educated, until whoever decides on resources and priorities in terms of people, health and protection, we will definitely not achieve what we want to achieve. *Zanele Muholi, conference delegate*

Research itself, its practices, its epistemologies need to be significantly questioned and transformed, so that new research practices emerge. But there are a number of other issues that need to be investigated as well...For example, the notion of Africanness is not a fixed category and it is undergoing significant transformation. This suggests that research offers a venue for practices of citizenship and political strategies around creating visibility, not only through the insertion of affirmative statements about a marginalised or minority group, but also through very deliberate acts of trying to change practices, to the point of questioning the very basic notions that I just call methodology.
*Robert Sember, conference delegate*

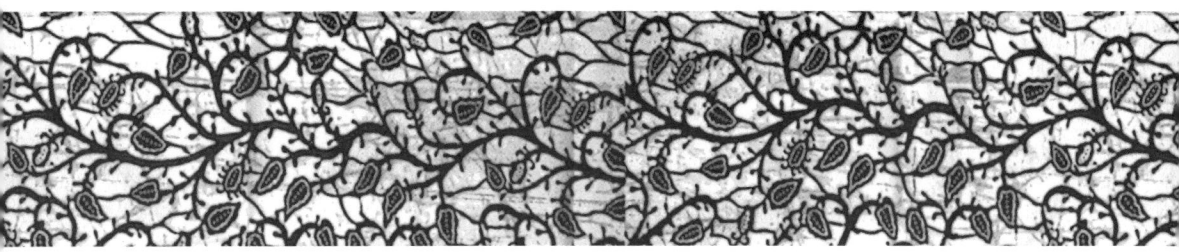

People are tired of getting researched and a lot of the fatigue has to do with the fact that people don't always see the benefit of what they do. I think that if you are going to do a research project and people can really see how they have contributed to bringing about some change, then people want to contribute. The other thing is that we tend to go out with pages and pages of questionnaires and we really need to think of how we are going to make this friendlier…If you can get some information in two pages, it could be much more valuable than a person writing one or two words for every answer in your ten-page questionnaire. And you can be original in how you get information. Interviews, for instance, take much more time and I know that they are more expensive, but often you need to do a one-on-one interview, go back, and do a second one. There are ways in which you can deal with that. *Ian Swartz, conference delegate*

There's a great need to assist our communities to understand the need for research, to engage with researchers and the questions developed towards that research being undertaken. But also, and even more important, there is a need to hold researchers responsible for the information that they send out after having engaged with the relevant communities. There's a whole lot of misinformation after researchers have engaged with us and it's about time that we mobilise against such issues. *Nonhlanhla Mkhize, conference delegate*

CHAPTER FOURTEEN

# Mobilising gay and lesbian organisations to respond to the political challenges of the South African HIV epidemic

Nathan Geffen, Zethu Cakata, Renay Pillay and Paymon Ebrahimzadeh

## The struggle for gay and lesbian rights in South Africa

The achievements of gay and lesbian organisations struggling for the rights of gays, lesbians, men who have sex with men (MSM), women who have sex with women (WSM), bisexuals, transgendered and other people who vary from the heterosexual norm in South Africa have been remarkable. The human rights struggle pursued by gay and lesbian organisations has led to the inclusion of sexual orientation in the equality clause of the South African Bill of Rights, repeal of discriminatory anti-sodomy laws, recognition of partnerships in same-sex relationships for immigration purposes, and for pension and medical benefits and, ultimately, the legalisation of same-sex civil unions and marriage.

Since at least the 1980s, gay and lesbian organisations have mobilised our communities against homophobic legislation and the HIV epidemic (Pegge 1995). The National Coalition for Gay and Lesbian Equality, with leaders such as Zackie Achmat, Mazibuko Jara and Jonathan Berger, and its successor, the Lesbian and Gay Equality Project, mobilised political demonstrations and Pride Marches throughout the 1990s and 2000s so that litigation at the Constitutional Court was backed by a popular movement. Simon Nkoli and others mobilised black gay men and lesbians and openly gay prisoners, and worked aggressively to demand the inclusion of the rights of gay men and lesbians in the newly created Constitution.

The formation of the National Coalition for Gay and Lesbian Equality managed to make gay rights part of a much broader political project. Its successes can be associated with submissions to the Constitutional Assembly which stressed that 'equality and non-discrimination are the fundamental and overriding principles of the interim constitution, furthermore discrimination against gays and lesbians, displays the same features as discrimination on the grounds of race and gender' (Cock 2003: 37–38).

Consequently, South Africa has an excellent sexual orientation legal framework. It is easier for middle-class gay men and lesbians to be more open in 2009 than it was in 1990 – and this is probably true for working-class communities as well, although not to the same extent. Service delivery, including HIV services for gay men and lesbians, in major cities has improved substantially over the last 17 years.

## The South African HIV epidemic

South Africa's HIV epidemic has been described as being hyper-endemic. (UNAIDS 2006). The Human Sciences Research Council's household survey in 2005 estimated that 10.8 per cent of people over the age of two years are HIV-positive (Shisana et al. 2005). An estimated 2 million people have died since the epidemic began (UNAIDS 2007). Although antiretroviral treatment (ART) is available in over 400 public health facilities across the country and over 300 000 people are on highly active ART in the public health system (DoH 2008), 500 000 people in need of treatment do not receive it (Dorrington et al. 2006).

Since HIV is predominantly heterosexually transmitted in South Africa, it is understandable that most interventions are geared towards heterosexuals. However, this has left MSM and WSW at risk of infection, with insufficient delivery and testing services addressing their specific needs. Despite major achievements in the gay and lesbian movement, both before and particularly after 1994, cultural, political and governmental obstacles have left MSM/WSW particularly vulnerable in many specific sectors of society. This is exacerbated by the depoliticisation of gay and lesbian community organisations that has taken place since the late 1990s.

This chapter is intended to address the role of government and gay and lesbian organisations in ensuring prevention strategies and service delivery. Examples are presented that show that MSM and WSW in South Africa continue to be adversely affected by the epidemic in ways that could be avoided. We argue that gay and lesbian organisations need to participate in and lead campaigns for a number of crucial health interventions, including public information campaigns on HIV: campaigns to increase the uptake of counselling and testing; to improve treatment of depression; to improve HIV education, treatment and prevention for prisoners; to decriminalise sex work; and to address discrimination against MSM and WSW in townships and working-class areas.

Organisations like the Triangle Project, the Durban Gay and Lesbian Community & Health Centre, and others, do excellent service delivery work for the gay and lesbian communities they serve. For example, the Triangle Project provides HIV counselling and treatment services and distributes educational material on HIV. The Durban Gay and Lesbian Community & Health Centre, uniquely amongst South African gay and lesbian organisations, has predominantly black clients and provides counselling and information on HIV. It also distributes pamphlets to Durban clubs on how to use condoms. It would be inaccurate to state that the work of these organisations is not political; both issue statements on political issues and participate in the activities of the Treatment Action Campaign (TAC), the organisation at the forefront of HIV human rights campaigning in the country. But we argue that the tempo and involvement of their political work needs to be increased substantially if the above interventions are to be successfully implemented.

## Failure of the South African government to respond appropriately to HIV/AIDS

The South African government's response to the HIV epidemic has been characterised by a pseudo-scientific AIDS denialist approach which has resulted in hundreds of thousands of avoidable deaths and infections. This has been well documented by Myburgh (2007), Nattrass (2007), Cameron and Geffen (2005) and Heywood (2004).

The struggle with the Department of Health's (DoH) delayed ART rollout and prevention of mother-to-child transmission (PMTCT) programme came to a climax in 2001 when the TAC took the DoH to court to ensure implementation of a comprehensive PMTCT programme. TAC's eventual victory at the Constitutional Court in 2002 compelled government to allow health workers to provide HIV-positive pregnant women with antiretroviral prophylaxis for PMTCT. Following this, TAC and its allies pressurised government into rolling out ART (Myburgh 2007; Nattrass 2007; Cameron & Geffen 2005). This culminated in the DoH's Operational Plan for Comprehensive HIV and AIDS Care, Management and Treatment for South Africa on 19 November 2003.

Despite rollout initiation, its delay had disastrous effects. As *The Price of Life* reveals:

> A largely untreated AIDS epidemic has profound implications not only for the people who are needlessly suffering and their loved ones, but also for the country as a whole...Rising levels of sickness and death place severe strain on the state, which is under growing pressure and a constitutional obligation to provide adequate forms of support to families affected by HIV/AIDS. There is also an increasing burden on the public health system, as people living with HIV/AIDS require repeated treatment of opportunistic infections. (AIDS Law Project & TAC 2003)

The epidemic has had a disproportionate effect on the gay and lesbian community, whose access to healthcare was already insufficient prior to the epidemic. Therefore, ensuring that individuals have access to treatment, particularly among MSM and WSW, must be a priority. However, ensuring access to treatment on the scale that will be required within South Africa cannot rely on individual service providers, but rather, a mass lobby demanding access to treatment is necessary.

Despite the need for increased lobbying, gay and lesbian organisations have become primarily focused on service delivery and, as a result, have been less able to engage with the serious political challenges of the epidemic. This is not, however, to undermine the progress that we have already discussed and praised. Rather, it is to reinforce that service delivery organisations will not and cannot meet the future needs of South Africa – including the needs of MSM and WSW (AIDS Law Project & TAC 2003). Only the state has the capacity to supply or finance service delivery on such a large scale. Service delivery organisations can set good examples for how scaled-up health interventions can be implemented, but if such delivery is unaccompanied by a political programme, only the relatively few people receiving service from the organisation will benefit. ART provides a good example of this. Before 19 November 2003, numerous service delivery organisations provided treatment to a few thousand people. Today, the public sector treats over 300 000 people (DoH 2008).

It is our contention that this lack of focused lobbying is exacerbated by the fact that many gay and lesbian activists have become too focused on the narrow issues of identity politics – an indulgence that removes attention from more important issues. In order for the gay and lesbian movement to effectively address the likely dimensions of the impact of HIV and AIDS in future, problems need to be corrected.

An example of the kind of mobilisation necessary comes from Lusikisiki – a town serving a rural and extremely poor district in the former Transkei in the Eastern Cape. Several years ago Médecins Sans Frontières helped establish ART in the district's public health facilities. Young people, mostly women, in Lusikisiki established TAC branches to campaign around issues of HIV treatment and to provide themselves, their friends and family with treatment education.

Now Lusikisiki has the biggest antiretroviral programme in the Eastern Cape and there have been unprecedented changes in the community and in the health services there as a consequence of that programme. TAC volunteer Akhona Ntsaluba has played a large role in this. She has been at the forefront of HIV education and campaigned for the Eastern Cape government to provide the area with the resources it needed to make the antiretroviral rollout work. She and others set up campaigns on gender, sexuality and domestic violence. A lesbian community has begun to develop in the area, providing an example of how a grassroots-based campaign can bring real change to working-class gay men and lesbians.

We now describe several further examples of where there is a dire need for the intervention of gay and lesbian organisations, but where insufficient work has been done until now.

## Where gay and lesbian organisations need to intervene

### Public information campaigns

In our view, the large-scale public information campaigns for HIV prevention in South Africa have been insufficient and appalling. The two largest organisations tasked with running these campaigns, loveLife and Khomanani, have run insipid programmes, the former characterised by obscure messages promoting an aspirant lifestyle out of the reach of most South Africans, and the latter characterised by some good advertisements – if only they were seen and heard more often. Only recently has loveLife's campaign consistently included people living with HIV. Furthermore, from our perspective, both campaigns all but ignore gay men and lesbians. In order for these campaigns to be effective in both their scope and intent, gay and lesbian organisations must demand that a significant portion of public messaging on HIV address issues directly affecting gay men and lesbians, as well as MSM at high risk of HIV infection. Gay role models as well as information on gay-friendly HIV services need to be prominently featured in public information campaigns.

## Testing campaigns

Testing campaigns are similarly inadequate in that they do not directly target MSM. Gay and lesbian organisations need to step up campaigns to encourage MSM to get tested and to encourage existing testing campaigns to actively include MSM in their target audience. MSM who are HIV-positive need to be encouraged to enrol in monitoring and treatment programmes.

## Counselling and care

Many men presenting for voluntary counselling and testing (VCT) or with AIDS symptoms in public health facilities have contracted HIV through homosexual sex. However, counselling for the specific needs of MSM is seldom included in VCT programmes. This allows for further spreading of the disease. In reality, the counselling component of the VCT programme tends to be inadequate and lacks standardisation, leaving it highly dependent on the competence and open-mindedness (or otherwise) of the counsellors. The lack of public information campaigns further exacerbates prejudice. Lesbian and gay organisations must advocate for HIV counselling training programmes to include a component on dealing with MSM.

## Depression

The effect of depression on MSM, WSW and people with HIV is one area that has been well documented (Bing et al. 2001). It has been shown that MSM with chronic untreated, or poorly treated, depression are more likely to engage in high-risk sex associated with transmission (Rogers et al. 2003). Yet public health facilities lack the medicines, skills and other resources to manage depression or psychiatric illness, thereby missing an opportunity to decrease infection rates. Lack of proper diagnosis, quality control and treatment makes depression in MSM/WSW communities particularly disturbing. These barriers not only prevent MSM/WSW from testing initially, but further prevent proper counselling and care. Some gay and lesbian organisations have sufficient expertise on depression which they could use to effectively lobby for improvements to mental health services in our community.

## Prisoners

The AIDS Law Project and TAC have been running a campaign to promote treatment for HIV-positive prisoners for nearly two years. They have focused primarily on the Westville Correctional Facility. Only recently, in preparation for a pending court case, did this prison introduce widespread condom distribution, though (as far as we understand) without the distribution of lubricants. The situation is likely to be much worse in most other South African prisons. Gay and lesbian organisations should begin to address the needs of prisoners, an issue which has been mostly disregarded by the gay and lesbian community, and demand proper condom and lubricant distribution in all prisons, as well as access to ART.

## Sex work decriminalisation

Sex workers are a key to both prevention and treatment in the HIV epidemic. As the UN describes, 'The risk of infection is highest where sex workers are most powerless and therefore unable to negotiate or insist on the use of condoms by their clients, or to resist violent and coercive sex'(UNAIDS 2007). In South Africa, the Sex Worker Education and Advocacy Taskforce (SWEAT) is running a campaign for the decriminalisation of sex work. The industry operates underground and openness is rare. It is consequently extremely difficult to provide adequate health services to sex workers. Vivienne Lalu of SWEAT explains:

> The continued criminalisation of sex workers has contributed to the stigma, isolation and violation of human rights of sex workers. Sex workers are forced to work in isolated and remote areas. These working conditions not only make them vulnerable to violence and abuse, but also make it very difficult for intervention projects to locate them to do prevention work. A significant number of sex workers are men offering services to MSM. (Lalu 2004)

Gay and lesbian organisations do provide services for male sex workers, but they also need to be at the forefront of SWEAT's decriminalisation campaign.

## Addressing discrimination, safety and facilities for MSM and WSW in townships

Many of the successes of the gay and lesbian movement have not yet reached townships and many other working-class communities. Many townships lack facilities and campaigns for addressing discrimination, stigma and violence towards, and lack of support for, MSM and WSW. Similarly, there is very little information on MSM and WSW practices in townships, and gay and lesbian organisations are rare. The Lusikisiki story above provides an example of what can be done, even in remote and conservative areas. Without adequate information and support particular to their needs, gay men and lesbians in poor areas are at higher risk of HIV infection or, if infected, less able to access health services.

## Lack of information

A lack of research on the prevalence of HIV infection among MSM affects all of the mentioned examples. Without proper understanding of the scope and course of HIV incidence and prevalence, prevention and treatment campaigns will be less effective and even misdirected and wasteful. A study analysing data of MSM worldwide concluded for sub-Saharan Africa that:

> In spite of ethnographic evidence, no quantitative data on the prevalence of male same-sex sexual activity in the general population were available for this region. There were, however, estimates of such prevalence among HIV/AIDS cases or prison inmates. This absence is likely due to the overwhelming heterosexual HIV epidemic as well as the widespread assumption of the non-existence of homosexual behaviour in Africa. Most of the available behavioural studies are conducted on young people or women and include no questions on the subject of MSM. (Cáceres et al. 2006)

## Looking ahead

There remain serious shortcomings in state policy and service delivery with respect to the HIV epidemic. The needs of MSM/WSW will not be addressed by the state unless gay and lesbian organisations actively campaign for improvements. Community organisation service delivery is important and helps a significant number of people, but it cannot reach the scale of a state-provided intervention. Gay and lesbian organisations need to bring more campaign politics into their work if we are to adequately improve service delivery for the vast majority of MSM/WSW.

**Postcript:** Since this chapter was written there have been some positive developments. In particular, two clinics aimed primarily at MSM with HIV and other STIs have opened up in Cape Town. Also, the chapter did not address the problem of hate-crimes against lesbians in townships, a serious shortcoming. Gay and lesbian organisations must prioritise a campaign against these heinous crimes.

## References

AIDS Law Project & TAC (2003) *The price of life: Hazel Tau and others vs GlaxoSmith Kline and Boehringer Ingelheim.* Johannesburg: AIDS Law Project & TAC. Accessed 17 February 2008, http://alp.org.za.dedi20a.your-server.co.za/images/upload/20030812_Price11-12.pdf

Bing EG, Burnam MA, Longshore D et al. (2001) The estimated prevalence of psychiatric disorders, drug use and drug dependence among people with HIV disease in the United

States: Results from the HIV Cost and Services Utilization Study. *Archives of General Psychiatry* 58(8): 721–728

Cáceres C, Chatterjee A, Konda K, Lyerla R & Pecheny M (2006) Estimating the number of men who have sex with men in low and middle income countries. *Sexually Transmitted Infections* 82 (Supplement 3): 3–9

Cameron E & Geffen N (2005) *Witness to AIDS*. London: Tauris

Cock J (2003) Engendering gay and lesbian rights: The equality clause in the South African Constitution. *Women's Studies International Forum* 26(1): 35–45. Accessed 7 November 2007, http://www.sciencedirect.com/science?ob=ArtcleURL&_udi=B6VBD-47XF5S8-4&

DoH (Department of Health) (2008) *South African ARV sites February 2008*. Accessed 16 February 2008, http://www.tac.org.za/documents/arvsitesfebruary2008.pdf

Dorrington R, Bradshaw D, Daniel T & Johnson L (2006) *The demographic impact of HIV/AIDS in South Africa: National and provincial indicators for 2006*. Cape Town: Medical Research Council

Heywood M (2004) Price of denial. *Development Update* 5(3): 93–122

Lalu V (2004) *Sex work, human rights and HIV/AIDS. A response to the United Nations' HIV/AIDS and human rights guidelines*. Accessed 5 January 2009, http://www.sweat.org.za/index.php?option=com_content&task=view&id=61&Itemid=28

Myburgh J (2007) *The Virodene affair (I – V)*. Accessed 17 February 2008, http://www.politicsweb.co.za/politicsweb

Nattrass N (2007) *Mortal combat: AIDS denialism and the struggle for antiretrovirals in South Africa*. Pietermaritzburg: University of KwaZulu-Natal Press

Pegge JV (1995) Living with loss in the best way we know how: AIDS and gay men in Cape Town. In M Gevisser & E Cameron (Eds) *Defiant desire: Gay and lesbian lives in South Africa*. Johannesburg: Ravan Press

Rogers G, Beilby J, Curry M, Oddy J, Pratt N & Wilkinson D (2003) Depressive disorders and unprotected casual anal sex among Australian homosexually active men in primary care. *HIV Medicine* 4(3): 271–275

Shisana O, Bhana A, Connolly C, Jooste S, Parker W, Pillay V, Rehle T, Simbayi L & Zuma K (2005) *South African national HIV prevalence, HIV incidence, behaviour and communication survey*. Cape Town: HSRC Press

UNAIDS (2006) *Fact sheet: Sub-Saharan Africa*. Accessed 16 February 2008, http://data.unaids.org/pub/GlobalReport/2006/200605-FS_SubSaharanAfrica_en.pdf

UNAIDS (2007) *Sex workers and client*. Accessed 16 February 2008, http://www.unaids.org/en/PolicyAndPractice/KeyPopulations

CHAPTER FIFTEEN

# Are South African HIV policies and programmes meeting the needs of same-sex practising individuals?

Laetitia Rispel and Carol Metcalf

The 2007 UNAIDS report shows that HIV prevalence and deaths have declined in some countries, but that the HIV pandemic remains a major socio-economic and public health challenge (UNAIDS & WHO 2007). Globally, every day, over 6 800 persons become infected with HIV, and over 5 700 persons die from AIDS, mostly because of inadequate access to HIV prevention and treatment services (UNAIDS & WHO 2007). Southern Africa remains the most seriously affected sub-region, accounting for 35 per cent of all people living with HIV (UNAIDS & WHO 2007). South Africa is the country with the largest number of HIV infections in the world, although antenatal clinic surveillance suggests that HIV infection levels might be levelling off, albeit at a high level of 29 per cent in 2006 and with considerable variation across provinces (DoH 2007a). National adult HIV prevalence was 16.2 per cent in 2005 (Shisana et al. 2005a).

UNAIDS suggests that there are two broad patterns to the epidemic: generalised epidemics sustained in the general populations of many sub-Saharan African countries, and concentrated epidemics among populations most at risk, such as men who have sex with men (MSM), injecting drug users (IDU), and sex workers and their sexual partners (UNAIDS 2006a). In South Africa, the emergence of the generalised heterosexual HIV epidemic eclipsed the HIV epidemic among MSM, although there is no evidence to suggest that there is no longer an HIV epidemic among MSM. There is also a dearth of information on the role of homosexual transmission in the generalised South African HIV epidemic.

This chapter provides an assessment of how well existing HIV policies and programmes meet the needs of same-sex practising individuals, and is based primarily on a review of relevant literature. For the purposes of this chapter, same-sex practising individuals include lesbians and/or women who have sexual relations with women; gay men and/or MSN; bisexuals; and transgender individuals. The first section of the chapter presents a framework for analysing current HIV policies and programmes, using an adaptation of the Country Harmonisation and Alignment Tool (CHAT) developed by UNAIDS (2007). This is followed by a brief analysis of current policies and programmes, with particular reference to the lesbian, gay,

# SOUTH AFRICAN HIV POLICIES AND PROGRAMMES

bisexual and transgender (LGBT) communities. The chapter concludes with the main observations emerging from the analysis and makes key recommendations for research and programme action.

## A conceptual framework for analysis

The CHAT tool developed by UNAIDS (2007) was adapted as a conceptual framework for analysis. This is shown in Figure 15.1 and highlights three dimensions of analysis: LGBT participation and engagement in the HIV response; the mapping of the epidemic, including information on key risk factors; and the presence of an enabling environment for service provision, including funding and human resource provision. Although the proposed dimensions are interconnected, they are considered separately to provide a framework for appraising policies and actions.

**Figure 15.1** Framework for analysing policy and programmes for same-sex practising individuals

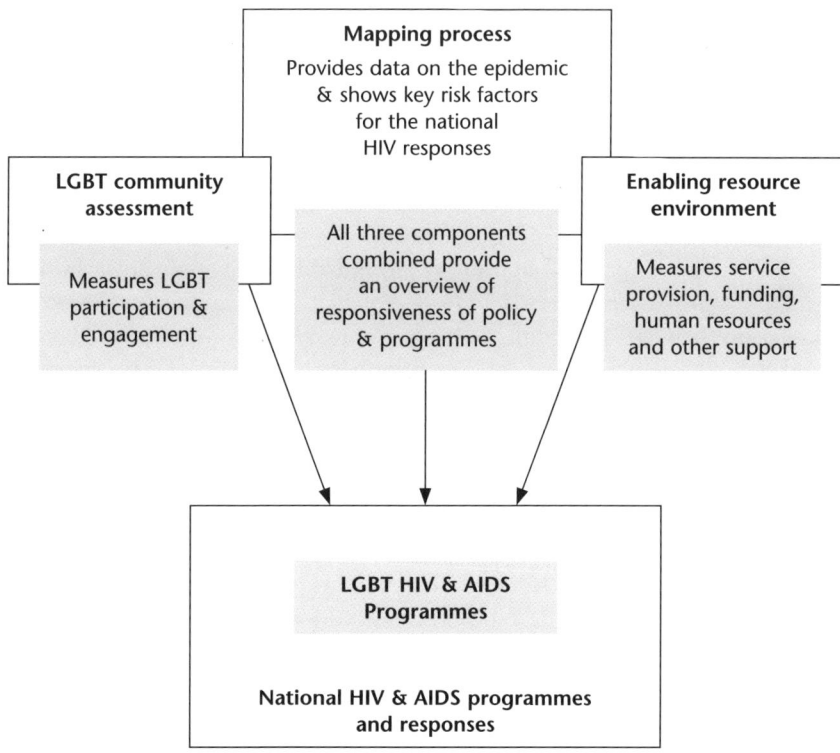

Source: Adapted from the UNAIDS CHAT tool (UNAIDS 2007)

## Analysing current policies and programmes

### LGBT participation and engagement in the HIV response

Community involvement is widely recognised as key to successful implementation of policies and programmes. However, if social movements and community empowerment are to fulfil their potential to promote inclusion, national governments must create and maintain the conditions necessary for genuine involvement of the people or groups that are the target of the policy, action or programme. People living with HIV (PLHIV) have fought for and, to some extent, won a place in national HIV planning activities, and most National AIDS Control Committees and other official HIV and AIDS-related bodies now include formal representation of PLHIV (Johnson 2007; UNAIDS 2006a).

Johnson's (2007) research on same-sex practising Africans, human rights protections, and HIV and AIDS programmes has found that gay and lesbian representatives and HIV specialists with an interest in HIV same-sex transmission or the provision of services, have not been involved. The author has argued that, 'There is a wall of silence that surrounds AIDS and same-sex practices that may prove to be a significant obstacle to conquering the disease.'[1]

The South African Constitution (Act 108 of 1996), prohibits discrimination on the grounds of sexual orientation. In 2006, the Civil Union Act extended marriage laws equally to all LGBT South Africans. However, social attitudes towards homosexuality lag behind legal protections against discrimination, and same-sex sexual relationships are still not widely accepted in the country (Rule & Mncwango 2006). In the 2003 South African Social Attitudes Survey conducted by the Human Sciences Research Council (HSRC), it was found that 78 per cent of a sample of more than 4 000 people surveyed indicated that it was '…always wrong to have sexual relations between two adults of the same sex' (Rule & Mncwango 2006). Gay men and lesbians, as well as gay venues, have been the target of hate crimes (Nel 2005).

The *HIV & AIDS and STI National Strategic Plan* (NSP) *2007–2011* (DoH 2007b) is useful for analysing our first criterion around LGBT participation and engagement in the HIV response. Widely considered a major success in bringing together all health stakeholders in the public and private sectors, as well as members of civil society, this five-year strategy to tackle the epidemic was drawn up after extensive consultations embracing a wide range of stakeholders, including the LGBT sector (Kapp 2007). A two-day consultative meeting in March 2007 provided stakeholders with the opportunity to make inputs to the NSP, and the final version was released at the launch of the South African National AIDS Council on 30 April 2007 (DoH 2007b). However, the consultation only happened after extensive civil society and stakeholder critique, lobbying and advocacy.

But until 2007, there had been no mention of the needs or involvement of same-sex practising individuals in national HIV policies and programmes. Although MSM in South Africa, as elsewhere, are generally considered a high-risk subpopulation (DoH 2007b; UNAIDS 2000), messages directed at MSM have been conspicuously absent from all the major national HIV prevention campaigns and treatment programmes.

The NSP acknowledges the omission of same-sex practising individuals in HIV policies, programmes and interventions, and recognises the need for specific programmes. These are hopeful signs, although the challenge is in the implementation of the NSP, the extent to which the LGBT community will be engaged in programme development, and the provision of dedicated funding for targeted programmes.

## Mapping the epidemic, including information on key risk factors

Scientists and policy-makers have put little effort into understanding the links between hetero- and homosexual HIV transmission and have been slow to acknowledge the possibility that sexual transmission among MSM is playing an important role in HIV transmission in Africa (Johnson 2007).

There is some evidence of an emerging epidemic of HIV infection among MSM in developing countries (Beyrer 2007). UNAIDS (2006b) advocates that HIV sub-epidemics among MSM should also be regarded as linked to the epidemic in the general population. However, the prevalence of HIV infection among MSM in developing countries is sometimes not closely related to the overall HIV prevalence in the general population, and estimates of HIV prevalence among MSM tend to exceed HIV prevalence among adults in the general population (Beyrer 2007; Girault et al. 2004; Van Griensven 2007; Van Griensven et al. 2005; Wade et al. 2005).

The first HIV prevalence study of MSM in Africa was conducted in Senegal in 2005 (Wade et al. 2005). The study found an HIV prevalence of 21.5 per cent among MSM, compared to an HIV prevalence of 0.2 per cent among adult males overall (Wade et al. 2005). Similarly, HIV prevalence studies among MSM conducted by the International AIDS Vaccine Initiative in Kenya found an HIV prevalence of over 40 per cent, compared to an HIV prevalence of 6.1 per cent among Kenyan adults aged 15 to 49 years (Johnson 2007). It has been speculated that HIV prevalence among MSM in South Africa may also exceed the HIV prevalence in the general population (Lane, cited in Johnson 2007).

Currently in South Africa, there is ongoing monitoring of the HIV epidemic by means of annual surveys of pregnant women attending antenatal clinics (DoH 2007a – see Figure 15.2) and national household surveys every three years (Shisana, Simbayi et al. 2002; Shisana, Bhana et al. 2005a).

**Figure 15.2** Prevalence of HIV infection among women attending antenatal care clinics in South Africa, 1990–2006

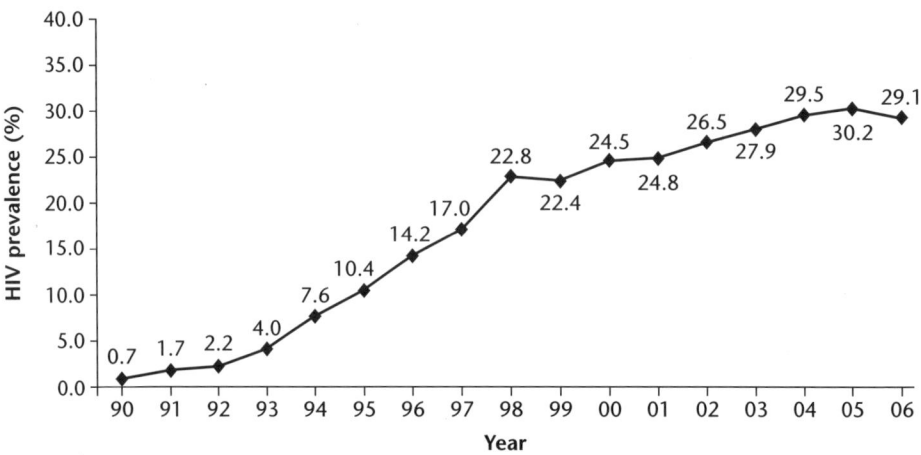

Source: DoH (2007a)

The prevalence of same-sex sexual behaviour in South Africa is unknown. Furthermore, HIV infection and AIDS remain highly stigmatised, exacerbating the challenge of understanding the HIV epidemic among the LGBT community in South Africa (Cloete et al. 2006). Information on the incidence and prevalence of HIV among MSM in South Africa, of risk behaviour, and of prevention strategies to minimise the risk of HIV infection, or of transmitting HIV to their sexual partners, is extremely limited. This is despite the fact that the country experienced a more limited HIV epidemic among MSM before the emergence of a generalised HIV epidemic in South Africa (Van Harmelen et al. 1997). Most of the early cases of AIDS diagnosed in South Africa were among white MSM who had travelled internationally, and who had a history of sexual contact with men from other countries (Sher 1985, 1986, 1989; Sher & Dos Santos 1985). In the 1980s, gay activists were among the first to draw attention to the HIV epidemic in South Africa, to mobilise support for PLHIV and to promote the adoption of less risky sexual behaviour.

Early research on HIV transmission in South Africa focused mostly on the sexual behaviour of gay men. One such study found that changes in sexual behaviour had occurred among gay men in the face of the increasing risk of HIV infection (Schurink & Schurink 1990). Another study examined gay and bisexual identity and the implications of the HIV epidemic for gay communities (Isaacs & McKendrick 1992). However, early studies on HIV among MSM in South Africa tended to be small and descriptive in character, and typically lacked the methodological rigour needed to make generalisable conclusions about the HIV epidemic among MSM.

**Table 15.1** Estimates of HIV prevalence among persons aged 15 to 49 years in South Africa

| Year | Source | Adults (15–49 years) | Adult men (15–49 years) | Adult women (15–49 years) |
|---|---|---|---|---|
| 2002 | Shisana et al. 2002 | 15.6% | 12.8% | 17.7% |
| 2005 | Shisana et al. 2005a | 16.2% | 11.7% | 20.2% |
| 2007 | ASSA (2003) | 18.8% | 15.5% | 22.0% |

There is a lack of information on the extent to which the HIV epidemic among MSM represents a separate epidemic in parallel with the larger generalised epidemic (see Table 15.1), or whether it is a subcomponent of the generalised HIV epidemic. A study of HIV among South African public school teachers found that the HIV prevalence among male teachers who reported having sex with men only, had a slightly higher HIV prevalence (14.4 per cent) than male teachers who reported having sex with women only (12.8 per cent), although this difference was not statistically significant (Shisana et al. 2005b).

National population-based surveys conducted by the Human Sciences Research Council (HSRC) in 2002 and again in 2005 have shown that HIV prevalence is high among both men and women in the general population, although it peaks at an older age among men than among women (Shisana et al. 2002; Shisana et al. 2005a).

A number of recent meetings and events in South Africa have highlighted the urgent need for information on the HIV epidemic among MSM, and the need to implement HIV prevention programmes directed at this group (see Table 15.2). LGBT organisations have attempted to address this gap through commissioned studies done under the auspices of the Joint Working Group. However, the information obtained is not representative and is primarily collected to inform service or programme activities.

Globally, there is lack of research and information on female-to-female HIV transmission (Canadian HIV/AIDS Clearinghouse 2002; CDC 2006). Women who identify as lesbian or who have sex with women may engage in risky behaviours and practices, including unprotected sex with men, IDU, and alternative insemination (Canadian HIV/AIDS Clearinghouse 2002). Same-sex practising women are at risk of sexually transmitted infections, and female-to-female transmission of HIV has been reported (Bailey et al. 2004; Kwakwa & Ghobrial 2003).

Same-sex practising women may be vulnerable to acquiring HIV infection as a result of an interlocking set of social inequalities, including a limited ability to refuse unprotected sex when having sex with men; human rights violations such as 'corrective' rape; discrimination and homophobia; and a lack of access to healthcare (CDC 2006; Johnson 2007).

**Table 15.2** Events that highlight the lack of information on HIV and MSM

| Date | Event |
| --- | --- |
| 2006 | Protests against South African Blood Transfusion service policies that prevent MSM from donating blood. |
| 2006–2007 | Recurrent requests to the Human Sciences Research Council (HSRC) for questions on same-sex sexual behaviour to be included in the 2008 national household survey, as part of second generation HIV surveillance. |
| March 2007 | The NSP acknowledges that little is known about the HIV epidemic amongst MSM in South Africa and that MSM have not been considered to any great extent in national HIV and AIDS interventions. The NSP identifies MSM as a priority population for surveillance and for interventions. |
| May 2007 | Joint HSRC, Columbia University, Durban Lesbian and Gay Community & Health Centre, OUT Same-Sex Sexualities Conference in Pretoria, highlights a need for further research on same-sex sexual practices and HIV in South Africa and for policies and programmes directed at same-sex practising individuals. |
| May 2007 | HIV among MSM identified as a research priority by leading South African researchers at a national meeting convened by the previous deputy minister of health, Nozizwe Madlala-Routledge, in Cape Town. The meeting focused on priority research areas to give effect to the NSP. |
| June 2007 | Delegates at the Third South African AIDS Conference in Durban raise concern at the lack of inclusion of resolutions relating to MSM in the conference declaration. |
| Sept/Oct 2007 | Need to report on UNGASS indicators for the 2007 country report highlights gaps in HIV information on most at-risk populations (MSM, commercial sex workers, IDU). |

## An enabling environment for service provision, funding and human resources

At the May 2006 Abuja Special Summit of the African Union (AU) on HIV and AIDS, African states released a statement advising members to prioritise vulnerable people, defined as MSM, women, young people, orphans, migrants, prisoners, sex workers, the disabled, people affected by conflicts, and IDUs (AU 2006). However, this commitment to citing the most vulnerable groups and stated targets was subsequently abandoned at the June 2006 UN General Assembly Special Session (UNGASS) meeting in New York (Johnson 2007).

Johnson (2007) has found that although there are some exceptions, few African governments' HIV programmes conduct specific outreach to sexual minorities or train staff to work effectively with same-sex practising individuals. In addition to a lack of specific HIV programming and services, same-sex practising men and women often face stigma and discrimination when accessing healthcare services (Johnson 2007; OUT 2007).

In South Africa, despite laudable transformation efforts in the health sector for over 10 years, the most progressive Constitution in the world, and one of the most extensive HIV and AIDS strategic plans, there are no targeted government HIV programmes to meet the needs of the LGBT community. LGBT organisations tend to be the main service providers, but such services are limited in scope and scale and often dependent on foreign donor funding. In a May 2007 submission to the South African Human Rights Commission on access to healthcare, OUT LGBT Well-being (OUT), a Gauteng community-based organisation focusing on the well-being of the LGBT community, stated that:

> Currently, in South Africa, targeted health care services for LGBT people are provided primarily by LGBT organizations, whose funding is for the most part dependent on foreign donors. To ensure that health facilities, goods and services are accessible to LGBT people, without discrimination, requires concerted and programmatic efforts in which the public sector becomes a leading agent. Shifts need to take place at both individual and institutional levels, to ensure accessible, tolerant, safe and inclusive health care services and programmes. (OUT 2007: 7)

The Third South African AIDS Conference also highlighted the lack of HIV targeted programmes and services for sexual minorities, and made a commitment to '…making counselling and testing available and accessible to vulnerable groups, including men who have sex with men, sex workers, truck drivers, and prisoners', and '…ensuring initiatives to promote prevention and care for HIV-positive people including men, MSM and sex workers'.[2]

Health workers do not receive training to respond to the specific physical and psychological needs of same-sex practising clients, while compassion and responsiveness in overall health service provision is often lacking. Little information is available on healthcare access and quality, although LGBT organisations have begun to address this gap in the last few years. The Triangle Project in Cape Town found that HIV-positive gay men expressed high levels of satisfaction with their medical practitioners (Crowe 2005). However, the findings are not generalisable, as individuals surveyed are already members of Triangle Project support groups, the sample consisted of 34 men only, and there were methodological problems with the study.

In a study conducted jointly by OUT and the University of South Africa's Centre for Applied Psychology, 8.4 per cent of black lesbians and 7.6 per cent of black gay men in Gauteng had been refused medical treatment as a result of their sexual orientation (Wells & Polders n.d.). Aspects highlighted in the Gauteng and KwaZulu-Natal surveys are summarised below (OUT 2007; Wells & Polders n.d.).

- Black same-sex practising individuals are more likely to use the public health sector for care.
- 30 per cent of KwaZulu-Natal respondents indicated that healthcare practitioners made them feel uncomfortable.

- Approximately double the sample of black compared to white participants in Gauteng indicated that the healthcare practitioner consulted had asked heteronormative questions.
- Around 12 per cent of respondents in both provinces reported delays in seeking treatment for fear of discrimination based on sexual orientation, with black people four times more likely to delay seeking care.
- 12 per cent of respondents in Gauteng reported delays in seeking care for haemorrhoids, rectal bleeding and genital infections for fear of their sexual orientation being discovered. Again, black people were more likely to delay seeking care for fear of their sexual orientation being made known.
- 76 per cent of the Gauteng sample reported satisfaction with healthcare services, with white respondents more likely to be satisfied with services.
- Disturbing levels of gender-based violence were reported in both provinces.

The South African government has now included MSM as a target group in its national response to HIV and AIDS, the NSP. To the credit of advocacy and lobbying by civil society in general, and the LGBT community in particular, the NSP includes a target of, 'Incremental roll-out of comprehensive customised HIV prevention package for MSM, lesbians and transsexuals including promotion of VCT [voluntary counselling and testing] and access to male and female condoms, and STI [sexually transmitted infections] symptom recognition' (DoH 2007b: 69).

## Recommendations

Our recommendations are premised on the critical role of government in ensuring the provision of sexual and reproductive health services for vulnerable populations in a supportive and non-discriminatory environment. We use our analytic framework to structure our recommendations, which are that government and other stakeholders:
- increase LGBT participation and engagement in their responses to HIV;
- conduct research to improve understanding of the HIV epidemic among LGBT communities;
- develop supportive programmes to improve access and coverage.

### LGBT participation and engagement in the HIV response

The NSP acknowledges past gaps in HIV policy and programme development for LGBT communities, and there is a commitment for LGBT inclusion in programme and funding priorities. This is largely unchartered terrain for government, but involvement and engagement of LGBT communities is critical, given the context and overt discrimination faced by these individuals. OUT has suggested that 'partnerships between public health programmes and LGBT service providers should be strengthened and integrated into a comprehensive framework for increasing the accessibility and relevance of appropriate health care services for LGBT people' (OUT 2007: 7).

Involvement will ensure that policies and programmes protect and respect LGBT people's right to privacy regarding their sexual orientation.

### Research to improve understanding of the epidemic

Research in other countries has shown that HIV is widespread among MSM and that without active surveillance and appropriate interventions, a hidden epidemic may flourish. Hence research should inform the social situations/contexts of HIV transmission among MSM, HIV prevention strategies among LGBT, and HIV prevention and care needs of this community (Cloete et al. 2007). Furthermore, research should provide insights into barriers to care, including funding constraints in the health services and attitudes of healthcare professionals.

### Supportive programme development

Due to the stigma experienced by LBGT populations, non-conventional channels are often used to obtain healthcare services. Creative strategies are needed to improve access to care, including outreach programmes by volunteers or professional social or health workers. Safer-sex campaigns and skills training, including the use of condoms, and the promotion of lower-risk sexual practices as alternatives to penetrative sex, are important. In other countries, peer education among MSM has proven to be very effective (UNAIDS 2000).

The education of healthcare professionals, including those working at the primary care level and within STI clinics, is essential to overcome ignorance and prejudices about same-sex practising individuals. Appropriate clinical guidelines should be developed, drawing on the rich experience of other countries. For example, in Asia and the Pacific region, clinical guidelines have been developed to assist clinicians, counsellors and other healthcare workers, especially doctors, nurses and counsellors who care for MSM and transgender people (IUSTI n.d.). The guidelines include principles and aspects of taking a confidential sexual history and doing an examination in a non-judgemental and respectful manner. Similarly, guidelines for dealing with the health concerns of lesbians have been developed by Brown University Health Services in America.[3]

## Conclusion

Using an adaptation of the CHAT tool developed by UNAIDS, we have shown that existing HIV policies and programmes in South Africa fall short of meeting the needs of same-sex practising individuals. Although there have been encouraging developments, there is inadequate engagement of the LGBT communities in HIV policy and programme development. In addition, there is a dearth of information on the prevalence of HIV among MSM in South Africa compared to the level of HIV in the general population; the social contexts in which HIV transmission is taking place among MSM; and whether prevention strategies among MSM are working. The information gap is even more pronounced in the case of same-sex practising women and bisexual and transgender individuals. Finally, we have shown that the country has some way to go in creating an enabling environment consisting of dedicated funding, adequately trained staff, and a non-discriminatory healthcare environment. As South Africa remains the country with the highest number of HIV infections, creative strategies are needed to ensure prevention of new infections among all subgroups of the population and to turn the tide of the epidemic.

## Acknowledgements

We thank Theo Sandfort and Vasu Reddy for comments on an earlier draft of this chapter. Nico Jacobs is thanked for administrative support. The views presented in the chapter are those of the authors and do not necessarily represent the decisions, policy or views of the institutions that employ the authors.

## Notes

1. Press release on *Off the Map*, (Johnson 2007) issued by the International Gay and Lesbian Human Rights Commission, 2007.
2. Durban II Declaration on HIV and AIDS Prevention, Treatment and Care, Third South African AIDS Conference held in Durban, 5–8 June 2007. Accessed December 2008, http://www.saaids.co.za/index.php?option=com_content&task=view&id=47&Itemid=35.
3. See http://www.brown.edu/Student_Services/Health_Services/Health_Education/general_health/home.htm (Accessed 6 January 2009).

## References

ASSA (Actuarial Society of South Africa) (2003) *Projections of HIV indicators abstracted from the Actuarial Society of South Africa (ASSA)*. Accessed 1 August 2007, http://www.assa.org.za/aids/content.asp?id=1000000449

AU (African Union) (2006) Africa's common position to the UN General Assembly Special Session on AIDS, Special Summit of the African Union on HIV/AIDS, Tuberculosis and Malaria, 2–4 May, Abuja, Nigeria

Bailey JV, Farquhar C & Owen C (2004) Bacterial vaginosis in lesbians and bisexual women. *Sexually Transmitted Diseases* 31(11): 691–694

Beyrer C (2007) HIV epidemiology update and transmission factors: Risks and risk contexts (16th International AIDS Conference Epidemiology Plenary). *Clinical Infectious Diseases* 44: 981–987

Canadian HIV/AIDS Clearinghouse (2002) *Are women who have sex with women at risk for getting HIV?* Fact sheet. Ottawa: Canadian Public Health Association

CDC (Centers for Disease Control and Prevention) (2006) *HIV/AIDS among women who have sex with women*. CDC HIV/AIDS fact sheet. Atlanta: CDC

CDC (2007) *HIV/AIDS among men who have sex with men.* CDC HIV/AIDS fact sheet. Atlanta: CDC

Cloete A, Simbayi LC & Kalichman SC (2006) Stigma and discrimination experiences of HIV positive men who have sex with men (MSM) and heterosexual men in Cape Town, South Africa. Poster presentation at the XVI International AIDS Conference, Toronto, 13–18 August

Cloete A, Henda N, Kalichman SC, Simbayi LC & Strebel A (2008) Stigma and discrimination experiences of HIV positive men who have sex with men in Cape Town, South Africa. *AIDS Care* 20(9): 1105–1110

Cloete A, Rispel L & Metcalf C (2007) Behind the mask: The need for research on HIV among men who have sex with men (MSM) in South Africa. Paper presented at the MSM seminar series for Pride 2007, Cape Town, South Africa

Crowe D (2005) *A descriptive report of selected data collected during the Living PoZitively support group survey conducted by the Triangle Project, July 2004.* Cape Town: Triangle Project

DoH (Department of Health) (2007a) *Summary report. National HIV and syphilis prevalence survey, South Africa, 2006.* Pretoria: DoH

DoH (2007b) *HIV&AIDS and STI national strategic plan for South Africa: 2007–2011.* Pretoria: DoH

Dorrington R, Johnson L, Bradshaw D & Daniel T-J (2006) *The demographic impact of HIV/AIDS in South Africa: National and provincial indicators for 2006.* Cape Town: Centre for Actuarial Research

Girault P, de Lind van Wijngaarden JW, Saidel T, Song N et al. (2004) HIV, STIs, and sexual behaviors among men who have sex with men in Phnom Penh, Cambodia. *AIDS Education & Prevention* 16(1): 31–44

Isaacs G & McKendrick B (1992) AIDS: The new homosexual crisis. In G Isaacs & B McKendrick *Male homosexuality in South Africa: Identity formation, culture and crisis.* Cape Town: Oxford University Press

IUSTI (The International Gay and Lesbian Human Rights Commission) (n.d.) *Clinical guidelines for sexual health care of men who have sex with men.* Asia Pacific: IUSTI

Johnson CA (2007) *Off the map: How HIV/AIDS programming is failing same sex practising people in Africa.* New York: International Gay and Lesbian Human Rights Commission

Kapp C (2007) South Africa unveils new HIV/AIDS plan. *Lancet World Report* 369(9573): 1589–1590

Kwakwa HA & Ghobrial MW (2003) Female-to-female transmission of Human Immunodeficiency Virus. *Clinical Infectious Diseases* 36(3): e40–41

Nel JA (2005) Hate crimes: A new category of vulnerable victims for a new South Africa. In L Davis & R Snyman (Eds) *Victimology in South Africa.* Pretoria: JL van Schaik

Niang C, Moreau A, Kostermans K et al. (2004) Men who have sex with men in Burkina Faso, Senegal and Gambia: The multi-country HIV/AIDS program approach. Poster presentation, 15th International AIDS Conference, Bangkok

Onyango-Ouma W, Birungi H & Geibel S (2005) *Understanding the HIV/STI risks and prevention needs of men who have sex with men in Nairobi, Kenya*. Horizons Final Report. Washington, DC: Population Council

OUT (OUT LGBT Well-being) (2007) *Health care for lesbian, gay, bisexual and transgender people: Issues, implications and recommendations*. Submission to the South African Human Rights Commission public inquiry into the right to have access to healthcare services. Accessed 6 January 2009, http://www.sahrc.org.za/sahrc_cms/downloads/OUT.doc

Ruan Y, Li D, Li X, Qian HZ et al. (2007) Relationship between syphilis and HIV infections among men who have sex with men in Beijing, China. *Sexually Transmitted Diseases* 38(4): 592–597

Rule S & Mncwango B (2006) Rights or wrongs? An explanation of moral values. In U Pillay, B Roberts & S Rule (Eds) *South African social attitudes: Changing times, diverse voices*. Cape Town: HSRC Press

Schurink E & Schurink WJ (1990) *AIDS: Lay perceptions of a group of gay men*. Pretoria: HSRC Press

Sher R (1985) AIDS in Johannesburg. *South African Medical Journal* 68(3): 137–138

Sher R (1986) Acquired Immune Deficiency Syndrome (AIDS) in the RSA. *South African Medical Journal* (Supplement) 23–26

Sher R (1989) HIV infection in South Africa, 1982–1988: A review. *South African Medical Journal* 76(7): 314–318

Sher R & dos Santos L (1985) Prevalence of HTLV-III antibodies in homosexual men in Johannesburg. *South African Medical Journal* 67(13): 484

Shisana O, Bhana A, Connolly C, Jooste S, Parker W, Pillay V, Rehle T, Simbayi L & Zuma K (2005a) *South African national HIV prevalence, HIV incidence, behaviour and communication survey*. Cape Town: HSRC Press

Shisana O, Peltzer K, Zungu-Dirwayi N & Louw JS (2005b) *The health of our educators: A focus on HIV/AIDS in South African public schools*. Cape Town: HSRC Press

Shisana O, Simbayi L et al. (2002) *Nelson Mandela/HSRC study of HIV/AIDS: South African national HIV prevalence, behavioural risks and mass media household survey, 2002*. Cape Town: HSRC Press

Teunis N (2001) Same-sex sexuality in Africa: A case study from Senegal. *AIDS and Behaviour* 5(2): 173–182

UNAIDS (2000) *AIDS and men who have sex with men: Technical update*. Geneva: UNAIDS

UNAIDS (2006a) *Report on the global AIDS epidemic*. Geneva: UNAIDS

UNAIDS (2006b) *HIV and sex between men: Policy brief*. Geneva: UNAIDS

UNAIDS (2007) *Country harmonisation and alignment tool (CHAT). A tool to address harmonisation and alignment challenges by assessing strengths and effectiveness of partnerships in the national AIDS response*. Geneva: UNAIDS

UNAIDS & WHO (2007) *AIDS epidemic update*. Geneva: UNAIDS & WHO

Van Griensven F (2007) Men who have sex with men and their epidemics in Africa. *AIDS* 21(10): 1361–1362

Van Griensven F, Thanprasertsuk S, Jommaroeng R et al. (2005) Evidence of a previously undocumented epidemic of HIV infection among men who have sex with men in Bangkok, Thailand. *AIDS* 19(5): 521–526

Van Harmelen J, Wood R, Lambrick M, Rybicki EP, Williamson AL & Williamson C (1997) An association between HIV-1 subtypes and mode of transmission in Cape Town, South Africa. *AIDS* 11(1): 81–87

Wade AS, Diallo PAN, Diop AK, Gueye K, Kane CT, Largarde E, Mboup S & Ndoye I (2005) HIV infection and sexually transmitted infections among men who have sex with men in Senegal. *AIDS* 19(18): 2133–2140

Wells H & Polders L (n.d.) *Gay and lesbian people's experience of the health care sector in Gauteng.* Research initiative of the Joint Working Group (JWG) conducted by OUT LGBT Well-being and UNISA Centre for Applied Psychology. Pretoria: OUT & JWG

Wolitski RJ, Valdiserri RO, Denning PH & Levine WC (2001) Are we headed for a resurgence of the HIV epidemic among men who have sex with men? *American Journal of Public Health* 91(6): 883–888

CHAPTER SIXTEEN

# Lessons learned from current South African HIV/AIDS research among lesbian, gay and bisexual populations

Dawie Nel

It is well known that the South African Constitution (Act 108 of 1996) promises equality on the basis of sexual orientation. Yet, this legal equality very seldom translates into full social equality. This also holds true for the HIV/AIDS arena, such as government HIV programmes targeting lesbian, gay and bisexual (LGB) people and research into LGB HIV/AIDS issues. LGB community structures have played an important role in addressing this situation. Their work takes place on many levels – they address legal discrimination, ensure appropriate services, and address wider societal prejudice and patriarchy. When it comes to HIV/AIDS research, however, these community structures cannot rely on any mainstream research. There is no national data available which offers insight and understanding into issues such as LGB HIV incidence and prevalence rates or factors contributing to risky sexual behaviour.

South African LGB structures have started filling some of the research gaps in HIV/AIDS issues. There are a few examples of national and local LGB research on the table, including coverage of HIV/AIDS issues. Such research is not enough – there are only a few studies and there are urgent gaps.

This chapter starts with a description of how mainstream South African HIV/AIDS research silences LGB issues. The focus, however, is on what HIV/AIDS research has been done, primarily by South African lesbian, gay, bisexual and transgender (LGBT) organisations. It describes research needs, how the research that has been done came about, and how the research is used programmatically. The relevant research findings, some analyses and research methodology are discussed. Based on this, conclusions and recommendations are offered for service providers, communities and researchers.

This chapter draws heavily on two presentations made at the Gender, Same-sex Sexuality and HIV/AIDS conference held in 2007 in Pretoria, the edited proceedings of which are contained in this volume. The presentations were titled 'Practical lessons learned from current South African HIV/AIDS research in general and among lesbian/gay/bisexual populations', and 'What kind of knowledge is needed and why? A service provider, community and research perspective'.

This chapter offers perspectives from a service provider within the LGB community. It focuses on research done within the context of our intervention programmes, and illustrates that, although limited, there are data upon which to build.

The chapter is informed by my own experiences as director of OUT LGBT Wellbeing (OUT), an NGO that has been in existence for more than 14 years. It is not based on a thorough scan of mainstream South African or international research, but on my knowledge of two studies we have been directly involved in. The chapter also only covers issues that affect open and self-identified lesbian women and gay men and does not include men who have sex with men (MSM) or women who have sex with women (WSW). I am aware that the complex issues surrounding MSM and WSW identities go much broader than gay men and lesbian women and that, ideally, one should cover all these categories. However, because of limited resources within the LGB sector and the need to prioritise LGB people in our work, this discussion only includes lesbian and gay people. Bisexual people are also not discussed, as this group is not a priority within the LGB sector's current agenda.

## Silencing of LGBT issues within mainstream South African research

LGBT issues are not included in mainstream HIV/AIDS research. The national antenatal prevalence studies by the Department of Health (DoH 2005), which focus on pregnant women, and the Human Sciences Research Council's national prevalence surveys (see, for example, Shisana et al. 2005), do not include the variable of sexual orientation. There are also no national data on HIV/AIDS and LGB people in large general population surveys. This holds true for all aspects, such as prevalence, informants of risky behaviours, and monitoring programmatic impacts and new tendencies, such as the rise of certain sexually transmitted infections (STIs) at specific times among certain groups. The mainstreaming of LGB HIV/AIDS research issues is an area that needs to be addressed. Stakeholders need to lobby to have these issues placed on mainstream research agendas. Probably the most urgent issue is to obtain valid and reliable data on prevalence and incidence rates among gay men and lesbian women. This type of baseline data will illustrate the extent of the problem.[1] Once prevalence rates are nationally monitored, further research should be undertaken on factors influencing risky behaviour, the impact or HIV-related intervention programmes and new tendencies.

## Context of some HIV/AIDS research within the South African LGB sector

The organised South African LGB sector is represented within the Joint Working Group (JWG), an alliance of roughly 20 structures. These are mainly LGB community structures, but also include other bodies such as university centres that have an interest in furthering LGB equality. The primary aim of the JWG is to combine resources to address common aims. The JWG has had two cycles of collaborative work – from 2003 to 2005, and from 2005 to the present. In the first cycle the focus was on combined products, namely collaborative research, a marketing booklet, and a conference for lesbians; in the second cycle, the focus was on the internal development of organisations, the development of the sector as a whole, and on more limited product and external programmatic work.[2]

On an organisational level, LGBT organisations can be roughly divided into emerging organisations and more established structures. The more established organisations have a full-time staff component, have usually been in existence for more than five years, and manage sustained programmes. The issues they address are broad and include advocating for legal reform within the sexuality, gender and human rights arena; strengthening human rights and progressive gender alliances; providing direct health and mental health services, including HIV prevention, testing and care; research; offering LGBT social spaces and hosting events such as film festivals; and mainstreaming of sexual orientation issues within selected agents, such as provincial government education departments. The scale of all these programmes is geographically limited and often only reaches selected target groups.

Turning specifically to HIV/AIDS programmes and research, there are three groups, namely OUT, the Triangle Project and the Durban Gay and Lesbian Centre, that have provided services over the last five years. They are based in Tshwane (Pretoria), Cape Town and Durban. These services include prevention programmes for selected target groups, testing, limited treatment, and care. The research done tends to relate mainly to needs analyses for programme interventions.

The JWG has completed three large quantitative studies on the levels of empowerment of lesbian and gay people in Gauteng (Wells & Polders 2004), KwaZulu-Natal (Wells & Polders 2005) and the Western Cape (Rich 2007). These studies were managed by OUT in close cooperation with the Centre for Applied Psychology at the University of South Africa (Unisa). In the case of the Western Cape, the study was done by the Unisa Centre for Applied Psychology and Triangle Project. This type of collaboration, between community structures and academic institutions, has been of great value, especially in directing academic expertise to programmatic needs within the community. These studies have clearly illustrated discrimination and its impact, informed programme planning and enabled the JWG to lobby for increased resources on the basis of clear evidence.

## Empowerment of gay and lesbian people

### Methodology and aims

Most other research in the area of HIV and AIDS and the LGBT community undertaken in South Africa has been largely of a qualitative nature. The few existing studies have dealt primarily with white middle-class men, and have excluded black people, lesbian women, and people from the lower socio-economic classes. The main aim of the JWG research was to gather data of a quantitative nature that was more broadly representative of the South African population as a whole (Wells & Polders 2004). The research was initially limited to Gauteng, with the possibility of repeat studies in provinces where services for lesbian and gay people are provided. The reason for this was to try to control variables that could potentially influence findings, such as urban/rural differences.

The scope of the research project was vast and included both macro and micro issues to serve as indicators for empowerment. The research was informed by theory as well as the needs outlined by LGBT organisations in South Africa.

The research included investigations into:
- social lifestyles;
- victimisation experienced;
- experience of the police and/or criminal justice system;
- health service satisfaction;
- health status;
- substance use;
- well-being;
- religious interest and discrimination;
- socio-demographics and LGBT people in Gauteng.[3]

The above issues were explored in relation to the influence of race, sex, age and socio-economic status. The sample was not split along racist and sexist lines; instead, clusters were identified (for example, young, black males or older, white females) for which interventions could be designed and targeted appropriately. Gay and lesbian respondents were selected through a purposive quota sampling technique. At least 30 respondents were to be acquired for each cluster. Thus, the total sample was to be comprised of at least 360 participants. Table 16.1 indicates the 12 clusters that were identified.

The final sample size was 487 respondents – 45 per cent female (160 black and 56 white women) and 55 per cent male (148 black and 117 white men). Forty-six per cent of the respondents were between 16 and 24 years, 48 per cent between 25 and 40 years, and 6 per cent were over 41 years. Altogether, 8 per cent of the respondents identified themselves as gay/lesbian and 14 per cent as bisexual (Wells & Polders 2004).

**Table 16.1** Clusters of respondents

|  | 16–24 years | | | | 25–40 years | | | |
|---|---|---|---|---|---|---|---|---|
|  | Black | | White | | Black | | White | |
|  | M | F | M | F | M | F | M | F |
| Under-resourced | ✓ | ✓ |  |  | ✓ | ✓ |  |  |
| Resourced | ✓ | ✓ | ✓ | ✓ | ✓ | ✓ | ✓ | ✓ |

Sources: Wells & Polders (2004)

## Results, analysis and discussion

This chapter will only describe the health status section of the research.

### Perception of health status

Approximately 80 per cent of the black and 90 per cent of the white respondents considered their health to be 'good' or 'excellent'. Only 2.5 per cent of black females identified their health as 'very poor'.

### Sexually transmitted infections

Respondents were asked if they had had an STI in the previous 24 months (see Table 16.2). The percentage of black females with STIs is similar to that of both black and white men; the number of black women who are unsure whether they have an STI or not is the highest in the overall sample. Due to the sensitive nature of the question and because the data are self-reported, it is possible that these figures are underestimated.

### HIV status

Regarding testing for HIV, 64 per cent of the sample had tested for HIV, with approximately half of the black and 80 per cent of the white respondents having tested. A limitation in this data is that no time frame was placed on this question, and it is not clear if this testing had taken place within the last six months (see Table 16.3).

Among the black respondents were some who did not collect or did not understand their test results, whereas these categories were non-existent for the white respondents. The number of HIV-positive lesbian women in the sample was high in comparison with international figures. This contradicts the belief that lesbian women are relatively risk-free. It should be noted that some lesbian women may also have male partners and/or experience high levels of rape.

**Table 16.2** Respondents that had a sexually transmitted infection in the previous 24 months

| Group | Yes (%) | Unsure (5) |
|---|---|---|
| Black females | 13.6 | 16.2 |
| White females | 3.7 | 3.7 |
| Black males | 13.7 | 8.2 |
| White males | 15.5 | 2.6 |

Source: Wells & Polders (2004)

**Table 16.3** Number of respondents who had tested for HIV

| Group | HIV+ (%) | Did not collect results (%) | Did not understand results (%) |
| --- | --- | --- | --- |
| Black females | 9 | 14 | 6 |
| White females | 5 | 0 | 0 |
| Black males | 15 | 4 | 3 |
| White males | 8 | 0 | 0 |

Source: Wells & Polders (2004)

## Study on the sexual behaviours of young gay men

### Methodology and aims

The study on the sexual behaviours of young gay men was conducted in 2005 by OUT in collaboration with the Centre for the Study of AIDS based at the University of Pretoria. The aim was to inform an online HIV prevention intervention, targeting young, resourced gay men using the internet to meet each other primarily for sexual contacts. An online questionnaire was put on the OUT website and on two other widely used gay websites, Mambaonline and G-Max. A total of 318 questionnaires were completed. All respondents were in the 18–35 age range and they were from all provinces in South Africa. The following areas were explored: internet usage; lifestyle issues; sexual behaviours, condom and lubrication use; HIV/AIDS; relationships; substance use; well-being.

### Results, analysis and discussion

The full results of the study are not discussed here. Rather, some findings are described in order to illustrate the extent of risk behaviours and some factors contributing to such risk.

Findings included the following:
- 19 per cent of the sample never use condoms when using alcohol and drugs; 15 per cent sometimes or mostly don't remember what they do when they use alcohol and drugs.
- 17 per cent of the sample have been pressured to have unprotected anal intercourse more than once in the last three months.
- 21 per cent of the sample said that they are not in monogamous relationships and have deliberately chosen to 'bareback'.
- Sexual risk decreases as age increases.
- 8 per cent of the sample are not 'out' to anyone and this correlates with increased sexual risk (Kruger et al. 2006).

From the above, it seems that approximately a fifth of the young, gay male respondents engaged in risky behaviours, be this unsafe sex when using substances or deliberately choosing to 'bareback'.

## Conclusion

There are many reasons why much-needed research on HIV/AIDS issues among LGB people is not available. In this chapter it was argued that it is silenced within mainstream HIV/AIDS research and within large-scale surveys among the general population. LGB issues have to be put on the agenda of mainstream research agents and this will be the task of activists, academics and other influential stakeholders.

The organised LGB sector has already begun filling some of the research gaps. However, this sector has limited capacity and many priorities. The research already done tends to be within a programmatic needs analysis framework. Increased collaboration on this type of research between community structures and academic institutions could be very useful.

Turning to the results, it is not yet possible to reliably estimate how many LGB people are HIV-positive. From the empowerment study discussed in this chapter (Wells & Polders 2004), it seems that there is reason to be concerned about the rates of HIV and STI among black lesbian women, where 9 per cent reported to be HIV-positive. Programmatically, it should be noted that there are issues for black LGB people around not fetching and/or not understanding HIV test results.

In the study on young gay men (Kruger et al. 2006) there are some indications of risky behaviours and factors that influence this. Approximately a fifth of respondents engaged in risky sex influenced by substance use and the practice of barebacking. Younger gay men are more at risk of engaging in risky behaviours, as are those who are not 'out' as a gay man. These are factors that should be considered programmatically by LGB HIV prevention agents. This study is a good example of how research could improve programmatic interventions.[4]

To sum up, collaborative efforts are crucial and collaborations between decision-makers, community workers and academics should be encouraged. Valid and reliable research has proven to be invaluable to community structures such as OUT. Research offers us opportunities to participate on public platforms and to raise LGBT issues in credible ways. In so doing, it creates spaces and opportunities to lobby for further resources and efforts to address discrimination and silencing. Valid and reliable research has been used to launch systematic work within government agencies, such as the departments of education and social development as well as within other mainstream service providers such as Lifeline. In addition, such data have drawn attention to where OUT programmes should be directed. Research could thus play a significant role in bridging the gap between legal and social equality that currently exists in South Africa.

## Notes

1. This point was illustrated in 2006 when the exclusion of gay men as blood donors by the South African National Blood Services (SANBS) was addressed by community organisations. In taking up this matter with the SANBS, community groups argued that South Africa, with a generalised HIV/AIDS epidemic, cannot simply rely on HIV prevalence rates among gay men in places like San Francisco, and then use these data to exclude this population as a high-risk group. In the absence of South African evidence-based data, this amounts to discrimination (see P Tau, 'Ban on gay's blood sparks row', *The Star*, 13/01/2006).
2. One highlight of collaborative programmatic work in the second cycle was securing the legalisation of same-sex marriage in 2006.
3. The analysis of socio-demographic variables will be used for more in-depth studies, and is not described in this chapter.
4. More information about interventions informed by the study can be viewed at www.men2men.co.za.

## References

DoH (Department of Health, South Africa) (2005) *National HIV and syphilis antenatal seroprevalence survey in South Africa*. Pretoria: DoH

Kruger T, Maritz J, Matroos S & Wells H (2006) *Sexual practices of young gay men*. Pretoria: OUT-LGBT Well-being

Rich E (2007) *Levels of empowerment among lesbian, gay, bisexual, transgender (LGBT) people in the Western Cape, South Africa*. Cape Town: Triangle Project

Shisana O, Bhana A, Connolly C, Jooste S, Parker W, Pillay V, Rehle T, Simbayi L & Zuma K (2005) *South African national HIV prevalence, HIV incidence, behaviour and communication survey*. Cape Town: HSRC Press

Wells H & Polders L (2004) *Levels of empowerment among lesbian, gay, bisexual, transgender (LGBT) people in Gauteng, South Africa*. Pretoria: Joint Working Group

Wells H & Polders L (2005) *Levels of empowerment among lesbian, gay, bisexual, transgender (LGBT) people in KwaZulu-Natal, South Africa*. Pretoria: Joint Working Group

## CHAPTER SEVENTEEN

# Observations on HIV and AIDS in Cape Town's LGBT population

Glenn de Swardt

Triangle Project is a well-established LGBT service organisation based in Cape Town; we celebrated our 25th anniversary year in 2006. The organisation aims to promote mental, physical and social health of LGBT people, and as such all aspects of our work include an emphasis on HIV-related prevention, management and care.

Current services provided by the organisation include the following:
- The Gay and Lesbian Helpline offers telephonic information and counselling seven days per week. Once activated, this service returns the caller's call and the organisation thus carries the costs of all telephonic counselling sessions. Counsellors are trained to provide safer-sex information and counselling.
- Trained and supervised community counsellors provide non-professional face-to-face counselling in Khayelitsha and the Cape Flats. This is a free service.
- Professional psychosocial, psychotherapeutic and psychiatric face-to-face counselling is offered in our clinic by our team of 16 social workers, psychologists and a psychiatrist. Some members of our team specialise in same-sex couple counselling, and we are also able to offer basic counselling related to nutrition. A fair amount of counselling is related to HIV, with individuals and to both seroconcordant and discordant couples. This service is free to anyone earning less than R3 000 per month, in which case we also reimburse travel costs incurred to access the service.
- We offer a range of support groups, including an empowerment group for gay men living with HIV. Participation in groups is free of charge.
- Our client relief service provides basic foodstuffs, vitamins and toiletries to clients in need of material aid.
- Internet support and HIV-related information is provided via the 'gay, lesbian and bisexual expert' forum on the websites Health24.com and via gaydar.co.uk
- A Gay Men's Sexual Health Clinic is conducted every Tuesday evening by our team of volunteer gay doctors. In addition to voluntary testing and counselling (VTC), using both rapid and laboratory screening, we diagnose and treat sexually transmitted infections (STIs) and provide sexual health counselling. Likewise, we offer a bi-weekly Lesbian Health Clinic. Medical services are supported by complementary health services, including massage and aromatherapy.

- We produce LGBT-related media, including specialised HIV prevention messaging and use the mass media to reach the broader community.
- We offer workshops, training courses and regular seminars to disseminate topical information. For example, the themes of two recent seminars were 'The interface between recreational drugs and ARV treatment', and 'Is reinfection just a myth?'
- Our community outreach workers are well versed in providing basic HIV-related information, and distribute our media products, with free condoms and water-based lubricant, to diverse geographical areas.
- Our legal service is able to offer HIV-related legal information.
- We conduct research, often in partnership with large research organisations such as the Medical Research Council and the Human Sciences Research Council. We have established a close partnership with the Desmond Tutu HIV Centre, resulting in the Mother City Men's Health Project which specifically addresses sexual health issues in the men who have sex with men (MSM) population.

The generalised, collective psychological response to HIV by lesbian women in Cape Town is, 'I am not at risk and therefore I don't need to test.' This is often based on the erroneous assumption that lesbians are magically immune from HIV because they do not have sex with men and therefore are not exposed to semen. Many lesbians themselves believe that Cape Town's lesbian population is arbitrarily isolated in having no sexual contact with men.

Many heterosexuals and gay men believe lesbians only express themselves sexually within committed and monogamous relationships and are somehow incapable of having anonymous sex or of being promiscuous.

Contrary to the above, we need to acknowledge the rich and diverse content of women's sexual identities and how these are expressed. The reality is that Triangle Project has indeed tested lesbian-identifying women as HIV-positive, and has mourned the loss of lesbian clients and volunteers to AIDS. It is a sad reflection on our society that in all such instances transmission occurred through rape or coerced sex with men. Indeed, it is generally known that lesbians – particularly those living in traditionally black township areas and in rural areas – are at an increased risk of rape on the grounds of their sexual orientation. 'Curative' or 'corrective' rape, based on the myth that a lesbian sexual orientation can be 'cured' through rape, has culminated in countless lesbians being infected with HIV. This represents a marked interface between social (myths, hate crimes, gender-based violence and prejudice), psychological (trauma) and health-related issues (HIV and lack of access to lesbian-friendly services).

In addition to many lesbians having been previously heterosexually married or otherwise in a sexual relationship where they were exposed to the male partner's HIV-positive status, many are socio-economically compelled to engage in sex with men in order, for example, to pay for rent or to ensure that they retain their jobs.

An increasing number of lesbian women are being counselled with regard to being HIV-positive. In many instances such women initially seek counselling services as opposed to our medical services, presenting with depression or relationship issues; only subsequently are they able to address previously being raped and being HIV-positive.

During 2006 we counselled our first seroconcordant HIV-positive lesbian couple, with the majority of couples being serodiscordant. Of particular concern, based on the assumption that woman-to-woman transmission of HIV is impossible, is that some HIV-positive lesbians choose not to disclose their status to their partners.

Our clinic has tested a very limited number of transgender individuals as being HIV-positive. In all such instances, transgender clients have engaged in commercial sex work where they often report experiencing physical assault and clients demanding unprotected intercourse.

Cape Town is a very interesting city in terms of addressing diverse sexual health issues. Besides accommodating a rich diversity of socio-cultural sexual identities, the city is a very popular destination for both international and domestic gay tourists. Northern-hemisphere sexual dynamics frequently 'land' in Cape Town and subsequently travel inland from here. Examples of this include not only actual sexual behaviours but also terms used to describe such behaviours (including 'felching', 'docking', 'snowballing' and 'slamming'). Whilst these sexual acts have long been practised in Cape Town, it is only recently that their northern-hemisphere labels started being articulated by local men in their sexual discourses.

One cannot address the HIV pandemic in the gay population of Cape Town without taking cognisance of the endemic use of recreational substances. In particular, Cape Town is experiencing alarming abuse of methamphetamine. An alarming number of gay men in Cape Town have incorporated the use of the drug into their sexual interactions. Interestingly, the complex discourse around sexuality in the city becomes manifest when discussing the use of methamphetamine – white gay-identifying men usually refer to the drug as 'crystal', while the drug is referred to as 'tik' when used by coloured people. There is less understanding of the use of the drug methcathinone (commonly referred to as 'khat' or 'kat') by the gay population, but anecdotal evidence suggests it is the sexual drug of choice for many. Some men discuss their choice of either crystal or khat according to whether they plan to 'top' or 'bottom' in their sexual encounters.

Anecdotal information suggests that crystal is often the primary drug used in venues such as Cape Town's steam bath and clubs, whilst khat features more prominently in home-based sexual interactions and parties. For many patrons of the gay village precinct in Cape Town, local car guards reportedly serve as the primary suppliers of recreational drugs.

There is clear evidence that abuse of crystal and other drugs by the gay population is a major contributing factor to ongoing HIV infection and STI transmission.

First-hand observations, based on face-to-face conversations, indicate that approximately 80 per cent of patrons visiting the steam bath over weekends are using recreational drugs.

'Barebacking' (consciously unprotected anal intercourse) is rife in Cape Town; alarmingly, anecdotal data suggest that more than 60 per cent of penetrative sex taking place in public spaces (a steam bath, a leather club and a gay porn venue and sex club) is high risk. In a similar vein, there is an apparent increase in the number of local gay men whose profiles on the popular cruising website *Gaydar* indicate that they consume recreational drugs 'socially'.

According to one theory, the collective psychological response to HIV by MSM in Cape Town is one of, 'I am at risk, but I remain negative until tested positive'.[1] The latter stance culminates in two disturbing factors, namely:
- many MSM avoid testing; and
- it 'allows' them to claim (to both their partner and themselves) to be HIV-negative when entering a sexual interaction, without causing too much psychological dissonance.

Further to this scenario, the cycle of risk is augmented by two additional consequences to the collective denial, namely:
- the collective defence (denial and deceit) makes it easier for MSM to accept *each other's* claims to be negative at face value, thereby becoming a collective collusion; and
- unless blatantly challenged by either partner, the denial facilitates an alliance to engage in barebacking.[2]

Paradoxically, barebacking thus becomes ritualised and serves as a defence against the fear of HIV and AIDS, creating a space where denial is absolute. The use of drugs such as crystal further seals the sexual space against any superego impulses that may cause psychological dissonance. Interestingly, very few gay men in Cape Town appear aware of the availability of post-exposure prophylaxis (PEP) yet they are able to access recreational drugs with utmost ease.

It is little wonder then that for some gay men semen has become a fetish and the exchange of this fluid through sexual interaction has become the primary determinant in terms of reaching sexual fulfilment. Clearly, advocating for condom use in this scenario is highly challenging and alternative messaging needs to be explored. Promoting the use of polyurethane female condoms for anal sex by MSM with a fetish for semen provides an interesting option in that it allows the receptive partner to literally 'collect' semen from his partner/s without exposing himself to risk. To date, we have received feedback indicating curiosity when promoting the use of female condoms to men visiting the local steam bath.

In order to circumvent the endemic denial of HIV, we are careful to label our weekly Gay Men's Sexual Health Clinic as a generic (as opposed to an HIV-centred) medical service. We provide both a confidential and anonymous service, using fake names and only professional gay counsellors are deployed. In a similar vein, our Women's Health Clinic is clearly not labelled as being specifically HIV-related, in order to negate the stigma surrounding HIV, and in reality conducts more pap smears than HIV tests.

**Table 17.1** Sex-positive paradigm

| Stage | Activity | Content | Aim |
|---|---|---|---|
| 1 | Recognise the ritualised meaning related to the client seeking VTC at this time | Counsellor indirectly determines whether the ritual is related to appeasing guilt about unsafe sex, a cleansing ritual, a punitive ritual, a ritual related to entering a new relationship or a combination of many factors | Establishing rapport |
| 2 | Recognise homophobia and internalised analphobia | Counsellor explains that HIV is not transmitted through any sexual act, but through the exchange of high-risk body fluids, notably semen and blood. If socio-culturally appropriate, counsellor might mention several sexual acts, such as rimming, fucking, kissing, sucking or fisting. Counsellor affirms that ideally MSM should not experience any shame or guilt related to their sexual expressions | Negating client's internalised guilt, shame or conflict about his internal fantasy world and behaviours and reducing psychological dissonance that impairs congruent and open discourse |
| 3 | Provide accurate information | Didactic input. Counsellor explains that HIV is transmitted through body fluids, explains the varying viral concentration in each fluid and focuses on semen and blood as being high risk. Counsellor needs to explain the different risks between pre-ejaculate and semen and confirm that saliva poses no real risk.[a] Explain to client that even non-sexual contact with semen or blood poses a risk and give examples | Provide client with sex-positive information on the biological transmission of HIV he can relate to in order to create greater insight into HIV transmission and the dynamics underlying safer-sex messaging |
| 4 | Support client to determine his own risk of contact with the HI virus, facilitating meaningful development of a risk-reduction strategy based on potential exchanges of bodily fluids | If socio-culturally appropriate, counsellor could explain that in terms of casual or anonymous sex, it is statistically likely that most gay men have interacted sexually with other men who are HIV-positive. Counsellor helps client determine his risks by exploring his exposure to various body fluids | Enable client to make informed assessment of risk, based on concrete biological factors that circumvent dynamics related to internalised analphobia and homoprejudice |

Note: a. Approximately 80 per cent of MSM counselled believe that there is a 'relative' risk associated with the exchange of saliva but this has not discouraged them from deep kissing.

In my experience the denial around HIV by gay men is further evidenced by their poor response to HIV-focused safer sex messaging in workshops, informal discussions and in internet chat rooms. I have frequently found it easier to engage gay men in discussion about *other* STIs, such as syphilis or gonorrhoea, possibly because such infections are likely to:
- present with short-term and possibly tangible symptoms; or
- negate their short-term sexual functioning or pleasure.

Whilst the perception of HIV and AIDS threatening life psychologically overwhelms many, they remain more likely to express real concern about the short-term health and actual appearance of their penis and anus. This could be an expression of the gay community's ongoing superficial emphasis on bodiliness and the objectification of the body, specifically centred on the penis.

Another factor that negates safe sex is the lack of suitable water-based lubricants. In spite of government-issue condoms being available, the vast majority of gay-identifying and sexually active men in Cape Town are unable to access commercial lubricants due to socio-economic realities. We hear of gay men using products such as butter, cooking oil and Vaseline to facilitate anal penetration, making condom use redundant. Attention has been focused on the availability of condoms in prisons, but sadly the availability of water-based lubricants has not featured in such discourse.

Recognising the realities of social homoprejudice and internalised analphobia in gay men, our pre-test counselling model is specifically designed to *desexualise* HIV transmission (De Swardt 2000). Many MSM experience a significant level of conflict between their internalised shame and their risk-taking behaviour and sexual fantasies in the context of social constructs of homosexuality and homoprejudice, within the framework of patriarchy.

In addition to addressing the generally accepted norms and protocol related to pre-test counselling, we address the above dynamics through a sex-positive paradigm, as summarised in Table 17.1.

All test-related counselling naturally includes reference to recreational drugs, barrier methods (condoms, gloves and dental dams), suitable lubricants and PEP. Serodiscordant couples are often provided with a script for PEP to keep at home for timely use in the event of high-risk exposure.

It is essential that we ask ourselves the question: who are we attracting for VTC? My personal observation is that the high-risk population of MSM, who engage in regular barebacking for example, continue to resist HIV testing until they are confronted with clear features of having seroconverted. In the light of the endemic and rigid denial of HIV and ritualised unsafe sex, it is perhaps understandable that VTC sites in Cape Town continue to attract MSM who could be categorised as 'high anxiety, low risk'.

Research conducted jointly by Triangle Project and the University of South Africa's Centre for Applied Psychology (Rich 2007), commissioned by the Joint Working Group, indicates that of the total number of people interviewed (N = 948):
- 12 per cent of men and 1 per cent of women are HIV-positive (self-reported);
- 15 per cent of men and 5 per cent of women had an STI in the preceding 24 months;
- 23 per cent of men and 31 per cent of women have never tested for HIV;
- in the age group 16–24 years, 44 per cent of respondents had never tested.

Significantly, the above data are reflective of the gay and lesbian population in the Western Cape province as a whole, and the research report does not highlight the objective realities of HIV infection among gay men in Cape Town who engage in anonymous sex. Estimates of the prevalence of HIV among the city's gay men (who are sexually active in diverse gay venues and via *Gaydar*) range from between 40 per cent and 80 per cent. It is noted with concern that such estimates are supported by Triangle Project clients who are themselves HIV-positive and who report frequently engaging in bareback sex. Indeed, there is anecdotal evidence of men socially known to be HIV-positive being rejected by potential bottom partners when they attempt to introduce condoms into the interactions.

This is reinforced by anecdotal information gleaned from specific gay-identifying men in predominantly coloured areas, such as the Cape Flats, where a gay identity is often infused with a feminine gender identity. As opposed to predominantly white, city-dwelling gay men who espouse a markedly masculine self-identity, these coloured gay men are more likely to present as feminine. Their desired sexual partners are invariably straight-identifying MSM who are happy to top the effeminate partners without needing to question their own heterosexual identities. In such situations, the straight-identifying men enjoy relative social power over the receptive gay-identifying partners, with the latter often colluding with an assumption that the more powerful partner is entitled to unprotected intercourse. As one client stated to me, 'I wanted him so badly and if I tried to get a condom he would be gone.'

Indeed, I assert that we still have a very limited understanding of the complex and varied power dynamics that play out between men engaging in sex and how such dynamics impact on both unsafe and safer sex. At one extreme this manifests in male-on-male rape – which I suggest has been neglected in research – but the power dynamics playing out between top and bottom, young and old, resourced and poor, racial groupings and gay-identifying and straight-identifying MSM, are worthy of further research.

The Triangle Project is meeting the above challenges by, inter alia, refining our services, attempting to ask relevant research questions, and through specific public education and training initiatives. New services planned include the use of a mobile VTC clinic, a support group for lesbian survivors of rape, training a group of skilled volunteers to form a 'safer-sex crew' to initiate discussion on HIV and recreational drug use among MSM, and rolling out our distribution of water-based lubricants. Research initiatives include an emphasis on better understanding the complex sexual and power dynamics impacting on our client populations and how these can be utilised to promote behaviour changes and better access to relevant services.

In order to extend access to LGBT-friendly health services, the organisation plans – in partnership with the city's health department – to train staff at selected community clinics in sexual identities and how such staff can challenge their own bias towards non-heterosexual diversity. Trained facilities will be rewarded with a plaque of accomplishment – similar to the grading system used to rank hotels – and the LGBT community will be informed of such 'gay-friendly' resources through the mass media.

In terms of the major research need regarding HIV and AIDS among Cape Town's LGBT population, we again call for an in-depth and detailed study of the impact of the disease on the LGBT population.

Until such time as a baseline study is able to provide hard data, it remains almost impossible to target specific prevention (both primary and secondary) messaging and other services, and to evaluate the impact of such services. In recognising the uniqueness of Cape Town's sexual and gender identities we are hopeful that any HIV prevalence studies conducted in the city will cater to our diversity by including clearly stratified sampling methods.

## Conclusion

This chapter has relied heavily on community-based observations of various elements of Cape Town's LGBT population. It has attempted to highlight the distinctly different challenges in addressing HIV and AIDS in lesbian and gay groupings, while focusing on the attitudes and behaviours of particularly high-risk MSM groupings. Any organisation with limited capacity needs to question where to focus its resources according to several dynamics, including the continuum of education–VTC–management–treatment, as well as the following:
- the anticipated feasibility of shifting attitudes and changing sexual behaviours; and
- the degree of vulnerability of population groupings according to their perceived access to information and barrier methods (including water-based lubricant), and their levels of empowerment to reduce their own risks of HIV infection.

In conclusion, then, this chapter postulates that we must be very wary of literally 'writing off' groupings of high-risk MSM, in spite of the many challenges this population presents, and instead we should attempt to gain further insights into dynamics that feed their attitudes and behaviours. This becomes increasingly significant when we remind ourselves that this high-risk group, as described in the chapter, is not arbitrarily boundaried and has an element of appeal to vast numbers of gay men. Indeed, by understanding MSM who engage in barebacking, we are better equipped to design programmes that could potentially avoid other men being absorbed into the culture of frequent high-risk sex.

## Notes

1. G De Swardt, 'Wake up queer Cape Town! We've become trapped in denial', *The Pink Tongue*, October 2007.
2. G De Swardt, 'A few thoughts about barebacking', *Detail*, June 2003.

## References

De Swardt G (2000) *The anal taboo, Part 1.* Accessed 27 April 2008, http://www.health24.com/sex/Gay_lesbian_bisexual_issues/1253-2462,36751.aap

Rich E (2007) Levels of empowerment among LGBT people in the Western Cape. Cape Town: Triangle Project & Centre for Applied Psychology, University of South Africa

## CHAPTER EIGHTEEN

# Some personal and political perspectives on HIV/AIDS in Ethekwini

Nonhlanhla 'MC' Mkhize

The isiZulu words *Ukukukhunjulwa kwabantu, ukubhekana nenzondo, ukuqhubekela phambili* mean: 'Remembering people, confronting homophobia, moving forward.' This description in some way captures and characterises the work done by the Durban Lesbian and Gay Community and Health Centre (referred to here as the Community Centre) since its formation in 2000.

The Community Centre plays an essential role in service provision in the province of KwaZulu-Natal (KZN), located in the eastern seaboard of South Africa. HIV and AIDS is a key area of intervention within the Centre's sexual health programme. HIV and AIDS is important in a province where rates of infection and mortality are still high. And if you consider the perceptions that HIV and AIDS is a gay disease, then the connection between homophobia and disease is a necessary fact that requires our intervention. In this province the perception is rife that being gay (less so if you are a lesbian) is un-African, in some instances un-Zulu, that being gay is a Western construct and an insult to 'African' identity and 'Zulu' culture. Deep-seated prejudice continues in the mindsets of many, despite far-reaching legal victories that benefit and should protect us. Despite the legal protections and a visible black and increasingly 'open' African lesbian and gay population, prejudice and hate crimes (especially against African lesbians) prevail. The provision of services and community development initiatives through the Community Centre helps to promote positive messages about being black and gay in our communities, and also helps to debunk many myths and negative stereotypes.

While the Community Centre's role is to facilitate healthy self-concepts for lesbian, gay, bisexual and transgender (LGBT) communities, directed largely at the black working-class communities, we maintain a vigilant activist focus and are actively involved in campaign work that promotes universal human rights for all. Through our work, we strive to remain relevant, appropriate and user-driven as we continue to provide a 'safe space' for people who are marginalised from the mainstream of our society. And, central to our work is an understanding that HIV and AIDS is a disease affecting all of us, that it is linked to our human rights, and that we have a right to proper information, prevention and treatment. But understanding the work of the Community Centre in relation to HIV and AIDS (including current gaps and future needs) cannot be considered without taking into account our history.

## Context and history

The history of the Community Centre is closely related to the National Coalition for Gay and Lesbian Equality (NCGLE). The latter was a voluntary association of 74 LGBT organisations in South Africa and, in the early 1990s, it was the only national organisation of its kind in South Africa with an explicit political agenda of mobilising gay and lesbian people. Formed in December 1994, the NCGLE successfully lobbied the Constitutional Assembly (the body that drafted the South African Constitution) for the inclusion of sexual orientation as one of the protected grounds for non-discrimination in the 1996 Constitution of the Republic of South Africa. The NCGLE was mandated to work for legal and social equality for its members, as determined by its annual national conferences.

Stalwarts of our struggle, such as Zackie Achmat, Sheila Lapinsky, Edwin Cameron, the late Simon Nkoli and Ronald Louw, reminded us of the political importance of our work. Phumi Mtetwa, Mazibuko Jara and many others also shaped the course of our history with their work in the NCGLE. The work included law reform, lobbying, litigation, advocacy, employment equity, leadership training and development (work that is now subsumed in the Lesbian and Gay Equality Project). The NCGLE made significant public and policy interventions in arenas such as the defence force, police services, immigration services, education and health services. For strategic reasons, much of the work of the NCGLE was carried out in Johannesburg and Cape Town. However, the NCGLE had a number of provincial branches, the most active, in our opinion, being the KZN Coalition.

Formed in April 1995, the KZN Coalition lobbied and advocated for lesbian and gay equality beyond the period of the adoption of South Africa's Constitution (Act 108 of 1996). Although its membership was primarily made up of individuals, affiliate members included local university gay and lesbian organisations, gay and lesbian churches, and principally young, black gay men and lesbians. The work of the KZN Coalition was undertaken exclusively by a core group of volunteers who met regularly at people's homes or in parks to plan activities.

Between 1995 and 1999, the KZN Coalition held public meetings and consultative forums in which many people from the Durban metropolis and rural areas participated, including people from Newcastle, Ladysmith, Richards Bay and Ulundi. The initial brief and mandate of the KZN Coalition was to lobby for the inclusion and retention of 'sexual orientation' in a clause of the Bill of Rights in the new Constitution. This goal was met when then-President Nelson Mandela signed the Constitution into law at Sharpeville on 10 December 1996. The second brief, emanating from constitutional recognition, was the process of decriminalising homosexuality – this involved developing legislation to remove discriminatory clauses from the statute books (for example, opening the way for adoption and custody rights, and rights to pensions and medical insurance for same-sex partners).

The post-1996 work of the KZN Coalition focused on public and political education and matters related to the decriminalisation of same-sex conduct. At the same time, gay and lesbian people in KZN expressed the urgent need for a service-driven community centre that would also provide a safe space for gay and lesbian people in Durban. The idea of establishing a community centre was unanimously adopted by participants at a KZN coalition consultative conference in the mid-1990s.

Vasu Reddy, our late comrade Ronald Louw and I established the Durban Community Centre on 9 August 2000, National Women's Day in South Africa, renting office space from the Treatment Action Campaign (TAC). It is telling that what is now the leading movement in HIV and AIDS in South Africa was a key partner and supporter of the Community Centre's work from the beginning. On the day we formed, we were joined by our loyal comrades, friends and volunteers at the time – Bongani Mthiyane, Bonga Emile Dlamini, Linda Mayekiso and the late McDivitt Hove. Justice Edwin Cameron and the deputy mayor (Councillor Logie Naidoo) of eThekwini Municipality officially opened the Centre in April 2001. We now operate as an independent organisation, with our own space in the central business district of eThekwini (popularly known as the City of Durban).

The history of the Community Centre's formation demonstrates our close relationship with social and human rights movements focused on HIV and AIDS and gender. It is no coincidence that HIV and AIDS work within the Community Centre was integrally linked to the influence and impact of the TAC. Some of our staff, including myself, are still actively involved in TAC's programmes.

A few months after April 2001, the Community Centre's application for funding from the AIDS Foundation of South Africa (AFSA) was approved by the then executive director (Gary Adler) who had previously been the director of our sister organisation, the Triangle Project (Cape Town). After Adler left AFSA, his successor and the current executive director, Debbie Mathew, continued to support the Community Centre in a number of our initiatives, particularly in counselling services (for both mental and sexual health). AFSA funding facilitated the establishment of the first gay and lesbian service-oriented community centre on the east coast of South Africa. Much of the political work of the KZN Coalition is now taken up by our Community Centre projects, which focus on capacity building in gay and lesbian communities, public education and training from a human rights perspective, lobbying and advocacy, sexual and mental health, and legal advice. Our vision is to empower the LGBT communities by providing services, training and support to enable them to claim their rights to equality, dignity and freedom within the context of transformation. Our work therefore translates into:
- direct services (personal, HIV and legal counselling and advice, research/resource, and information services);
- support (individual and group support through counselling; sexual health services through prevention, treatment workshops and material, condom/

femidom distribution; human rights campaigning and advocacy; gay and lesbian tourist advice);
- training (internally through weekly staff development seminars, discussions and LGBT movies; and externally through community outreach workshops, diversity training (primarily for the business industry) and edutainment activities.

In the area of HIV and AIDS education and support, the Community Centre offers services for LGBT communities including the following: awareness workshops; HIV individual and group counselling; HIV-positive living workshops; information on sexually transmitted infections (STIs), HIV and tuberculosis testing and treatment; HIV buddies; and home-care services.

## The communities we serve

To reinforce our vision, we implement our mission which is directed towards promoting diversity, particularly sexual diversity that challenges inequality, oppression and discrimination, within mainstream society. LGBT communities in Durban are diverse. The Community Centre's focus has been predominantly focused on black, Indian, coloured and historically disadvantaged communities, although this latter category is slowly changing as our democracy evolves. Our focus goes beyond the cityscapes, and includes surrounding townships as well as small towns in KZN. We work in areas such as Chatsworth (predominantly Indian), Wentworth (predominantly coloured) and Lamontville (predominantly African), addressing class and race issues that are often overlooked in gay and lesbian work. By working with people from these largely working-class areas in community halls, schools and churches, our organisation remains committed to working with black and poor lesbian and gay communities.

Unsurprisingly, mainly the youth seem to access our services. Many youth who visit our Community Centre are also unemployed. Some have been expelled from their homes because of their sexual orientation. This is at times compounded by poor conditions of education and health. In the eight years of operation in Durban and surrounds, the Community Centre has already made a significant impact on the communities that we serve, and has also begun making inroads into the rest of KZN. The positive impact has been largely within the STI and HIV and AIDS programme, through our condom distribution, safer-sex talks, and seminars on power balance in relationships. Our diversity/sensitivity training, which promotes the 'knowing your rights so as to be able to claim them' message, has also had a major impact. However, as we continue to learn (in large part through the death of Ronald Louw, who failed to have an HIV test and as result learnt of his status two months before he died in 2005), we know that a lot of work remains to be done in encouraging LGBT communities and society at large to *test frequently and to get early treatment for STIs and HIV*. Launched in Ronald's memory in 2005, the Ronald Louw 'Get Tested, Get Treated' memorial campaign is mainstreamed in the Community Centre's work.

The campaign is a vivid reminder of what we can learn from Ronald's life and work, and how best we can negotiate our own lives as lesbians and gays by learning from Ronald's failure to be tested early.

As may be deduced, a clear political and educative aspect informs our work. Our aim is to nurture communities through providing them with access to information on a range of issues, while simultaneously helping our target group develop healthier self-images. Our work challenges people to raise questions concerning their identity, and to respond to the homophobia of the hegemonic heterosexual population. By confronting issues of classism, sexism and racism in the context of homophobia (through regular interactive workshops), we are beginning to offer an internal critique of the diversity and differences that characterise our heterogeneous communities. We recognise and address the important issues of racism and classism in gay and lesbian communities. We also recognise and address the damage these realities have caused to people.

The mission statement of our organisation emphasises the view that service provision is a political 'coming in' (as opposed to 'coming out') to society. We believe that the provision of services is informed by the same logic that informed gay and lesbian liberation (the freedom from homosexual oppression), and therefore constitutes further development of our freedom as South Africans. The extension of services, therefore, is a refined development of rights in the legal sense. If we accept that rights are products of social relations and historical circumstances, then we also hold that services reinforce the ideal of citizenship, which may be broadened to include *social* as well as *civic* rights. In order to fully grasp what 'services' imply, I will explain some of the strategies we use.

Our initiatives promote systematic social change as a strategic process to challenge homophobia. This is informed by an overall strategy to challenge anti-discriminatory practices. To reinforce this, our organisation fosters strategic partnerships and networks with organisations that are working within a human rights framework (such as the Gender Aids Forum, TAC, other gay and lesbian service providers, and broader South African human rights organisations). As a result, we are currently actively involved in the Joint Working Group (JWG) (a loose coalition of lesbian and gay organisations) on a number of strategic areas related to research, advocacy and networking. At the time of writing (late 2008), the JWG was in the process of formulating a programme for rollout to lesbians and gay men on HIV and AIDS. Human rights lobbying, training and gender equality are driven by our campaigns coordinator. The lobbying work of the Community Centre ranges from issuing a press release on homophobia or a particular issue, to coordinated campaigns around an identified priority, such as our campaign to challenge the common law definition of marriage.

Another strategy is to offer direct services to the gay and lesbian community as a way of empowering individuals within that community. This entails direct visits to targeted communities within and outside the city centre. These visits focus on developing our organisation by building the leadership capacity of black gay men and lesbians. Our organisation will continue with this broad mission to work with poor lesbians and gay men.

## The road ahead: HIV and AIDS barriers and challenges

The Community Centre is fully aware that service provision in the context of programming (where HIV and AIDS is a factor) requires research-based interventions. We understand that 'research' is a broad concept and can vary depending on the context in which one is located. While we engage in basic research to assist us with our programmes, we recognise that our programmes could also benefit from a better understanding of HIV and AIDS in relation to same-sex sexuality in our country.

Homosexuality is criminalised in many African countries – for example, Zimbabwe, Nigeria, Cameroon and Kenya have instituted discriminatory laws that negatively affect LGBT communities. Apart from making human rights work difficult in Africa, criminalising same-sex sexual activity has resulted in the exclusion of LGBT, men who have sex with men (MSM) and women who have sex with women (WSW) communities from healthcare programmes and HIV prevention campaigns in their own countries. In environments where the state fails to protect and promote equal rights for its citizens to live, access safety and security services, education, housing, and healthcare services, HIV infection rates among people worsen. While we in South Africa have protections, we nevertheless face hate crimes and discrimination, mainly from 'straight' society. It is also widely acknowledged that we have no detailed prevalence studies conducted in South Africa that profile MSM and WSW and, because of the lack of such data, we do not have appropriate interventions that fully address prevention of HIV among these populations. We understand that MSM and WSW communities exist (they often 'live' and socialise within various communities, but do not want to be visible).

At the service provision level we recognise that:
- There are numerous attempts to attend to the *known* needs of LGBT communities (for example, service provision, education, advocacy, policy formation, and materials development and distribution).
- There is some support (organisational, clinics, professionals, individuals) for HIV-infected LGBT communities.
- There are some LGBT-specific HIV programmes within specific organisations and institutions.

We would like to see:
- Greater understanding and addressing of LGBT, MSM, WSW needs (for example wider availability of preventative measures).
- The existence of more, and the full utilisation of, support systems for HIV- and AIDS-affected and infected individuals (for example, we need sensitised

healthcare workers, better access to healthcare, better quality healthcare provision, better access to knowledge and information from healthcare institutions).
- More accessible HIV programmes beyond counselling, education, voluntary counselling and testing and support.

We think what may be needed is the following:
- The implementation of needs-orientated programmes (for example, services, campaigns and policies) as these contribute to a community's acceptance, appreciation and even proper utilisation of the programmes.
- Support for HIV-positive LGBT, MSM and WSW (for example, the inclusion of LGBT health issues in curricula, research studies, public healthcare, welfare services, and in accessing information, prevention and treatment).
- More LGBT-, MSM- and WSW-specific HIV programmes beyond HIV prevention, testing and treatment.

While there may be no national data on the prevalence of HIV and AIDS among the LGBT populations, based on the Community Centre's *Oral Sex Survey 2003: A Snap Shot* (Livingston & Mkhize 2003) and our 2004/05 sexual practices qualitative research study (Ebden & Mkhize 2004), we have reason to believe that the HIV and AIDS prevalence rate among LGBT people might be higher than is generally assumed. This is based on the number of condoms distributed versus the numbers of self-reported rates of condom use, and self-reported rates of STI (Livingstone & Mkhize 2003).

The seven-month *Oral Sex Survey 2003* explored whether people engaged in protected or unprotected oral sex, an aspect far too often overlooked when dealing with sexual health issues (Livingstone & Mkhize 2003). Based on a sample of 844 responses, only 754 (89.3 per cent) could be used. These responses reflected the following:
- 63 per cent of respondents were males and 37 per cent females;
- the overall age average was 25.5 years;
- the average age for males was 27.3 years and 22.4 years for females;
- in terms of racial demographics: 54.2 per cent of respondents were African, 23.7 per cent were white, 11.7 per cent were Indian, 6 per cent were Asian, and 4.4 per cent were coloured;
- 50.4 per cent self-identified as straight (heterosexual), 27.7 per cent gay, 11.0 per cent bisexual, 7.2 per cent lesbian, 3.3 per cent 'questioning' and 0.4 per cent transgender.

The survey revealed that 55.2 per cent of the respondents did not use any form of protection during oral sex. Of these:
- 67.5 per cent were male and 32.5 per cent female;
- the majority were between the ages of 22 and 27 years (40.9 per cent), while nearly a quarter (24.5 per cent) fell between the ages of 16 and 21 years;
- 45.9 per cent of respondents self-identified as straight, 29.6 per cent gay, 12.3 per cent bisexual, 8.9 per cent lesbian, 2.6 per cent 'questioning' and 0.7 per cent transgender;

- in terms of racial demographics: 44.7 per cent were African, 30.3 per cent were white, 14.2 per cent were Indian, 5.8 per cent were Asian, and 5.0 per cent were coloured.

At a research level, the current situation is such that we would like to see:
- Research into the *specific* needs (same-sex sexual activity and sexual health) and issues (hate crimes, gender-based violence) of LGBT, MSM and WSW communities, and at all social, economic and political levels.
- A central, accessible register of all research done on gender, same-sex sexualities and HIV.
- Continuous *informed* research towards addressing the challenges and attending to the needs of LGBT, WSW and MSM, as communicated by various research reports.

At the risk of belabouring the point, in most African societies same-sex sexuality is regarded as 'unnatural' and 'un-African'. Despite these perceptions, same-sex sexual practice exists. It is therefore essential that research takes into account the variety of same-sex sexual practices and the contexts in which they are expressed. But at a community level we must also take into account that:
- There are lesbian and gay parents, those with HIV, and those with children whose needs and issues remain unknown, are not understood, and in most cases not addressed.
- There is limited private and public knowledge on the sexual health of LGBTs.

## Conclusion

It is important to acknowledge that the HIV epidemic is multilayered and complex. This is also the case when trying to understand sexuality in all its diverse expressions. Therefore there is a need for holistic research, programme strategising at service provision level, and political awareness at community education level. The Community Centre believes that there is a need for an emphatic, intensive, holistic approach to research on same-sex sexualities and HIV at different social, economic and political levels within the context of:
- what benefit this has on the knowledge pool (available, accessible, and accurate information and literature);
- the spin-off this has on the implementation of better and specific needs-orientated service provision (specific programmes, counselling, prevention, treatment, care);
- advocacy work;
- policy-making processes.

In all of this we also place a premium on the importance of:
- Research that prioritises women (especially their specific vulnerabilities and effective long-term interventions).

- Research into and service provision of training and media production that attends to the sexual health needs and issues of LGBT, WSW, MSM and other same-sex sexualities with disabilities.
- Studying and understanding the impact of HIV in sexual identities beyond same-sex sexualities identified as LGBT (in other words WSW and MSM are important populations to prioritise).
- Identifying opportunities to use various forms and methods of research, public organising and messaging (such as photography and video) in addressing the challenges faced in accessing accurate information towards better understanding sexual identity, sexual expression and sexual behaviour.

As indicated earlier, the death of Ronald Louw of AIDS-related complications in 2006 served as a turning point for much of the work we had collectively commenced as a strategic team in 2000. As he lay dying at Westville Hospital, Ronald expressed the desire that, should he recover, he would begin a campaign for early testing. In 2006, the Community Centre launched the Ronald Louw Get Tested, Get Treated Memorial Campaign. This campaign is the Community Centre's flagship and will be sustained in all our prevention work in coming years. Our work will always be informed by the need to use knowledge (and to probe that which we do not know) to ensure HIV/AIDS is reduced in our communities and to ensure social change in our society.

## References

Dlamini N & Mkhize N (Eds) (2005) An exploration of sexual practices rendering Durban lesbians and women who have sex with women vulnerable to sexually transferred infections. Research commissioned by the Durban Lesbian & Gay Community & Health Centre

Ebden T & Mkhize N (Eds) (2004) Negotiating duality and discrimination: An exploration of the meaning of sexual practices in the lesbian, gay and bisexual communities of Durban. Research commissioned by the Durban Lesbian & Gay Community & Health Centre

Livingston J & Mkhize N (2003) *Durban oral sex survey 2003: A snap shot.* Durban: Durban Lesbian & Gay Community & Health Centre

CHAPTER NINETEEN

# Health for all? Health needs and issues for women who have sex with women

Vicci Tallis

> Lesbian women are often a silent and invisible majority within the broader definition of marginalised sexuality. (Wells et al. n.d.: 1)

Despite a progressive Constitution and legislation, lesbian women face double marginalisation in South Africa: both as women and as women who have sex with women (WSW) living in a patriarchal, heterosexist society. Some lesbian women face deeper marginalisation, for example because of race, class, ethnicity or HIV status. Multiple marginalisation impacts on different aspects of women's lives, including their health. Women's health in general, and the health needs of WSW in particular, does not seem to be high on the agendas of health service providers and researchers.

The advent of HIV and AIDS in the late 1970s and early 1980s forced LGBTI (lesbian, gay, bisexual, transgender and intersex) health issues into the spotlight. Initially conceived of as a 'gay disease' and named accordingly as GRID (Gay Related Immune Disease), lesbian women or WSW were included in the category 'high risk' by virtue of the fact that they were having same-sex sex. Once it became apparent that WSW were not, in fact, high risk, the focus on lesbian women shifted again and lesbians, and HIV-positive lesbians in particular, as well as lesbian health issues in general, once again disappeared from the agenda. Even though much rhetoric is dispensed about the gender dimensions of HIV and AIDS and (heterosexual) women's vulnerability, HIV and AIDS and women have been under-researched. For example, women are often in the minority in treatment/clinical trials, and when they are well represented, little attention is paid to the gender differences in prognosis and treatment of HIV and AIDS (Tallis 2001). Furthermore, the issues of WSW and HIV are often completely ignored despite the fact that, although woman-to-woman transmission is low, there are many lesbian and bisexual women who are living with HIV.

It is useful to locate lesbian health issues within the context of women's health debates: health has long been an issue for gender activists and feminists globally. A gendered approach to health does not only include addressing biological factors but also considers the critical roles that social and cultural factors play in promoting, protecting or impeding health (Garcia-Moreno 1999). Gender inequality impacts on every aspect of health and illness. This includes differences in vulnerability to illness and disease, prevention strategies, the response of the individual to symptoms, the organisation and delivery of healthcare, the politics of diagnosis, questions asked by clinicians and researchers, and knowledge and understanding of disease and treatment (Lorber 1997). Given the subject position of WSW, the negative gendered aspects of healthcare are felt more acutely, with WSW being largely invisible in the healthcare sector.

Medical research is profoundly gendered. It is often determined from a male perspective, and for the most part is about profit margins. Pre-clinical and clinical trials are expensive, but if a product is proven to be efficacious, then the possibility of massive economic gain is high. Women's health issues, both general and around sexual health and rights, are not seen as lucrative (a recent example is microbicides, a potential women-controlled HIV prevention technology, which is in research and development phases but is still not funded by the major pharmaceutical companies).

Sexual health rights broadly cover having control and autonomy over one's own body; having sex when, with whom and how one wants; making decisions about one's own sexuality and sexual orientation; experiencing sexual enjoyment; having the means to protect oneself from the risk of the consequences of sex, such as pregnancy and sexually transmitted infections (STIs), including HIV; and having access to non-judgemental, responsive services which help deal with sexual health concerns. Reproductive health rights include access to safe and appropriate contraceptives; access to termination of pregnancy; ability to plan if and when to conceive; assisted pregnancy for women who require it; and safe, accessible ante- and postnatal services. Access to the full range of sexual and reproductive health services and rights is essential for lesbian women yet common problems experienced by women tend to receive little attention when they are *not* seen as part of women's reproductive role.

Where the same disease affects both men and women, many researchers have ignored possible differences in diagnosis, symptoms, prognosis and the relative effectiveness of different treatments. Women's exclusion from research is often justified on the grounds that cyclical hormonal changes make it difficult to interpret results and/or the fact that women may become pregnant and put the foetus at risk. This shows the heterosexist bias in the assumption that all women may become pregnant. Women are treated on the basis of information gathered from research on drugs that have not been tested on women's bodies, for diseases which may not have been studied in women and in which women's experience of illness and treatment has not been adequately explored (Doyal 1995; Lorber 1997).

Further marginalisation occurs with the many and varied health issues of WSW. Lesbian health issues encompass general health, women's health issues, as well as sexual and reproductive health issues specific to WSW. For the purpose of this chapter, the focus will be on sexual and reproductive health issues, with a focus on HIV and AIDS as a major issue facing all women in South Africa and globally.

Although the terms 'lesbian', 'bisexual' and 'WSW' are used interchangeably in this chapter, they do not necessarily mean the same thing. WSW may or may not identify with the label 'lesbian' or 'bisexual'. Studies on identity show that many WSW do not self-identify as lesbian or bisexual. Morgan and Wieringa (2005) noted that the experience of many WSW includes having had relationships with men (in fact, they note there is a 'great deal of heterosexuality') for a range of reasons, including enforced heterosexuality, social pressure to be heterosexual and bear children, and personal choice. Some of the women interviewed in their research identified as lesbian, whilst others preferred not to label themselves or used other terminology, including 'bisexual' and 'dyke', and one woman in a lesbian relationship labelled herself as 'straight'.

The provision of appropriate health services for lesbian and bisexual women or WSW should be based on adequate knowledge of these complexities and issues. There is a huge gap in our understanding of sexuality, including sexual behaviour and practices. This chapter argues that lesbian health issues, as with most issues and experiences of the LGBTI community, have not received adequate attention from researchers.

## The research agenda: Where are women who have sex with women?

In South Africa, as on the continent in general, virtually no research has been conducted on the experiences of LGBTI people. There are huge gaps in knowledge about sexual practices and preferences, including the frequency of same-sex conduct, the number of people who claim same-sex identities, violence against the LGBTI community, as well as research into the more positive aspects of LGBTI life.

The advent of HIV and AIDS has resulted in many sex and sexuality studies in different populations and different countries. These studies present golden opportunities for collecting data on LGBTI behaviour and experiences and on attitudes towards the LGBTI community, but such questions are constantly neglected in research studies. If questions about same-sex identity, behaviour and experience are never asked, data will never become available (Johnson 2007). We have limited knowledge about lesbian and bisexual sex and sexuality and little research has been done on the health issues of WSW, including general health issues, HIV and AIDS and its impact on WSW, and sexual and reproductive health issues. The voices, experiences and issues of lesbian and bisexual women are glaringly absent from the research agenda.

NGOs are at the forefront of commissioning or conducting research in the LGBTI sector, often with small budgets and limited research capacity. Recent studies include the Joint Working Group (JWG) study (Wells et al. n.d.) – a collaborative effort between OUT LGBTI Well-being (OUT) and the Durban Lesbian and Gay

Community and Health Centre – which provides invaluable information on the lives and experiences of lesbians of different ages, races and relationship status in KwaZulu-Natal and Gauteng. The International Gay and Lesbian Human Rights Commission study on HIV and AIDS and same-sex practising people in Africa highlights many gaps in research, programming and policy which negatively influence the vulnerability of the LGBTI community (Johnson 2007). Such studies are often not taken seriously by policy-makers and other researchers.

Very few academic and research institutions have focused programmes on the issues facing the LGBTI community – it is clear that the issues facing same-sex practising men and women do not attract interest, focus or funding. In the few institutions that have an active commitment to researching the lives of the LGBTI community, programmes are often driven by individuals who have a personal interest in the issues, and the programmes are often not sustained when the individuals leave.

The issue of resources for research is a critical one: most LGBTI organisations are involved in service provision, advocacy and lobbying or capacity building, rather than research. And while more and more NGOs are becoming knowledge-creating organisations, this will seldom be their main focus. A study initiated in 2004 by the Association for Women's Rights in Development entitled 'Where is the money for women's rights?' surveyed over 2 000 women's rights organisations globally about their experiences in raising funds for different issues and activities (AWID 2006). Respondents were asked about specific subject areas, including HIV and AIDS and LGBTI rights. Comparing their experiences at the time of the research to their experiences five years previously, the organisations surveyed indicated whether it was more or less easy to raise funds for their specific issue. Whilst 72 per cent of women's organisations found it easier to raise funds for HIV and AIDS in 2005, only 26 per cent noted it was easier to raise money for sexual and LGBTI rights. In regard to raising money for research activities, compared to previously, 43 per cent of organisations found it harder, whilst 25 per cent noted the same level of difficulty. It is clear from the study that money for LGBTI work is less accessible from donors and that research is not high on donor agendas, especially where women's rights are concerned. Lobbying of donors for more funds and commitment, both for LGBTI programmes and for research, is needed.

The dearth of research resulted in the need to look for alternative sources of information for this chapter and I have therefore also drawn on my personal experiences as a feminist, lesbian and HIV and AIDS activist.

## What does research show?

Sexual orientation and one's feelings about one's own sexuality impact on health in different ways: there are specific health issues that are a direct result of behaviours linked to one's sexual orientation and what that means; the fear of discrimination and discomfort (for example, assumptions of heterosexuality and negative attitudes) and/or outright denial of care in healthcare settings based on sexual orientation may inhibit health-seeking behaviour; and women may not reveal their sexual orientation, resulting in withholding of complex life issues that may be of relevance. All these factors may lead to compromised health.

Access to health information and services needs to be seen in the context of lesbian or WSW lives. Given the dearth of research, it is difficult to get a full picture of the diverse experiences of lesbian lives in post-apartheid South Africa. Despite the 1996 Constitution protecting the rights of and asserting equality for the LGBTI community, many lesbians in South Africa still experience oppression on a day-to-day basis. Homophobic attitudes are still prevalent: a 1995 survey revealed that 48 per cent of the South African public were 'anti-gay' (a definition of anti-gay was not given), and over 68 per cent of people opposed letting gay and lesbian people adopt children (cited in Cock 2003).

Violence has reached endemic proportions, with murders of lesbian women not being uncommon. The Forum for the Empowerment of Women, working with black lesbians in Gauteng, found that WSW are systematically targeted for abuse, abduction and murder (Johnson 2007). On 7 July 2007, the murder of two lesbian activists, Sizakele Sigasa and Salome Massoa, in Meadowlands Soweto, shocked the lesbian community globally. Yet hate crimes aimed at black lesbians in South Africa are common and so-called corrective rape is rife. A six-country study of female same-sex practices in Africa facilitated by Morgan and Wieringa (2005) showed that the rape of WSW was most prevalent and violent in South Africa.[1]

## Health and women who have sex with women

The JWG research on lesbian lives in KwaZulu-Natal and Gauteng, conducted by OUT and the Durban Lesbian and Gay Community and Health Centre, throws some light on the experiences of almost 400 lesbian and bisexual women (Wells et al. n.d.). The study highlights the oppressive nature of religion, heterosexism, prescribed gender roles, and patriarchal norms, resulting in hate crimes, pressure and force being a feature of lesbian life. The multiple unequal power relations experienced by lesbian women impacts on many levels, including access to sexual and reproductive health information, services and rights. There is a lack of commitment to addressing HIV and AIDS, assisted pregnancy, and access to basic sexual health prevention, such as regular pap smears for WSW. Reproductive health is not seen by healthcare providers as an important issue for lesbian women, denying WSW rights to reproduce should they so wish, and perpetuating stereotypes that WSW are not 'women' and do not have the same needs and desires as other women.

## Health-seeking behaviour

Research shows that the health-seeking behaviour of women in general is mainly based on their reproductive role (either as a pregnant woman or as a mother with a sick child), and is usually what brings women into the healthcare arena (Garcia-Moreno 1999; Koblinsky et al. 1993). This focus on reproductive health of women is highly problematic and has implications for women's access to other health services. Young women, menopausal and post-menopausal women, and women who decide not to have children (all of whom could be WSW) may be denied access to adequate and appropriate healthcare during important periods in life. Other factors that impact on women's health-seeking behaviour include: time, mobility, access to funds/resources, fear of healthcare providers/facilities, and other social constraints which discourage them from attending healthcare facilities (Koblinsky et al. 1993). Access to health is also affected by the languages spoken (or not spoken) at clinics, hours of operation and attitudes of healthcare workers.

The OUT study revealed that 4 per cent of lesbian women interviewed had been refused health treatment because of their sexual orientation. Almost half of the women had experiences of healthcare practitioners asking heterosexist questions. The impact of these experiences was that 11 per cent of the women interviewed delayed seeking treatment for fear of discrimination, and this trend was more prevalent in young lesbian women under 25 years of age (Wells et al. n.d.). Trippet and Bain (cited in Richardson 2000) found that lesbians were particularly reluctant to seek help on menstrual, STI and breast problems.

Exposure to negative and discriminatory responses from healthcare professionals, the centrality of discussions of sexuality and sexual practices, and consequent pressure to 'come out', are significant factors in discouraging lesbians from seeking healthcare.

## HIV and AIDS

Women are more vulnerable to HIV infection than men, partly due to physiology but also due to their often limited ability to protect themselves from infection. This is heightened by a lack of women-controlled barrier mechanisms and the socially constructed 'rules' of heterosexual sex, where men tend to claim the power to decide when, where and how sex takes place. In the same way as much of the care that women receive is linked to their reproductive role, much of the research into women and AIDS focuses on the prevention of mother-to-child transmission. We know relatively little about HIV and AIDS in women, even less so in developing countries, and almost nothing about lesbians and HIV and AIDS. This obviously impacts on prevention, care and treatment.

No one knows how many lesbians or bisexual women are infected with HIV or have AIDS globally (Richardson 2000). Based on anecdotal reports, however, it appears that a substantial number of lesbian women in South Africa are living with HIV. Many women living openly with HIV and AIDS self-identify as lesbian. According to the OUT report, 'the high rates of HIV amongst lesbian and bisexual women in South Africa can in part be attributed to rape, unsafe transactional sex with men and sexual violence' (Wells et al. n.d.: 5). Obviously more accurate statistics need to be based on women testing for HIV – and many lesbian women are unlikely to go for an HIV test as they are generally deterred from talking about and seeking sexual healthcare. The OUT study revealed that just over 50 per cent of the women interviewed had undergone an HIV test, although the reasons for testing were not clear and could include routine testing (where an HIV test is done as one of a battery of tests, often without proper counselling or without informed consent). However, 9 per cent of the women who had tested did not return for their results. Reasons given for not testing included not thinking it was necessary (linked to the myth that lesbians are 'safe') and being afraid to test (Wells et al. n.d.).

Are lesbians aware of HIV and AIDS? Most of the women interviewed in the various countries in the Morgan and Wieringa study (2005) were aware of HIV and AIDS, yet very few of them, apart from the women living with HIV and AIDS, are practising safe sex. They explained they have no need to do so as they trust their partners to be monogamous, despite knowing of their partners' history of sex with men. The testing patterns of the women in the OUT study demonstrate that many women have a consciousness about HIV and AIDS, although some women are in denial about their risk (Wells et al. n.d.).

Aside from the obvious gaps in research around WSW, HIV and AIDS and, stemming from this, a lack of knowledge and understanding, there are few, if any, programmes in South Africa that specifically address lesbian women's issues.

Risk of HIV infection is about sexual practices. Women engage in a wide variety of sexual practices with other women, some of which may carry risk of HIV exposure: the slogan coined in the 1980s by lesbian organisations, 'low risk is not no risk', is still relevant today. Prevention programmes ignore the potential risk of women-to-women transmission, and the fact that many WSW also have sex with men. There are prevention technologies such as dental dams and finger cots, amongst others, that could be used by WSW. Such technologies are not part of the South African national prevention plan – despite active advocacy and lobbying by lesbian and gay organisations. Dental dams are distributed by some NGOs, for example the Gender AIDS Forum bought a small supply for distribution, but they are imported from the USA and are costly, and such small-scale distribution is in no way sustainable or effective. Analysis of the Department of Health's (DoH) approach to female condoms (from the DoH pilot projects in 1997 to 2008) reveals that accessibility to dental dams has hardly increased, and thus the chances of these being procured and distributed are highly unlikely. The use of microbicides for lesbian women has not been explored, but in the future if the technology is found to be efficacious, this could provide WSW with a prevention option.

Mainstream AIDS organisations do not have programmes that include or address WSW. In the response to HIV and AIDS lesbians have been ignored, and this marginalisation is based partly on misinformation and partly on a lack of knowledge about the complexities of lesbian lives.

## Setting our own agenda

As explored above, there are huge gaps in our knowledge and understanding about female same-sex practices. Lesbian women's health issues are not on research agendas. Research is urgently needed. Over and above research needs, policy that will ensure services and programmes that address the realities of WSW is vital. Part of addressing the lack of services is to get the commitment from government, (national and provincial health departments) and from NGOs and community-based organisations, to provide services to address the health issues of WSW.

There are three critical questions that must be addressed. Firstly, who sets the research agenda? It is obvious that in the past the agenda has been pushed by the LGBTI community and this must continue. However, even within the LGBTI community there may be a bias toward men setting the agenda and a focus on 'male' issues. We need to be aware of and counter such bias. Also, there needs to be active advocacy and lobbying to ensure that other groups, such as women's rights and HIV and AIDS activists, do not overlook the health needs of WSW. It is vital that WSW themselves determine the research agenda, but that other sectors do not marginalise, but rather include, the issues facing lesbian and bisexual women.

A key part of advocacy and lobbying for a lesbian research agenda will be to secure substantial funding from national and international donors for extensive, well-planned and executed and credible research projects. Partnerships between LGBTI organisations and research institutions will not only ensure that more substantial research is conducted, but also that the issues facing WSW are integrated into other agendas.

The second question is, what is the research agenda? Given the paucity of qualitative and quantitative research, there are many unanswered questions and unexplored areas. As suggested above, lesbian organisations should be at the forefront of defining the agenda.

Having said that, there are certain areas I would like to put forward as possible arenas for future research.
- Research into the experiences of WSW life: despite the recent research into the lives and experiences of WSW (Morgan & Wieringa 2005; Wells et al. n.d.), we still do not have a clear picture of the rich and diverse experiences of WSW in South Africa. It is vital that we make distinctions between lesbian and bisexual women, understanding that they occupy different positions socially and historically (Richardson 2000). Different experiences need to be documented, acknowledged, understood and acted upon.
- We need a deeper understanding of sexuality: sexuality is complex: there is no simple relationship between behaviour and identity, although sexual behaviour is often equated with sexual identity. It is important to address different elements of sexuality, including sexual behaviour, sexual identity and sexual drive, and understand that they mean different things and are experienced in multiple ways by women (Richardson 2000).

- It is also important that we get a clearer picture of sexual practices and what is seen as risky. What are lesbians' perceptions of risk? There have also been suggestions that we do not fully understand women-to-women transmission of HIV and other STIs, and that further work needs to be done (Johnson 2007; Richardson 2000).
- The OUT study points to gross discrimination at healthcare facilities. This needs to be further investigated and could include an analysis of women's experiences; healthcare workers' beliefs, attitudes and behaviours; and government health policy.

The final question is: what are the implications of WSW not being on the research agenda? Quite simply, the invisibility and marginalisation of lesbian and bisexual women is leading to the sexual and reproductive health needs of WSW not being adequately met. This is especially true when one looks at HIV and AIDS – there is an urgent need for programmes that address WSW in order to reduce their vulnerability. Safer-sex messages should include lesbian women, bisexual women and WSW, and provision should be made for the distribution of prevention technologies for women.

## Conclusion

Policy change will not happen based on anecdotal accounts of discrimination against WSW. We need to build on what is already known, ensure that research is thorough and vigorous and depicts the realities and diversity of lesbian life, and then we need to ensure that our research findings are implemented into effective programmes and services.

### Note

1   For a discussion on violence against lesbians, see also Wells et al. (n.d.).

### References

AWID (Association for Women's Rights in Development) (2006) *Where is the money for women's rights? Assessing resources and the role of donors in the promotion of women's rights and the support of women's organizations.* Toronto & Mexico City: AWID

Cock J (2003) Engendering gay and lesbian rights: The equality clause in the South African Constitution. *Women's Studies International Forum* 26(1): 35–40

Doyal L (1995) *What makes women sick? Gender and the political economy of health.* London: MacMillan

Garcia-Moreno C (1999) *Gender and health: A technical paper.* Geneva: World Health Organization

Johnson CA (2007) *Off the map: How HIV and AIDS programming is failing same-sex practising people in Africa.* New York: International Gay and Lesbian Human Rights Commission

Koblinsky M, Gay J & Timyan J (1993) *The health of women: A global perspective.* Boulder CO: Westview Press

Lorber J (1997) *Gender and the social construction of illness.* New Haven CT: Sage

Morgan R & Wieringa S (2005) *Tommy boys, lesbian men and ancestral wives: Female same-sex practices.* Johannesburg: Jacana Media

Richardson D (2000) The social construct of immunity: HIV risk perception and prevention among lesbians and bisexual women. *Culture, Health and Sexuality* 2(1): 33–49

Tallis V (2001) Treatment issues for women. Paper commissioned by the Treatment Action Campaign

Wells H, Kruger T & Judge M (n.d.) *Experiences and dimensions of power: Discussions with lesbian women.* Pretoria: OUT LGBTI Well-being. Accessed December 2008, http://www.out.org.za/images/library/pdf/Lesbian_Power_Research_Findings.pdf

# CONCLUSIONS

Issues of safety and violence, I think that is the subject that I have spent the most of my time worrying about when doing this research. As a researcher it is always the challenge for me: how do we balance moving forward with the research and how far can we go before it becomes a liability to the people we are studying. Maybe, for example, the media picks what we are doing, publishes a story and that inflames public opinion and it becomes a punitive response. These are the kinds of things that have often kept me up at night. And there have been times when I felt like I have had to appeal to some of my colleagues to restrain or pull back and reflect on this as well. But at the same time I am always continuously surprised that when we do this research and we do it well, I am always surprised at how it is received. Even in countries like Kenya and Senegal and I think openness and trust goes a long way. *Scott Geibel, conference delegate*

I would like to cite a proverb. In my culture they say, 'one mind is not a mind'...No matter how brilliant you are, if you don't interact with other minds you don't have a mind. We are starting to build a collective mind that will help to resolve the problems we are facing today. *Cheikh I Niang, conference delegate*

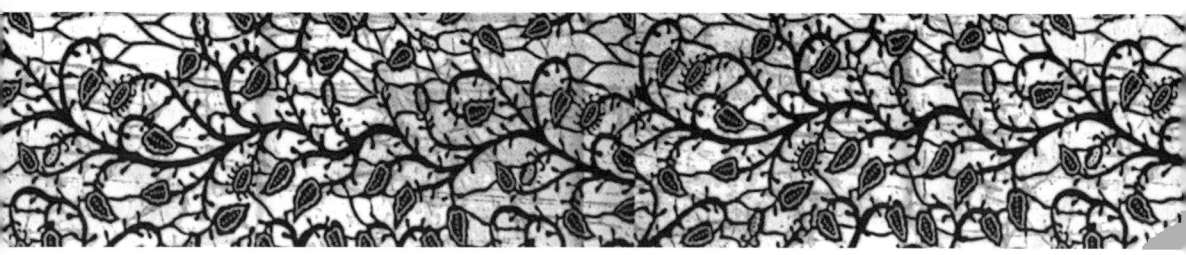

There's something extraordinary about the need to deconstruct the term 'heterosexual'. Heterosexuals are not a homogeneous group. Their sexualities are extraordinarily complicated and fragmented as well…Heterosexuality is constructed in relation to homosexuality, and the idea that you don't know what's happening under the term homosexuality means that you cannot by definition know what's happening in any true sense with heterosexuality [either]. So I think there's potential for a kind of liberation for straight people, and for research on straight people, through this work as well. *Robert Sember, conference delegate*

## CHAPTER TWENTY
# Taking research and prevention forward

Theo Sandfort, Vasu Reddy and Laetitia Rispel

*From Social Silence to Social Science* maintains that important conditions need to be met to be able to move research and prevention forward so as to improve our understanding of how homosexual transmission could be fuelling the existing HIV/AIDS pandemic. Several chapters have convincingly demonstrated that research to develop an appropriate and evidence-informed approach to programmes on HIV prevention for same-sex practising individuals is important to effect behaviour changes.

Other issues covered in the volume focus on understanding lesbian, gay, bisexual, transgender and intersex (LGBTI) communities through sexual networks and sexual cultures in the context of their heterogeneity; the methods to be employed when conducting research; terminology; the nature of collaboration between researchers, programme implementers and policy-makers; the purposes and value of research, including the relevance of research to service delivery; as well as the importance of political mobilisation in combating HIV/AIDS. The volume offers an understanding of sexuality (same-sex sexuality in particular) through the difference that HIV/AIDS makes to arguments about understanding the epidemic. All of these issues help us to move forward to future work.

As repeated so often in the arguments by service providers, researchers and activists, the South African HIV/AIDS epidemic is one of the most devastating worldwide (see specifically Chapters 6 and 15 in this volume). It is well documented how this epidemic has been developing. Given the crucial role of homosexual transmission in the worldwide epidemic, it seems reasonable to expect that in South Africa a lot would be known about HIV/AIDS and same-sex sexuality. Yet this is not the case.

In Chapter 10 of this volume, Cary Alan Johnson has cogently articulated what has been a central concern for a number of authors: same-sex sexuality is virtually 'off the map' in several African countries (see also Johnson 2007). Same-sex sexuality could therefore be theorised as having been erased from current understanding of how the HIV epidemic is unfolding in southern Africa. However, while several studies about same-sex sexuality and HIV/AIDS in Africa have been published especially since 2007 (Allman et al. 2007; Cloete et al. 2008; Geibel et al. 2007; Jewkes et al. 2006a; Kajubi et al. 2008; Lane et al. 2008; Lorway 2006; Niang et al. 2003; Onyango-Ouma et al. 2005; Parry et al. 2008; Sanders et al. 2007; Sandfort et al. 2008 Sharma et al 2008; Teunis 2001; Van Griensven & Sanders 2008; Wade et al. 2005), South Africa still lags behind. Fortunately, there are indications that the situation is changing.

In this conclusion, we briefly summarise what is known about same-sex sexuality in the South African HIV/AIDS epidemic. Based on the perspectives contained in the various chapters, we outline what the next steps should be, and address ethical aspects and issues of relevance. 'Same-sex sexuality' in its historical context of gay activism prior to 1994 is analysed by Mandisa Mbali in Chapter 7 in this volume. We now turn to some historical points articulated in the epidemiological literature that should help us chart another starting point for future work.

## Same-sex sexuality in the South African HIV/AIDS epidemic

The first cases of HIV infection and AIDS in South Africa, reported in 1983 and 1985, revealed that, at that time, infections were largely confined to white men who had sex with men or MSM (Anderson et al. 1983; Puren 2002; Ras et al. 1983; Sher & dos Santos 1985; Spracklen et al. 1985). In 1985, the prevalence of HIV among homosexual men in Johannesburg was estimated to be between 10 and 15 per cent. The concern among some medical professionals was great, as illustrated by a brief discussion paper in the *South African Medical Journal*, which included recommendations for precautions in sexual activity, the importance of the existence of a gay community, and the need for rapid revision and change in South Africa's healthcare support system (Isaacs & Miller 1985). In 1988, Schoub and colleagues reported with cautious optimism that the rate of expansion of the (white) homosexual epidemic in South Africa shows preliminary signs of being checked (Schoub et al. 1988).

By the late 1980s, however, a second, independent epidemic was recognised in South Africa. This epidemic appears to have come from central Africa and involved a different subtype of HIV (Van Harmelen et al. 1997; Williamson & Martin 2005) with differential survival rates (Maartens et al. 1997). The dominant mode of transmission of this second epidemic was heterosexual intercourse (Ijsselmuiden et al. 1988).

From its early detection, this epidemic was seen as potentially devastating. Presenting an overview of the seroepidemiology of human immunodeficiency viruses in Africa, Fleming (1988) concluded with alarm that, 'Even at existing seroprevalence, decimation or worse of the most productive age groups is inevitable during the next few years in certain countries. Similar alarming concerns were raised by other researchers (Padayachee & Schall 1990; Schoub et al. 1988). These scholars maintained that the black population would become the most affected group by the epidemic (Schall et al., 1990; Schoub et al. 1990). Schall and Padayachee (1990) predicted in 1990 that it was quite probable that millions of South Africans would die from AIDS in the next decade, since about 400 000 black South Africans are expected to be infected with HIV by 1992. While the current HIV prevalence rates in South Africa seem to be levelling off (Abdool Karim & Abdool Karim 2005), UNAIDS/WHO estimated 18.8 per cent prevalence in those aged 15–49 years old at the end of 2005 (the high and low estimates were 16.8 per cent and 20.7 per cent respectively) (UNAIDS 2006). This would imply that around 5.5 million South Africans were living with HIV at the end of 2005, the majority of them black people (Shisana et al. 2005; UNAIDS 2008).

In examining recent epidemiological data, one might get the impression that only a heterosexual epidemic exists in South Africa, and that the AIDS epidemic has completely disappeared among gay men. One of the most recent seroprevalence studies in which same-sex sexuality as a transmission route was reported, and that we were able to identify with a Medline, Pubmed, and Google Scholar search, stems from 1990 (Martin et al. 1990). It concerned a seroepidemiological surveillance study to monitor the prevalence of HIV-1 infection among 6 631 attendees at clinics for sexually transmitted diseases and at family planning clinics in Johannesburg, which had started at the beginning of 1988. While the data were seen as a confirmation of the entry of HIV infection into the black population in South Africa – 1.2 per cent of the black females and 0.8 per cent of the black males were positive – HIV prevalence was still highest among white homosexual males (20.4 per cent; 1 per cent in the heterosexual male group). The black participants' sexual orientation, self-identification or sexual practices were not reported.

We were not able to find any more recent references to the prevalence of HIV among gay men or the role of homosexual transmission in the overall epidemic in South Africa. One exception is the large national study among 17 088 South African teachers, which indicated that about the same proportion of male teachers who had sex with men tested HIV-positive compared to men who had sex with women only – 14.4 per cent and 12.7 per cent respectively (findings were not presented by race).

The absence of data about the prevalence of HIV among MSM is paralleled by a lack of understanding of the structural, cultural, interpersonal, and individual factors that affect protective practices in same-sex sexual activities in South Africa (for example, the introduction and Chapters 1, 2, 4, 8 and 19 in this volume address some of these issues, either directly or indirectly, in their arguments).

Other target groups (such as women, children and teachers) are receiving attention in the South African public health and behavioural sciences literature about HIV/AIDS, either in risk behaviour determinant studies or intervention studies (see for example Jewkes et al. 2006b; Petersen et al. 2006; Rehle et al. 2005; Simbayi et al. 2006). In these studies, sexual partners are assumed to be of the opposite sex, while sex workers are virtually always assumed to be female (cf. Dunkle et al. 2004). As indicated in the introduction to this volume, the absence of same-sex sexuality in social-scientific HIV/AIDS research stands in sharp contrast to scholarly work in law, anthropology, history, gender studies, cultural studies and other humanities-oriented disciplines, where same-sex sexuality is the focus of a significant body of literature (cf. Dunton & Palmberg 1996; Epprecht 2004; Germond & De Gruchy 1997; Gevisser & Cameron 1994; Isaacs & McKendrick 1992; Luirinck 2000; Morgan & Wieringa 2005; Reddy 2005; Reid 2007; Spurlin 2006).

On evaluating the current situation in terms of the social-scientific literature on HIV/AIDS, we conclude that there is little understanding of the scope of the problem: to what extent are MSM affected? Which men and women are affected? What are the treatment needs of MSM? What is the role of homosexual transmission in the overall HIV/AIDS epidemic in South Africa? Without such knowledge it is difficult to argue for the necessary resources. Also, there are no benchmarks that can be used to assess progress that is being made in addressing same-sex sexual transmission. Furthermore, the lack of understanding of the dynamics that contribute to unsafe sex practices and the further spread of HIV makes it impossible to develop and implement evidence-based interventions. This is a serious and urgent problem, because existing evidence strongly suggests that health promotion interventions are more effective if based on sound theory and empirical evidence that understands the needs of the affected (as motivated by Chapters 6 (Lane), 8 (Matebeni), 10 (Johnson), 11 (Nyadani), 12 (Matsikure), 13 (Fiereck), 14 (Geffen et al.), 15 (Rispel & Metcalf), 17 (De Swardt), 18 (Mkhize) and 19 (Tallis) in this volume).

While the focus in many chapters has been on men, a similar argument could be made about women who have sex with women (WSW). Although there are differing opinions about the nature and extent of HIV infection risk for WSW, there are indications that among some groups of women, HIV prevalence is high (Sandfort et al. 2008). It is not yet known how these women get infected. Given the implausible although not completely impossible transmission of HIV between women, it is likely that these infections are due to heterosexual intercourse. They could also result from so-called corrective rape and sex work. The lack of understanding of the background of these infections and the prevention needs of WSW – positive as well as negative or untested women – leave health policy developers in the dark (Tallis raises some similar concerns in Chapter 19 in this volume).

Although this should be investigated more fully, there are various reasons for the current lack of research attention for same-sex sexual transmission. The most plausible one is the fact that in South Africa, unlike in most Western, industrialised countries, heterosexual intercourse is the dominant mode of HIV transmission, while the scale of the South African epidemic is much larger. South Africa has a generalised epidemic with more women infected than men. There are other reasons as well. One of them is the idea that same-sex sexuality is un-African and therefore not supposed to occur among the predominantly black population in South Africa (Reddy 2002; Reid & Dirsuweit 2002). It should also not be forgotten that under apartheid, same-sex sexuality was criminalised (Gevisser & Cameron 1994; Ratele 2001; Reddy 2005).

## The road ahead

From a social justice perspective, the lack of attention to same-sex sexuality in the HIV/AIDS epidemic is unacceptable. This, we believe, is an overwhelming argument put forward by our authors. From a public health perspective, limited attention for same-sex sexual transmission might undermine the overall fight against HIV and AIDS in South Africa. It is obvious that much work needs to be done, and the conference on which this volume is based, and the chapters presented in this volume, all contribute to the goals that we outlined in the introduction. Chapters featured in this collection give a detailed sense of the broad arguments that respond to the organising questions: (1) How are same-sex sexual expressions and practices organised and networked? and (2) What is the prevalence of HIV among same-sex practising populations, and what is the contribution of homosexual transmission to the South African epidemic? The conference conversations also elicited various suggestions about how to move forward, many of which we abstract here by drawing on insights from the chapters in this volume, and the transcript of discussions from the conference.

There was general consensus among conference participants that, in relation to HIV/AIDS, research is needed that not only acknowledges but also fosters an understanding of the diversity in same-sex sexual practices. Same-sex involvement is not necessarily exclusive and there are various ways in which sexual and gender identities are integrated. Furthermore, labels that are being used do not necessarily have identical meanings for the persons involved. Understanding diversity implies acknowledgement of the fact that the organisation and expression of same-sex sexuality is tenuous: the use of identity labels changes as men and women's self-understandings change. This is the result of increasing exposure to different ways of expressing same-sex sexuality within South Africa as well as more globally. Research is also part of this process and is likely to contribute to it. Whatever future studies will be conducted about same-sex sexuality and HIV/AIDS, there is a great need for understanding the meanings attached to identities and practices (see for example Chapters 4 (Sandfort & Dodge), 6 (Lane) and 8 (Matebeni) in this volume).

A second point of agreement among conference participants was that HIV cannot be understood, and also cannot be effectively addressed, without interrogating the context and issues that affect men and women with same-sex sexual desires. This is in line with current thinking about HIV/AIDS which emphasises that in addition to the role of micro-level factors, attention should be given to structural factors as well. This implies the socioeconomic and cultural circumstances in which same-sex sexuality is practised, including the stigma attached to same-sex sexuality must be addressed – while South Africa currently has the most liberal Constitution as far as homosexuality is concerned, the Constitution contrasts sharply with the level of acceptance of homosexuality in South Africa (Inglehart & Welzel 2005). Discrimination and violence resulting from the stigma attached to same-sex sexuality affect how MSM and WSW shape, structure and experience their sexual practices, including the risks they take. Understanding stigma further requires an exploration of the meaning attached to gender, masculinity and femininity; same-sex sexuality is usually constructed in terms of masculinity and femininity by persons with same-sex desires as well as by others (Chapters 1 (Aggleton) and 8 (Matebeni) in this volume are strong on these points). Instead of exclusively focusing on individual determinants of risk, research should also account for *how* sex is expressed in social relationships, calling attention to power dynamics and structures. Understanding the potential spread of HIV also requires looking beyond individual behaviour, and exploring social and sexual networks. Examples of other issues suggested by conference participants were alcohol and drug use, and health literacy.

## Ethical aspects of research

The representation of various practical and scholarly disciplines at the conference also reinforced a discussion of ethical aspects of research – the core of Pierre Brouard's arguments in Chapter 5 of this volume. In discussion, participants expressed a strong need for constant reflection upon what researchers are doing: why are specific research questions asked? What could the consequences be of the outcomes of the studies we initiate? Is there acknowledgement of the context in which the work is being done?

In addition, research about same-sex sexuality and HIV/AIDS needs to follow specific ethical guidelines. To start with, directly affected communities (notably the LGBT communities) should be involved in as many parts of the research process as possible. Such participation should not be limited to the recruitment of study participants, but should also include the development of research questions, the methodology, as well as the dissemination of results. Inclusion of the community will facilitate research that resonates with the reality of the target group and will promote the use of study findings once available. Furthermore, researchers should be aware of the needs that might be elicited by their studies and make services available to address the needs identified. It was also suggested that researchers should take the responsibility for providing proper and adequate feedback to the target group once a study is finished.

In all of this, researchers need to reflect upon their social position as researchers and the role of research. This implies an understanding of the political dimensions of the work they are doing and the power dimensions involved. This also includes an awareness of the fact that in research, issues can be framed in various ways and that the way an issue is being framed is also embedded in politics. Researchers must ask the question: does my study and the terminology used do justice to the reality of the persons involved?

## Diverse functions of research: Consensus issues and some barriers

While we know that research is supposed to further our knowledge of a problem, issue, and a field, in relation to HIV/AIDS (as may be the case for other fields), there is an applied aim to research as well: research should help us prevent further transmission of HIV, make sure that affected people receive the support they need, and counteract stigma attached to HIV/AIDS. Consequently, the aim of most HIV/AIDS research is to develop and evaluate interventions, and respond to policies and develop new ones where existing policies fail. The research questions and issues raised in this volume respond in part to the policy framework of the *HIV & AIDS and STI National Strategic Plan for South Africa 2007–2011* (DoH 2007) in which the category of same-sex populations and their vulnerability to HIV/AIDS features for the first time in South African HIV policy (for discussion of the policy context see Chapters 6 (Lane) and 15 (Rispel and Metcalf) in this volume).

Research about same-sex sexuality and HIV/AIDS could have several additional functions. One of these functions may seem basic, yet the political implications are vast in the context of silence and denial: research can deliver proof that homosexuality in Africa exists, simultaneously dispelling through an evidence-based framework the myth that homosexuality is un-African. As espoused in, for example, the introduction (Reddy, et al.) and Chapters 8 (Matebeni) and 18 (Mkhize) in this volume, any discussion of same-sex sexuality must include the relevance of identity politics that confronts homophobia and bigotry. Several activists have expressed the view that science (through its institutions and its research endeavours) could be used to challenge homophobia, as well as to advocate for increasing the visibility of same-sex sexuality. In parallel, research can have a legitimising function for people who engage in same-sex practices. Science is furthermore needed to urge political attention towards problems and to advocate for the release of resources for prevention. The inclusion of same-sex sexuality in mainstream population studies, such as the 2008 South African national HIV prevalence survey (forthcoming), is likely to promote acknowledgement of same-sex sexuality and increase its visibility.

There is a strong consensus that what should be prioritised in South Africa is research which brings about *change* that has an impact on a variety of levels, and that can be used by various stakeholders. These stakeholders include policy-makers, LGBTI communities, healthcare workers, and persons with same-sex sexual desires and practices. Different stakeholders will of course have different research needs. In this sense, the *value* of collaboration has received overwhelming support by stakeholders. But while there is consensus, stakeholders have also highlighted a number of limitations.

While most researchers, community leaders and activists acknowledge a strong need for research on same-sex sexuality and HIV/AIDS, there is also an awareness of the various barriers to the kind of research proposed. One major barrier is the difficulty of gaining access to relevant populations, partly resulting from a reluctance to participate in research due to a homophobic climate. Another factor making research interesting but also complicated is the diversity of expressions of same-sex sexuality. While research should acknowledge this diversity, and even make it an object of study, this diversity will also limit the possibility of developing generalisable conclusions. Further structural barriers include the scarcity of financial and material resources and the lack of a social-scientific research infrastructure in South Africa focused on same-sex sexuality.

## Research questions and research approaches for the road ahead

The list of questions related to same-sex sexuality and HIV/AIDS that require research attention is extensive and it is hard to set priorities. The research questions requiring attention can be organised into various categories, as outlined below.

Firstly, there are several epidemiological questions. Research is needed to assess HIV prevalence among MSM and WSW and to understand the role of homosexual transmission in the South African HIV/AIDS epidemic. The political need for epidemiological data is to be able to legitimise attention for HIV prevention aimed at MSM and WSW and to claim needed resources to do so. Understanding homosexual transmission of HIV also requires determining who is having sex with whom, and what people are actually doing together in their social and sexual networks. Are people having sex with persons from within their social network or do sexual networks exist relatively independently of social networks? Understanding sexual networks will help to determine what the best places are to intervene to prevent the further spread of HIV (see Friedman et al. 2006). Epidemiological research also requires sophisticated sampling approaches that allow for the generalisation of study findings. Integrating homosexuality in general population surveys would give researchers an opportunity to make comparisons, and to put findings regarding same-sex sexuality into perspective.

A second group of research questions should help to successfully address the prevention and care needs of persons who engage in same-sex sexuality. This involves the exploration of the various factors associated with unsafe sex as well as with the adoption of preventive strategies. Also relevant in this context is to understand how sexual interactions come about: what kind of sexual communication takes place, and how are desires negotiated? Beyond the individual level, research focused on communities might be helpful: how are communities being built and how do such communities support safer-sex practices? Other questions deal with access to healthcare, including voluntary counselling and testing and treatment for HIV: what kind of barriers exist and how could these barriers be removed?

Understanding risk behaviour only makes sense if a broader context is taken into account. 'Risk' as a concept is potentially dangerous and could have ambiguous meanings, depending on how it is being deployed. Risk often has moral implications, and when used in relation to sexuality and sexual practices, these meanings have to be carefully unpacked. Given the reality that same-sex sexual practices already operate in a stigmatised and specifically homophobic environment, the meanings of 'risk' in relation to such sexual practices must be first understood by people who self-identify with same-sex sexual practices. More importantly, to address populations effectively it is of crucial importance to understand what same-sex roles, identities and practices mean to individuals and communities. What kind of understanding do people have of same-sex sexuality? How are these understandings changing and as a consequence of what kind of factors?

In order to promote adequate political attention to same-sex sexuality and HIV/AIDS, we also need to understand the history of policy-making. Why did it take so long for same-sex sexuality to be included in South Africa's National Strategic Plan? Such questions should be studied in the context of South Africa's general HIV/AIDS policy, taking into account the social meaning attached to homosexuality, and the role that should be played by lesbian and gay organisations in mobilising around HIV/AIDS (an argument strongly articulated in Chapter 14 in this volume). Other questions that would fall under the rubric of policy research deal with current decision-making processes: what attention is being paid to same-sex sexuality in policy and how can research-based advocacy influence this?

A final set of questions addresses programmatic needs and programme evaluation. Even though solid evidence is lacking for the development of interventions aimed at people with same-sex practices, such interventions are being implemented, predominantly by LGBTI organisations and community centres (notably Triangle Project in Cape Town; OUT LGBT Well-being in Pretoria, and the Durban Lesbian and Gay Community & Health Centre). It is also important to determine whether these interventions are having an impact. Part of the evaluation involves ongoing monitoring of the quality of programme implementation and the target populations' responses to the programme. Ongoing questions that remain are: what facilitates the implementation of programmes and what are the obstacles to programmatic success?

While we have repeatedly talked about same-sex sexuality in this book in a way that has emphasised MSM, we re-articulate the importance of appropriately defined gendered research with a focus on women. Gender as a relational concept is often sidestepped and overlooked by AIDS practitioners and researchers, as we are reminded by the plea in the ground-breaking study by Baylies and Bujra (2000). By gendered research we mean an investigation of the social, cultural and political dimensions shaping sexuality. The usual response to such a plea is that there is little transmission risk among women and that research focusing on WSW and HIV/AIDS is a waste of resources. While opinions may differ on this aspect, we argue that such research should be evaluated in a local context, through better-informed qualitative and quantitative data to demonstrate what we do not know (Chapter 19 in this volume makes a clear plea for this type of research). Available data suggest that in South Africa there are WSW who are HIV-positive (Sandfort et al. 2008). Furthermore, not all WSW are exclusively lesbian. Future research must take into account the concerns of WSW regarding HIV/AIDS, explore the sexual histories of infected women, and explore how WSW deal with their infection in their situated and diverse contexts.

## Conclusion

Based on the insights of our authors, we deduced at the beginning of this conclusion that the situation regarding same-sex sexuality and HIV/AIDS in South Africa is changing. Several activities have been set in motion. The first figures about risk behaviour and HIV infection in South African gay and lesbian populations are becoming available (see Sandfort et al. 2008). A major seroprevalence study among MSM is being carried out, while new initiatives are in the making. As indicated earlier, MSM are mentioned for the first time in the *HIV & AIDS and STI National Strategic Plan for South Africa 2007–2011* (DoH 2007). In this plan, it is stated that there is 'very little currently known about the HIV epidemic amongst MSM in the country' and that 'MSM have also not been considered to any great extent in national HIV and AIDS interventions' (DoH 2007: 38). The strategic plan further argues that behaviours of MSM are wide-ranging and also include bisexuality, implying that 'the HIV epidemic amongst MSM and the heterosexual HIV epidemic are thus interconnected' (DoH 2007: 38).

As implied in our introduction, *From Social Silence to Social Science* should be viewed as a first comprehensive stocktaking of HIV/AIDS through the lens of same-sex sexuality. The volume puts in motion a set of ideas by key players. Our authors hold important positions in various domains (mostly in research, social movements, community organisations, and in programme planning) and we believe their views are influential. All views coalesce around interventions that direct us to change at both the individual and societal levels, urging us to take note of current gaps and future prospects that also recognise social injustices and violations that fuel the epidemic. We believe this volume will help to make certain that same-sex sexuality becomes and remains an integral part of South African HIV/AIDS research, policy, prevention and movement building in coming years.

## References

Abdool Karim SS & Abdool Karim Q (Eds) (2005) *The future of the HIV epidemic in South Africa*. New York: Cambridge University Press

Allman D, Adebajo S, Myers T, Odumuye O & Ogunsola S (2007) Challenges for the sexual health and social acceptance of men who have sex with men in Nigeria. *Culture, Health & Sexuality* 9(2): 153–168

Anderson R, Eftychis HA, Prozesky OW, Swanevelder C, Simson IW & van der Merwe MF (1983) Immunological abnormalities in South African homosexual men. *South African Medical Journal* 64(4): 119–122

Baylies C & Bujra J with the Gender and AIDS Group (Eds) (2000) *AIDS, sexuality and gender in Africa: Collective strategies and struggles in Tanzania and Zambia*. London & New York: Routledge

Campbell C (2003) *Letting them die: Why HIV/AIDS intervention programmes fail*. Oxford: James Currey

Cloete A, Henda N, Kalichman SC, Simbayi LC & Strebel A (2008) Stigma and discrimination experiences of HIV positive men who have sex with men in Cape Town, South Africa. *AIDS Care* 20(9): 1105–1110

DoH (Department of Health) (2007) *HIV & AIDS and STI National Strategic Plan for South Africa 2007–2011*. Pretoria: Department of Health

Dunkle KL, Brown HC, Gray GE, Jewkes RK, McIntryre JA et al. (2004) Transactional sex among women in Soweto, South Africa: Prevalence, risk factors and association with HIV infection. *Social Science & Medicine* 59(8): 1581

Dunton C & Palmberg M (1996) *Human rights and homosexuality in southern Africa*. Uppsala: Nordiska Afrikainstituet

Epprecht M (2004) *Hungochani: The history of a dissident sexuality in southern Africa*. Montreal: McGill-Queen's University Press

Fleming AF (1988) Seroepidemiology of human immunodeficiency viruses in Africa. *Biomedicine & Pharmacotherapy* 42(5): 309–320

Fourie P (2006) *The political management of HIV and AIDS in South Africa: One burden too many?* Houndsmill, Basingstoke: Palgrave Macmillan

Friedman SR, Bolyard M, Flom PL, Goltzman P, Maslow C, Mateu-Gelabert P, Pawlowicz MP, Rossi D, Sandoval M, Singh DZ & Touze G (2006) Some data-driven reflections on priorities in AIDS network research. *AIDS Behaviour* 11(5): 641–651

Geibel S, Davies A, Graham SM, Getambu EM, King'ola N, Luchters S, McClelland RS, Peshu N, Sanders EJ & Van der Elst E (2007) Are you on the market? A capture-recapture enumeration of men who sell sex to men in and around Mombasa, Kenya. *AIDS* 21(10): 1349–1354

Germond P & De Gruchy S (Eds) (1997) *Aliens in the household of God: Homosexuality and Christian faith in South Africa*. Cape Town & Johannesburg: David Philip

Gevisser M & Cameron E (Eds) (1994) *Defiant desire: Gay and lesbian lives in South Africa*. Johannesburg: Ravan Press

Ijsselmuiden CB, Buch E, Padayachee GN, Schoub BD, Steinberg MH, Strauss SA et al. (1988) AIDS and South Africa: Towards a comprehensive strategy. *South African Medical Journal* 73(8): 455–460

Inglehart R & Welzel C (2005) *Modernization, cultural change, and democracy: The human development sequence*. New York: Cambridge University Press

Isaacs G & McKendrick B (1992) *Male homosexuality in South Africa: Identity formation, culture and crisis.* Cape Town: Oxford University Press

Isaacs G & Miller D (1985) AIDS: Its implications for South African homosexuals and the mediating role of the medical practitioner. *South African Medical Journal* 68(5): 327–330

Jewkes R, Dunkle K, Duvvury N, Jama N, Khuzwayo N, Koss M, Levin J, Nduna M & Puren A (2006a) Factors associated with HIV sero-positivity in young, rural South African men. *International Journal of Epidemiology* 35(6): 1455–1460

Jewkes R, Dunkle K, Duvvury N, Jama N, Khuwayo N, Koss M, Levin J, Nduna M, Puren A & Wood K (2006b) A cluster randomized-controlled trial to determine the effectiveness of Stepping Stones in preventing HIV infections and promoting safer sexual behaviour amongst youth in the rural Eastern Cape, South Africa: Trial design, methods and baseline findings. *Tropical Medicine and International Health* 11(1): 3–16

Johnson CA (2007) *Off the map: How HIV/AIDS programming is failing same-sex practising people in Africa.* New York: International Gay and Lesbian Human Rights Commission

Kajubi P, Chen S, Kamya MR, Mandel JS, McFarland W, Raymond HF & Rutherford GW (2008) Gay and bisexual men in Kampala, Uganda. *AIDS Behaviour* 12(3): 492–504

Lane T, McIntyre J, Morin SF & Shade SB (2008) Alcohol and sexual risk behaviour among men who have sex with men in South African township communities. *AIDS Behaviour* 12 (Supplement 1): 78–85

Lorway R (2006) Dispelling 'heterosexual African AIDS' in Namibia: Same-sex sexuality in the township of Katatura. *Culture, Health & Sexuality* 8(5): 435–449

Luirinck B (2000) *Moffies: Gay life and lesbian life in southern Africa.* Cape Town: David Philip

Maartens G, Byrne C, O'Keefe E & Wood R (1997) Independent epidemics of heterosexual and homosexual HIV infection in South Africa: Survival differences. *QJM: An International Journal of Medicine* 90(7): 449–454

Martin DJ, Lyons SF, McGillivray GM, Padayachee GN, Schoub BD, Smith AN et al. (1990) One year surveillance of HIV-1 infection in Johannesburg, South Africa. *Transactions of the Royal Society of Tropical Medicine & Hygiene* 84(5): 728–730

Morgan R & Wieringa S (Eds) (2005) *Tommy boys, lesbian men and ancestral wives: Female same-sex practices in Africa.* Johannesburg: Jacana Media

Niang CI, Castle C, Diagne M, Gomis D, Moreau AM, Niang Y, Tapsoba P, Seck K, Wade AS & Weiss E (2003) 'It's raining stones': Stigma, violence and HIV vulnerability among men who have sex with men in Dakar, Senegal. *Culture, Health & Sexuality* 5(6): 499–512

Onyango-Ouma W, Birungi H & Geibel S (2005) *Understanding the HIV/STI risks and prevention needs of men who have sex with men in Nairobi, Kenya.* Nairobi: The Population Council

Padayachee GN & Schall R (1990) Short-term predictions of the prevalence of human immunodeficiency virus infection among the black population in South Africa. *South African Medical Journal* 77(7): 329–333

Parry C, Carney T, Dewing S, Kroeger K, Needle R, Petersen P & Treger L (2008) Rapid assessment of drug-related HIV risk among men who have sex with men in three South African cities. *Drug Alcohol Dependence* 95(1–2): 45–53

Petersen I, Bell C, Bhana A, Mason A & McKay M (2006) Mediating social representations using a cartoon narrative in the context of HIV/AIDS: The AmaQhawe Family Project in South Africa. *Journal of Health Psychology* 11(2): 197–208

Puren AJ (2002) The HIV-1 epidemic in South Africa. *Oral Diseases* 8 (Supplement 2): 27–31

Ras GJ, Anderson R, Hamersma T, Prozesky OW & Simson IW (1983) Acquired immunodeficiency syndrome. A report of 2 South African cases. *South African Medical Journal* 64(4): 140–142

Ratele K (2001) The sexualization of apartheid. PhD thesis, University of the Western Cape

Reddy V (2002) Perverts and sodomites: Homophobia as hate speech in Africa. *Southern African Linguistics and Applied Language Studies* 20(3): 163–175

Reddy V (2005) Moffies, stabanis, lesbos: The political construction of queer identities in southern Africa. PhD thesis, University of KwaZulu-Natal

Rehle T, Colvin M, Glencross D & Shisana O (2005) *HIV positive educators in South African public schools: Predictions for prophylaxis and antiretroviral therapy.* Cape Town: HSRC Press

Reid G (2007) How to be a 'real' gay: Emerging gay spaces in small-town South Africa. PhD dissertation, University of Amsterdam

Reid G & Dirsuweit T (2002) Understanding systemic violence. *Urban Forum* 31(3): 99–126

Sanders EJ, Davies A, Graham SM, McClelland S, Muhaari A, Okuku HS, Peshu N, Price M, Smith AD & Van der Elst E (2007) HIV-1 infection in high risk men who have sex with men in Mombasa, Kenya. *AIDS* 21(18): 2513–2520

Sandfort TGM, Nel J, Reddy V, Rich E & Yi H (2008) HIV testing and self-reported HIV status in South African men who have sex with men: Results from a community-based survey. *Sexually Transmitted Infections* 84(6): 425–429

Schall R & Padayachee GN (1990) Doomsday forecasts of the AIDS epidemic. *South African Medical Journal* 78(9): 503

Schall R, Padayachee GN & Yach D (1990) The case for HIV surveillance in South Africa. *South African Medical Journal* 77(7): 324–325

Schoub BD, Johnson S, Lyons SF, Martin DJ, McGillivray G & Smith AN et al. (1988) Epidemiological considerations of the present status and future growth of the acquired immunodeficiency syndrome epidemic in South Africa. *South African Medical Journal* 74(4): 153–157

Schoub BD, Johnson S, Lyons SF, Martin DJ, Padayachee GN & Smith AN et al. (1990) Considerations on the further expansion of the AIDS epidemic in South Africa – 1990. *South African Medical Journal* 77(12): 613–618

Sharma A, Bukusi E, Cohen CR, Gorbach P, Holmes K, Kwena Z & Muga C (2008) Sexual identity and risk of HIV/STI among men who have sex with men in Nairobi. *Sexually Transmitted Diseases* 35(4): 352–354

Sher R & dos Santos L (1985) Prevalence of HTLV-III antibodies in homosexual men in Johannesburg. *South African Medical Journal* 67(13): 484

Shisana O, Rehle T, Simbayi LC, Parker W, Zuma K, Bhana A et al. (2005) *South African national HIV prevalence, HIV incidence, behaviour and communication survey, 2005*. Cape Town: HSRC Press

Simbayi LC, Cain D, Cherry C, Jooste S, Kalichman SC & Mathiti V (2006) HIV/AIDS risks among South African men who report sexually assaulting women. *American Journal of Health Behaviour* 30(2): 158–166

Spracklen FH, Becker ML, Becker WB, Holmes CM, Potter PC & Whittaker RG (1985) The acquired immune deficiency syndrome and related complex: A report of 2 confirmed cases in Cape Town with comments on human T-cell lymphotropic virus type III infections. *South African Medical Journal* 68(3): 139–143

Spurlin WJ (2006) *Imperialism within the margins: Queer representation and the politics of culture in southern Africa*. New York: Palgrave Macmillan

Teunis N (2008) Same-sex sexuality in Africa: A case study from Senegal. *AIDS and Behavior* 5(2): 173–182

UNAIDS (2006) *Report on the global AIDS epidemic*. Geneva: UNAIDS

UNAIDS (2008) *Report on the global AIDS epidemic*. Geneva: UNAIDS

Van Griensven F & Sanders EJ (2008) Editorial: Understanding HIV risks among men who have sex with men in Africa. *Sexually Transmitted Diseases* 35(4): 355–356

Van Harmelen J, Lambrick M, Rybicki EP, Williamson AL, Williamson C & Wood R (1997) An association between HIV-1 subtypes and mode of transmission in Cape Town, South Africa. *AIDS* 11(1): 113–116

Wade AS, Diallo PAN, Diop AK, Gueye K, Kane CT, Largarde E, Mboup S & Ndoye I (2005) HIV infection and sexually transmitted infections among men who have sex with men in Senegal. *AIDS* 19(18): 2133–2140

Williamson C & Martin DP (2005) Origin, diversity and spread of HIV-1. In SS Abdool Karim & Q Abdool Karim (Eds) *HIV/AIDS in South Africa*. New York: Cambridge University Press

# Contributors

**Peter Aggleton**, PhD, is Professor in Education in the Thomas Coram Research Unit, Institute of Education, University of London. The author or editor of over 20 books on sexuality and the social aspects of AIDS (including two series published by Taylor and Francis/Routledge in the UK), he is the editor of the journal *Culture, Health and Sexuality* and senior editor of *Global Public Health*. Peter currently directs the external evaluation of the Global Dialogue for Sexual Health and Well-Being supported by the Ford Foundation, and has been a senior adviser to UNAIDS, UNESCO, UNICEF, WHO and a wide range of bilateral and international organisations.

**Pierre Brouard** is the Deputy Director of the Centre for the Study of AIDS (CSA) at the University of Pretoria. From the late 1980s he has played a role in raising the standard of HIV/AIDS counselling in South Africa and developing a human rights culture around HIV/AIDS. He has been an expert witness for the AIDS Law Project at the University of the Witwatersrand, until recently sat on the board of the LGBTI organisation OUT LGBT Well-being (Pretoria), and currently oversees the work of two stigma and human rights projects of the CSA.

**Zethu Cakata** was a Senior Researcher and doctoral intern at the Gender and Development Cross-cutting Research Unit of the Human Sciences Research Council. She is now a researcher at the University of Pretoria. She has a master's degree in Research Psychology. Her areas of interest include psychology, gender, sexuality, education, African literature, feminism and body politics.

**Glenn de Swardt** resigned from the Triangle Project in February 2008. He is currently the Psychosocial Manager and project co-leader of Health4Men, a project of the Perinatal HIV Research Unit, funded by PEPFAR and USAID in partnership with the Western Cape Department of Health. Health4Men provides free comprehensive sexual health services to men who have sex with men, including access to free antiretroviral treatment, and is developing a model of care for rollout throughout South Africa in accordance with the national strategic plan on HIV and AIDS.

**Brian Dodge**, PhD, is Assistant Research Scientist in the Department of Applied Health Science and Associate Director of the Centre for Sexual Health Promotion at Indiana University (Bloomington). He is a core faculty member of the Public Health Unit and Affiliated Faculty at the Kinsey Institute for Research in Sex, Gender, and Reproduction.

**Paymon Ebrahimzadeh** is an international Treatment Action Campaign (TAC) volunteer and is completing his master's in Public Health in Epidemiology at the University of California (Los Angeles). On completion, he hopes to rejoin his friends, colleagues and mentors at TAC.

## CONTRIBUTORS

**Kirk Fiereck** is currently a PhD candidate studying Medical Anthropology in the Department of Sociomedical Sciences at the Columbia University Graduate School of Arts and Sciences.

**Nathan Geffen** is Treasurer of the Treatment Action Campaign. He has published extensively on issues around access to HIV treatment. He co-authored two chapters of Edwin Cameron's book *Witness to AIDS*, which jointly won the 2006 *Sunday Times* Alan Paton Award.

**Cary Alan Johnson** was recently appointed Executive Director of the International Gay and Lesbian Human Rights Commission (IGLHRC). Prior to this he was Senior Specialist for Africa (IGLHRC) based in South Africa. He holds a master's degree in International Relations from Columbia University and is author of *Off the Map: How HIV/AIDS Programming is Failing Same-Sex Practising People in Africa* (IGLHRC 2007).

**Busi Kheswa** has been working at the Gay and Lesbian Memory in Action (GALA) for the past six years. Busi is an experienced facilitator, and has facilitated workshops with OUT LGBT Well-being and the South African Department of Education. Her work at GALA also includes working on exhibitions and filming interviews and events to increase video archival holdings.

**Tim Lane**, PhD, is an Assistant Professor at the University of California, San Francisco Center for AIDS Prevention Studies, who specialises in qualitative research on gender, sexuality and HIV risk in sub-Saharan Africa. He has conducted research with men who have sex with men in Soweto and Mamelodi in collaboration with the Perinatal HIV Research Unit and OUT-Tshwane. He currently serves on the board of directors of the International Gay and Lesbian Human Rights Commission.

**Zethu Matebeni** is a doctoral fellow at the Wits Institute for Social and Economic Research (WISER), Johannesburg. Her PhD research works towards an understanding and exploration of black lesbian identities and sexualities in post-apartheid Johannesburg. Zethu is actively involved in various lesbian, gay, bisexual, transgender and intersex (LGBTI) organisations and projects promoting the lives and rights of LGBTI people.

**Samuel Matsikure** is the Programme Manager for Health at Gays and Lesbians of Zimbabwe.

**Mandisa Mbali** is a South African Rhodes Scholar and doctoral candidate at the Wellcome Unit for the History of Medicine at St Antony's College, University of Oxford.

**John Meletse** is Deaf, gay, HIV-positive and proud. He has worked as the Deaf Oral History Project and Outreach Officer at the Gay and Lesbian Memory in Action for the past four years.

**Carol Metcalf**, MBChB, MPH, is a Chief Research Specialist and epidemiologist in SAHA (Social Aspects of HIV-AIDS research programme) at the Human Sciences Research Council. She has a background in epidemiology, public health and international health. Her interests include HIV and STI prevention, HIV surveillance, HIV counselling and testing, and programme implementation based on research findings.

**Nonhlanhla 'MC' Mkhize** is the Director of the Durban Lesbian and Gay Community & Health Centre. She is currently completing her master's in Anthropology at the University of KwaZulu-Natal (Howard College) with a dissertation entitled 'The Female Condom: From Practice to Policy'.

**Ruth Morgan**, PhD, was the director of Gay and Lesbian Memory in Action (GALA) from 2002 until 2008. She is an anthropologist who has focused on life-story research for the past 17 years and has been collecting life stories on same-sex sexuality within an African context for GALA for the past 10 years. She is the co-author of the books *Tommy Boys, Lesbian Men and Ancestral Wives: Female Same-sex Practices in Africa* 2005) and *Deaf Me Normal: Deaf South Africans tell their life stories* (2008).

**Dawie Nel** has been the Director of OUT LGBT Well-being (a Pretoria-based NGO) since 2000. He completed a master's degree in Education at the University of the Witwatersrand in 2003, which focused on the experiences of lesbian and gay people in Gauteng schools.

**Juan Nel**, DLitt et Phil, is currently Associate Professor at the University of South Africa and Director: Centre for Applied Psychology. He has volunteered his services since 1995 as a psychologist at OUT LGBT Well-being, of which he is a founding member, chairperson from 1997–2000, and Board member since 2001. He furthermore represents the Psychological Society of South Africa on the International Network on Sexual Orientation-related Matters and Gender Identity Concerns in Psychology.

**Daveson Nyadani** is the Director at the Centre for the Development of People, an NGO that addresses the needs and challenges of minority groups in Malawi in the context of human rights, health and social development. He has a postgraduate degree in Publishing Studies and is a part-time lecturer in Media for Development at Chancellor College, University of Malawi.

**Renay Pillay** is an Assistant Director, Directorate: Research Co-ordination, Monitoring and Evaluation at the National Department of Education in Pretoria. Prior to this she was a Researcher in the Gender and Development Cross-cutting Research Unit of the Human Sciences Research Council. She holds an MA in Sociology and her areas of interest include gender and development, gender and transport, sexualities, education and feminism.

# CONTRIBUTORS

**Vasu Reddy**, PhD, is a Chief Research Specialist at the Gender and Development Cross-cutting Research Unit within the Policy Analysis and Capacity Enhancement research programme of the Human Sciences Research Council (HSRC). He is also an Honorary Associate Professor of Gender Studies in the School of Anthropology, Gender & Historical Studies (University of KwaZulu-Natal), where he continues to supervise master's and PhD students. In the early to mid-1990s he was part of the National Executive Committee of the National Coalition for Gay & Lesbian Equality (NCGLE), which successfully lobbied for the inclusion of a sexual orientation clause in the South African Constitution. After the NCGLE merged with the Lesbian & Gay Equality Project, he served two terms as Board member. In addition, he has served as a Board member of OUT LGBT since 2001 and is currently the Chairperson of the Board. In Durban, together with Nonhlanhla Mkhize and the late Ronald Louw, he co-founded the Durban Lesbian & Gay Community & Health Centre in 2000, where he serves as a Board member.

**Laetitia Rispel**, PhD, has been an Adjunct Professor at the Centre for Health Policy, School of Public Health at the University of the Witwatersrand, Johannesburg, since February 2008 and is the current President of the Public Health Association of South Africa. Prior to 2008, she was the Executive Director of the Human Sciences Research Council's Social Aspects of HIV/AIDS and Health (SAHA) research programme for two years.

**Theo Sandfort**, PhD in the Social Sciences, is Associate Professor of Clinical Sociomedical Sciences (in Psychiatry) at Columbia University and a Research Scientist at the HIV Center for Clinical and Behavioral Studies at the New York State Psychiatric Institute and Columbia University. He has written or edited 25 books, has over 100 publications in peer-reviewed journals, and has made over 25 English contributions to edited books. He is on the editorial board on various major sexuality journals, including *AIDS Care; Archives of Sexual Behavior; Culture, Health and Sexuality; Journal of Homosexuality; Sexualities* and *Sexuality Research and Social Policy*. He has served as elected President of the Dutch Society for Sexology and the International Academy of Sex Research. In 2008 he received the John Money Award from the Society for the Scientific Study of Sexuality for his work in the field of sexuality and health.

**Robert Sember** is a member of Ultra-red, a sound art collective concerned with anti-racism, migrant rights, fair housing and sexual rights. He is co-editor (with Richard Parker and Rosalind Petchesky) of *SexPolitics: Reports from the Front Lines* (2008).

**Vicci Tallis**, PhD, is an activist who has been involved in addressing the gender dimensions of HIV and AIDS since 1986. She is currently the Programme Manager for HIV and AIDS at the Open Society Initiative for Southern Africa.

# Index

**A**

Achmat, Zackie 10, 17, 92, 95, 168, 172, 208
activism, gay/lesbian/transgender 4, 12, 16–17, 23, 26–27, 35, 37, 39, 44, 59, 71, 74, 101
    apolitical/non-militant 80–81, 85, 87, 91, 95
    in deaf community 78, 118, 120–122
    Durban Lesbian & Gay Community & Health Centre 44, 173, 181*tab,* 192, 207–212, 215, 219–220, 236
    Forum for the Empowerment of Women 220
    Gay Association of South Africa 27, 83–84, 87–88, 91–92
    Gay and Lesbian Organisation of the Witwatersrand 85, 90–92, 97n16
    and gay law reform movement 22, 83–84, 93–94, 190, 192, 208
    Gay Pride marches 89, 94–95, 97n16
    Gays and Lesbians of Zimbabwe 143
    historical perspective on 81–85, 95
    International Lesbian and Gay Association 84
    KwaZulu-Natal Coalition for Gay and Lesbian Equality 208–209
    Lesbian and Gay Equality Project 14, 17, 172
    Lesbian Organisation of the Witwatersrand 81
    Organisation of Lesbian and Gay Activists 81, 85, 93–94
    OUT LGBT Well-being (OUT) 43–44, 128, 131, 183–184, 192, 195–196, 219–222, 224, 236
    Rand Gay Organisation 27, 97n17
    The Saturday Group 84, 97n16
    Triangle Project 44, 87, 117, 173, 183, 192, 198–199, 204–205, 209, 236
activism, HIV/AIDS gay
    and advocacy/lobbying/mobilisation 4, 17, 44, 61, 64, 81, 83, 89, 133, 141, 154, 157, 168–170, 178, 184, 192, 208–211, 214, 219, 222–223, 228, 236
    and AIDS Consortium 81, 93, 96
    AIDS Law Project 177
    Association for Bisexuals, Lesbians and Gays 92, 94, 97n16
    black-led 80–81, 84, 89–92, 95
    during apartheid 89–90, 94
    GASA 6010 84, 87–89
    Gay Men's Health Crisis 132
    and gay rights charters 81, 93–96
    Joint Working Group 23, 61, 191–192, 204, 211, 218–220
    Lesbian AIDS Project 132
    Mobilise Against Aids 89
    Mother City Men's Health Project 199, 202
    in prisons 177
    and public information/education campaigns 171, 204, 209
    and sexual health services 209–210, 212, 214
    tactic of disclosure 81, 89, 94–95, 118
    Township AIDS Project 90–92, 117
    Treatment Action Campaign 92, 95, 169–171, 173, 177, 209
    in the US 85, 89
    and voluntary testing and counselling 176, 193, 199, 201–204, 209–211, 214–215
    *see also* Gay and Lesbian Memory in Action Archives
African Christian Democratic Party 17–18, 22
Altman, Dennis 82, 91
anti-apartheid struggle 14, 27, 70–71, 80–81, 83–84, 87–89, 95–96
    and United Democratic Front 84
apartheid era 15–17, 19–20, 22, 24–25, 27, 40–41, 66, 84, 85
    censorship 94

**B**

Botswana 44, 69, 127–128
    African Youth Alliance of 127
Burkino Faso 5

**C**

Cameron, Edwin 17, 22, 81, 84, 93, 104, 208–209
class 10, 100, 172–173, 175, 210–212
    inequality 11, 14, 182
colonialism 14, 16, 19

# INDEX

**D**
decriminalisation of same sex practices 19–20, 69, 150, 168, 208–209
Doll, Lynda 53

**E**
Epprecht, Mark 8, 82–84, 87, 126, 149, 159, 231

**F**
Federation of Gay Games 35
feminism 37–38, 47, 100, 104, 106, 216

**G**
gay *see* identity, gender/sexual
gay-affirmative therapy *see under* health and same sex sexuality
Gay and Lesbian Memory in Action Archives 89, 117, 122n1
  oral history and outreach project 117–122
gay movement *see* activism, gay/lesbian/transgender
gender discrimination 2–3, 10, 18, 20, 23–25, 27, 33, 35–36, 40, 44–45, 47, 63, 69, 72, 74–75, 81, 83, 85, 95, 118, 120, 127, 138–139, 141, 144–145, 152, 87, 89, 93–94, 101, 132, 138, 140–141, 145, 148, 150, 155–156, 158–159, 161, 168–169, 173–174, 178, 182–184, 197n1, 208, 210–212, 219, 221, 233
  and blood donation 66, 87, 181*tab*, 197n1
  and heterosexism 15, 34, 40, 44–46, 102, 216–217, 220–221
  and homophobia/homoprejudice 10, 15–16, 40, 45–46, 69, 83, 85, 87–89, 91, 95, 100, 102, 118, 126, 132, 138, 141, 143–145, 159, 168, 182, 202*&tab*, 203, 207, 211, 220, 234–236
  and inequality 25, 28, 210, 216, 220
  lesbian/lesbophobia 10, 91, 182, 219
  marginalisation/exclusion 29, 35–36, 39, 43–45, 68, 78, 91, 113, 129–130, 132, 158, 207, 212, 216–217, 222–224
  and Marriage Alliance 22
  in the military 8, 24
  stigmatisation 10, 25, 32, 36, 47, 53, 63–64, 69, 72–73, 82, 85, 95, 118, 120, 126–128, 138–139, 141, 143–144*&tab*, 145, 148, 150, 155–156, 158–161, 173, 182, 185, 232–233, 236
  transphobia 10, 40
  victimisation 45, 47, 103, 210
  workplace 23, 155
  *see also* sexual violence/rape
gender equality 15, 20, 23, 28, 33
  Commission on Gender Equality 20
  and European Union 37
  Lesbian and Gay Equality Project 14, 17, 19, 24
  in LGBTI sector 34–35, 37–38, 40, 145, 220
  National Coalition for Gay and Lesbian Equality 20, 24, 92, 96, 172, 208
  *see also* gender discrimination; identity, gender/sexual; labelling in cross-cultural context; sexual and gender rights; sexuality: and gender awareness/diversity training
Gevisser, M 18, 26–27, 67, 71, 81, 83–84, 87–88, 90, 94–95, 96n5, 100–101, 104, 231
Ghana 69, 129–130, 134, 147–156
  National AIDS Control Program 128

**H**
health and same sex sexuality
  and American Psychological Association 33–34, 36–37
  gay/LGBTI-affirmative approaches 32, 37–39, 43, 45–47
  and International Network on Sexual Orientation-Related Matters and Gender Identity Concerns in Psychology 37
  and marginalisation of WSM 43–44, 174, 216–224, 231
  and medical research 217
  in the Netherlands 37, 43
  and provision of healthcare 32, 34, 36–37, 39–40, 42–45, 47, 59, 68, 72, 74, 118, 120, 128, 131, 134, 143–144, 151, 155, 159–160, 173–174, 176, 182–185, 192, 198–199, 207, 212–213, 223
  and Psychological Society of South Africa 37
  Sexual Health Charter 43
  Standards of Care 39
  in the USA 37
  World Professional Association for Transgender Health 39

*see also* HIV/AIDS interventions/treatment; research on sexuality and gender: behavioural/psychosocial; sexuality: education/psychosocial training/gender awareness
Heher, Jonathan 19
HIV/AIDS
 and AIDS Advisory Group 86–88
 and AIDS Foundation of South Africa 209
 ANC government response to 17, 25, 94, 140, 170–171
 in Asia 126, 133–134
 denial 201–203, 222
 education/public awareness 90–92, 94–95, 102, 112, 117–122, 140–141, 143–145, 173, 185, 204, 210, 214, 222
 heterosexual and mother-to-child transmission of 67, 98n24, 170, 221
 impact on tertiary education 58
 incidence/prevalence/infection patterns 32, 66–68, 73, 80, 84, 86–87, 95–96, 98n24, 130, 140, 156, 169, 176, 179–181*&tab*, 191, 213, 229–231, 237
 International HIV/AIDS Alliance 128, 131, 133
 lesbian/WSW/female to female transmission of 6, 91, 102, 109–114, 131–133, 134n6, 148–149, 159, 182, 193, 196, 199–200, 216, 221, 224, 231, 235
 LGB/same sex prevalence 185–186, 190–191, 228, 230–232
 media response to 85–87, 97n7,8&9, 141
 MSM transmission 66–72, 126–131, 137, 143–145, 176, 179–181&*tab*, 185, 201, 229–230, 235
 National AIDS Convention of South Africa 81, 93, 96
 people living with 16–17, 62–64, 95, 173, 178, 180, 210, 216, 221–222
 Political Declaration on 3
 and poverty/unemployment 43
 South African National AIDS Council 178
 stigmatisation/discrimination 10, 58–59, 63, 74–75, 95, 118, 120, 144–145, 180, 202
 transgender transmission of 200
 UNAIDS 127, 134n5
 UN Declaration of Commitment on 2–3

 *see also* activism, HIV/AIDS gay; Gay and Lesbian Memory in Action Archives; HIV/AIDS research
HIV/AIDS interventions/treatment 6, 9, 11, 43, 58–61, 64, 68, 70–75, 81, 92–93, 95, 128–134, 140–141, 143–147, 158, 160–161, 169–174, 176, 179, 181*&tab*, 184–185, 191–192, 195–196, 198–199, 205, 207–210, 212–216, 221, 228, 230–231, 234–237
 and antiretrovirals 118, 169–171, 173, 199
 and burden on healthcare system 42–43, 170, 229
 and depression 70, 169, 172, 200
 International AIDS Society Conference on Pathogenesis, Treatment and Prevention 13
 and microbicides 9, 217, 222
 and post-exposure prophylaxis 201
 and safer sex/condom use 6, 9–10, 69–70, 75, 81, 89–91, 102, 109–114, 118, 131–134, 141, 143, 145–146, 148, 151–153, 157–159, 161, 166, 169, 180, 184–185, 194–196, 201–205, 209–210, 213–214, 217, 222, 224, 230–231, 235
 and testing/counselling 58–59, 69, 74–75, 114, 118, 140, 144*tab*, 146, 169, 172, 183, 192, 194–196, 198–199, 201, 203, 210–211, 213, 215, 222, 235
HIV/AIDS policies and programmes
 monitoring 179
 National Strategic Plan 68–69, 178–179, 181, 183–184, 234, 236–237
 and relevance to LGBT 176–178, 181–185, 190, 223, 236–237
HIV/AIDS research
 and American Foundation for AIDS Research 133
 and Association for Women's Rights in Development 119
 and Centre for the Study of AIDS 58–59, 61, 63–64, 65n1, 120, 195
 donor-driven 60
 epidemiological/behavioural/social 6–7, 9–12, 53, 58–60, 62, 66–67, 70, 80, 86–87, 133, 141, 152, 161, 180, 229–230, 235
 feedback/presentation 64, 124, 134n1, 233
 and Guttmacher Institute 127
 Horizons Program 127, 131, 134n5

# INDEX

and International Gay and Lesbian Human Rights Commission 219
and internet 195
on LGBTI 219, 235
management 63–64
methodology 61–63, 72–75, 180, 192–193&*tab*, 195
on MSM/gay men 66, 69, 71–74, 126–131, 133–134n5, 178, 181–186, 195–196, 204–205, 229, 235
policy-driven 9, 60
and seroprevalence 129–133, 140, 149, 156, 160, 179, 182, 229–230, 237
and South African Institute of Medical Research 86–87
in sub-Saharan Africa 147–161, 174, 176, 228
UCSF Center for AIDS Studies 128, 130–131
on WSW/lesbian women 131–132, 148, 182, 186, 216–217, 219–220, 223–224, 235–237
HIV/AIDS risk/vulnerability factors 3, 11, 36, 41, 47, 127–128, 141, 144*tab*, 177&*fig*, 182–184, 190–191, 202*tab*, 205, 219, 234–236
bisexual 53, 132
and drug use 6, 73, 132, 148, 176, 181*tab*, 182, 200–201, 205
heterosexual 6, 216, 221
MSM/gay 3, 7–10, 29, 41, 53, 66–73, 95, 127, 129, 131, 133–134n5, 140, 147–148, 156, 158–159, 161, 169, 172, 174, 176, 179–181*tab*, 185, 195–196, 201, 203, 205–206, 233, 237
and sex workers 158–159, 173, 176, 181*tab*
WSW/lesbian 6–7, 41, 81, 91, 102, 110, 112–114, 131–133, 140, 148, 169, 174, 182, 194, 199, 214, 216–217, 222, 224, 233, 236–237
homoprejudice *see under* gender discrimination
homosexuality *see under* identity, gender/sexual
Hook, D 32–33
human rights
of citizenship 2, 9, 15–16, 18, 22–24, 27–28, 35–36, 138, 207, 211
Commission on Human Rights 2
Human Rights Watch 10, 32
International Covenant on Economic, Social and Cultural Rights 2
and poverty struggles 27, 29
and sexual orientation *see* sexual and gender rights
and South African Bill of Rights 14, 32, 81, 93, 101, 168, 208
and South African Human Rights Commission 19, 183
Universal Declaration of 2
UN Economic and Social Council 25
women's 4, 24–25, 100, 219, 223
*see also* sexual and gender rights
Hunter, M 154, 158

## I

identity, gender/sexual 2–4, 10, 15, 32–33, 38–39, 41–42, 53, 55, 61, 69, 78, 161, 165, 200, 211, 223, 236
bisexual 7, 11, 43, 51–54, 59, 69, 82, 145, 218
changing/evolving 80–83, 95, 200, 204–205, 236
feminine 5–6, 38–39, 70, 107, 204, 233
globalisation of 8, 10, 37, 71, 149, 153, 157, 161, 232
heterosexual/traditional 5–7, 38–39, 42, 59, 82, 226
homosexual/gay 3–8, 11, 13, 15, 22–23, 29–34, 38, 41, 55–56, 59, 63, 74, 86, 101, 130, 139, 145, 191, 204, 226
LGBTI 35, 40–42, 218
masculine 4–7, 38–39, 107, 204, 233
MSM 8, 55–56, 59, 67–68, 70–75, 82, 128, 157, 151, 163, 191
politics 27, 37, 46, 54, 59, 80, 175, 234
transsexual/transgender 11, 23, 35, 39–40, 59, 82
*see also* lesbianism; sexual orientation: and self-identification
India 7
Issack, Wendy 14–16, 27

## K

Karim, Abdool 96, 98n24
Kenya 5, 69, 127–131, 134&n5, 147, 149–153, 158, 179, 212, 226
Kheswa, Busi 118, 120, 122

## L

labelling in cross-cultural context
  in Africa/South Africa 51–53, 55, 59, 96n3, 157, 161, 200, 232
  in Asia 5
  and cross-dressing 52
  among MSM/WSW 4, 6, 8, 11, 42–43, 46, 51, 53–56, 58–59, 71, 78, 82, 100, 106–107, 110, 124, 218
  in the West 53–54, 59
  *see also* identity, gender/sexual: bisexual, homosexual/gay; sexual orientation: and self-identification
Labour Relations Act 23–24
Lalu, Vivienne 173
Lane, Tim 130–131, 179
legislation, anti-gay 101
  and sodomy laws 16, 19–20, 23–24, 27, 84, 90, 94–95
lesbianism
  black 41, 83, 92, 100–112
  and desexualisation 104, 110
  and identity 4, 6, 11, 34, 38–39, 41, 52–53, 59, 81–82, 100–105, 113, 191, 199, 218, 222–223
  and woman-identified experience 103–104, 110
  and WSW 52, 104, 110, 191, 116, 218–219, 237
  *see also* health and same sex sexuality
*Link/Skakel* (later *Exit*) 84, 88
Louw, Ronald 82, 208–211, 215
Lusikisiki antiretroviral campaign 171, 173

## M

Malawi, same sex sexuality in 137–141
  AIDS policy 140
  National Aids Commission 139–140
Mali 69, 131
marriage 7
  compulsory/forced 7, 44, 132, 138, 144*tab*
Mbeki, Thabo 67
McGeary, Barry 92–93, 117
Meletse, John 78, 118, 120–122, 122n1
Mellors, Shaun 81, 93–94
Metz, Jack 87
Mexico 5
Milk, Harvey 89
Mokgethi, Paul 118, 122

Moreau, Amadou 127
Morgan, Ruth 118, 122n1, 218, 220, 222
Morocco, Association de Lutte Contre le SIDA in 128
MSM *see under* identity, gender/sexual; HIV/AIDS; HIV/AIDS research; HIVAIDS risk/vulnerability factors; labelling in cross cultural context
Mugabe, Robert 15, 82, 143
Murphy, John 20

## N

Namibia 4–5, 44, 59, 148
national liberation *see* anti-apartheid struggle
Ngaunje, Marjorie 140
Ngcobo, Linda 81, 95
Nigeria 51, 53, 69, 129, 147–152, 155, 159, 212
Njinge, Mpumi 117
Nkoli, Simon 17, 80, 84, 87, 89–90, 92, 95, 96n6, 117, 208
Ntsaluba, Akhona 175
Nujoma, Sam 15, 82

## O

Open Society Institute for Southern Africa 122, 130

## P

patriarchy 15, 28, 33, 41, 44, 47, 101–102, 190, 203, 220
Pegge, John 85, 87, 88–89, 172
Philippines 5
political transition era 14, 66, 80, 91, 96
  neo-liberalism in 15
  secularism in 14–15, 18
post-colonialism 16, 153
pre-colonial societies 15, 82

## R

race/racial 47, 86, 100–101, 210
racism/racial discrimination 15, 22, 27–29, 41, 83–85, 91–92, 126, 153, 211
rape *see* sexual violence/rape
Reid, Graeme 52, 62, 78, 82
research on sexuality and gender
  behavioural/psychosocial 14, 32–35, 39, 41–42, 45–47, 51, 54–56, 59, 64, 67, 70, 72, 78, 82, 105–113, 127, 139–140, 147, 149, 183–184, 228–229

# INDEX

Centre for Applied Psychology, UNISA 192, 204
Centre for the Development of People (Malawi) 139–140
challenges/limitations/blindspots recommendations 60–63, 74–75, 129–130, 141, 146, 148–149, 160–161, 166, 184–186, 190, 212–215, 218–219, 223–224, 230–235
community-based 60–61
and Human Sciences Research Council 26, 169, 181*tab*, 182, 191, 199
monitoring 236
and organised LGB sector 74, 190–196, 197n1, 199, 204, 212, 213–214, 218–221, 223–224, 236
politics of 28–29
*see also* activism, HIV/AIDS gay: Joint Working Group; HIV/AIDS research
Rich, Adrienne 100, 103–104, 192, 204

## S

same sex sexual practices/behaviour 9–11, 41–42, 59, 61–63, 68–69, 78, 82, 95, 129–131, 218, 232, 236
  denial/notion of being 'un-African' 15, 29, 40, 82, 87, 101, 126, 138–139, 144*tab*, 170, 207, 212, 214, 231, 234
  female 41, 100, 103, 107–112, 131–132, 148–149, 199, 222–223
  inter-racial 84, 86–87, 95, 118
  male 148–151, 157, 195–196, 200–202, 204–206, 223, 235
  *see also* HIV/AIDS: risk/vulnerability factors; HIV/AIDS interventions/treatment; sex work
same sex sexuality 2–4, 6, 8, 10–11, 29, 180
  in Africa/South Africa 8, 69, 82, 95, 126–130, 133, 147–158, 212, 214, 219, 228
  ambiguity/complexity of 4–5, 223, 235
  criminalisation of 19, 25, 40, 45, 96n5, 133, 137–138, 144*tab*, 231
  in migrant labour compounds 70–71
  in prisons 8, 68, 70, 177, 203
  and power relations/dynamics 4, 158–159, 173, 204–205, 210, 220–221
  religious/moral attitudes to 2, 15, 28, 40, 138–139, 145, 163
  and sangomas 83
  subcultures 10, 37, 46–47
  *see also* decriminalisation of same sex practices; Malawi; same sex sexual practices/behaviour; decriminalisation of same sex practices
Satchwell, Kathy 20
Senegal 5, 69, 127–131, 134&n5, 147–153, 159–160, 179, 226
  National AIDS Control Program 128
sex work 9, 25, 29, 40, 130–131, 140, 154, 158, 177, 199
  and commercial and exchange sex 148, 153–155, 158–159, 161
  and decriminalisation campaign 174
  Sex Worker Advocacy and Education Taskforce 177
sexism 28, 91, 100, 211
sexology 32, 34, 42
  rights-based 35
  World Association for Sexology 3
sexual and gender rights 2, 32, 43, 122, 140–141, 159, 192, 207, 211, 216
  and adoption 20–21, 23, 208, 220
  ANC government policy/legislation on 17–18, 21–24, 26
  and health 2, 11, 25, 32, 35–36, 43–44, 68, 93, 96, 183, 207, 217
  and immigration 20
  and partnership/marriage 2, 15–18, 20–23, 25, 35–36, 70–71, 83, 164, 197n2, 211
  in post-apartheid context 14–16, 24
  and privacy 3, 19, 25
  resolution on Human Rights and Sexual Orientation 2
  and social transformation 28
  and the South African Constitution 14–19, 21–23, 24–25, 27–28, 32, 43–45, 75, 80, 93–94, 96, 101, 168, 178, 190, 208, 220
  threats to 29, 43, 138–139, 144*tab*, 145
  transgender 45
  and Yogyakarta Principles 2
  *see also* activism, gay/lesbian/transgender; gender discrimination; gender equality; Labour Relations Act; South African Police Service; White Paper on Social Welfare
sexual assault *see* sexual violence/rape

251

sexual orientation 3, 13, 24–25, 31–35, 38, 41–42, 44–45, 75, 81, 86, 94, 96n1&2, 183, 192, 208, 210
  legal framework 172
  and self-identification 54–56, 59–60, 74, 105–106, 157, 221
sexual violence/rape 2, 7, 19, 32, 36, 39–40, 43, 68, 96, 101–102, 112, 122, 128, 130–131, 133, 148, 155–156, 158–159, 161, 171, 173, 184, 193, 199, 220–221, 226, 233
  corrective rape 41, 81, 91, 101–102, 118, 182, 199, 204, 220–221
sexuality 25, 32–34, 39–40, 42, 82
  education/psychosocial training 43–46, 120, 140–141, 185, 192, 205
  and gender awareness/diversity training 36–37, 44, 46, 82, 120–122, 141, 185, 205, 210, 232
  heteronormative 7, 126–127
  lesbian 100, 103–104, 107–108&*tab*, 109&*tab*, 112–113
  and oppositional duality 104
  in post-apartheid South Africa 101–102
  *see also* health and same sex sexuality
sexuality, socially constructed 39, 80, 82, 86–87, 157, 161, 203
  Foucault's theories on 82, 87, 161
Sher, Ruben 85–88, 180
Skweyiya, Lewis 21
socioeconomic status 47, 68, 172, 203, 232
South African Law Reform Commission 22
South African Police Service 24

**T**
Taiwan 5
Tanzania, National AIDS Control Programme of 127
Termination of Pregnancy Bill 26–27
Thailand 4–5, 133, 137, 157
Toms, Ivan 80, 89, 95
traditional 'African' culture 14–16, 28
Transgender DynamiX 45
Tunisia 128

**U**
Uganda 5, 69, 128

**W**
Wade, Abdoulaye 129, 147–153, 155–156, 160, 179
White Paper on Social Welfare 23
World Conference on Women 25, 43
World Health Organisation 2–3, 34–35
WSW *see under* HIV/AIDS; HIV/AIDS research; HIVAIDS risk/vulnerability factors; labelling in cross cultural context; lesbianism

**Y**
youth, gay and lesbian 6–7, 18, 78, 100, 102, 107, 127–128, 210, 171, 174, 193, 196–196, 208

**Z**
Zimbabwe, same sex sexuality and HIV/AIDS in 143–145, 212
  recommendations 145–146